D1084609

Conscious and Unconscious Processes

CONSCIOUS AND UNCONSCIOUS PROCESSES

Psychodynamic, Cognitive, and Neurophysiological Convergences

Howard Shevrin, James A. Bond, Linda A. W. Brakel,
Richard K. Hertel, and William J. Williams

THE GUILFORD PRESS
New York   London

© 1996 The Guilford Press
A Division of Guilford Publications, Inc.
72 Spring Street, New York, NY 10012

All rights reserved

No part of this book may be reproduced, stored in a retrieval
system, or transmitted, in any form or by any means, electronic,
mechanical, photocopying, microfilming, recording, or otherwise,
without written permission from the Publisher.

Printed in the United States of America

This book is printed on acid-free paper.

Last digit is print number: 9   8   7   6   5   4   3   2   1

Library of Congress Cataloging-in-Publication Data

Conscious and unconscious processes: psychodynamic, cognitive, and
    neurophysiological convergences / Howard Shevrin . . . [et al.].
        p.   cm.
    Includes bibliographical references and index.
    ISBN 1-57230-091-4
    1. Subconsciousness.   2. Consciousness.   3. Psychology,
Experimental.   I. Shevrin, Howard.
    [DNLM   1. Psychotherapy—methods.   2. Consciousness.
3. Unconscious (Psychology)   4. Neurophysiology.   5. Cognition.
6. Psychological Theory.   WM 420 C754 1996]
BF315.C685   1996
154.2—dc20
DNLM/DLC
for Library of Congress   96-1714
                                                                    CIP

DISCARDED

WIDENER UNIVERSITY
WOLFGRAM
LIBRARY
CHESTER, PA.

Dedicated to the memory of

Charles Fisher

who led the way in exploring the unconscious
in the laboratory as well as from the couch.

Acknowledgments

Psychoanalysts, psychologists, psychiatrists, biomedical engineers, and computer specialists have actively collaborated to produce the research results reported in this book. The research group is divided into clinical and laboratory teams both headed by the senior author. Serving on the clinical team were James A. Bond, Ph.D., Linda A. W. Brakel, M.D., and Richard K. Hertel, Ph.D. Over the course of the research a number of other clinicians made contributions to the clinical team: Robert Hatcher, Ph.D., John Hartman, Ph.D., Susan Miller, Ph.D., and Dwarakanath Rao, M.D. Serving on the laboratory team were Ramesh Kushwaha, Ph.D., Robert E. Marshall, M.E.E., John Michael Snodgrass, Ph.D., and Philip S. Wong, Ph.D. Dorothy Holinger and Michael Kopka assisted in the collection of laboratory data. William J. Williams, Ph.D. headed the development and execution of the biosignal analyses, assisted by Leonides D. Iasemides, Hitten P. Zaveri, and E. J. Zheng. Beverly Knickerbocker diligently, laboriously, and accurately transcribed interview and testing tapes. Ila Atwood was responsible for typing the manuscript. The research has received support in its early stages from the MacArthur Foundation and more recently from the Ford Motor Co., and the National Science Foundation (Grant BCS 9110571), in addition to ongoing support from the Department of Psychiatry, University of Michigan Medical Center. The research has benefited greatly from generous donations by Robert Hunt Berry to the Ormond & Hazel Hunt Event-Related Potential Laboratory. We gratefully acknowledge the special contribution of John Michael Snodgrass, Ph.D., who performed all the statistical analyses cited in this book.

Contents

1. Introduction   1

Part I. Theory   11

    2. Psychoanalytic Theory   13
    3. Cognitive Theory   38
    4. Psychophysiological Theory   58

Part II. Methods   67

    5. The Psychodynamic Clinical Method and Word
       Selection Procedure   69
    6. The Subliminal Cognitive Method   91
    7. The Psychophysiological Method   109

Part III. The Experiment   131

    8. Experimental Procedures and Results   133

Part IV. Clinical Cases   145

    9. The Case of Mr. A   149
    10. The Case of Mr. B   187
    11. The Case of Mr. C   231

Part V. Conclusions   **259**

    12. Implications and Future Directions   261

Appendix A: Word Selection Algorithms   **281**

Appendix B: Time–Frequency Distributions   **283**

References   285

Index   295

Introduction

The notion of an unconscious mental life has been a source of controversy for more than a century. At issue is nothing less than how the mind should be conceived. Two opposing views, taking various forms over the years, have confronted each other down to our own day. During much of the latter half of the 19th century, in clear contradistinction to the speculative position taken by a number of philosophers in favor of an unconscious mental life, psychologists defined psychology as the science of consciousness. James, in his classic *Principles of Psychology* (1890), scoffed at the notion of an unconscious, marshaling ten arguments against it. The final argument was aimed at the then-novel idea of unconscious motivation, introduced by Freud. Not long after the turn of the century, behaviorism took up the cudgels not only against an unconscious, but against consciousness as well, limiting psychology to what could be observed and measured. Psychoanalysis remained the one advocate and defender of the concept of an unconscious mental life.

Hovering in the background of the controversy and enflaming it further in the minds of the opponents of the unconscious, was Freud's belief that psychoanalysis was a revolutionary science with an illustrious pedigree going back to Copernicus and Darwin. Copernicus had shattered long-standing illusions about humanity's habitation, the earth, reducing it to a satellite around the sun. Darwin decentered humanity itself as a special creation. Psychoanalysis, Freud believed, decentered consciousness as the sole source of individual experience and control. After the discovery of the unconscious, Freud argued, no one could continue to believe that the consciousness each of us possesses is the self-evident instrument by which we control ourselves and our lives.

Freud's claim continues to be disputed by many scientists and scholars. The most recent attack appeared in a well-known intellectual periodical (*New York Review of Books*) and was authored by Frederick Crews (1995), a literary critic and historian. Fundamentally, the charge of these critics can be summarized in one word: unproven. Until recently, psychoanalysis advanced its claim on the basis of clinical case histories and theoretical considerations. In the minds of many critics, anecdotal clinical evidence does not stand up too well in the court of scientific discourse. With the advent of the subliminal method drawn on in this book, a way has been opened for bringing unconscious processes into the laboratory and obtaining objective data that can stand up to searching scientific certainty.

Closer to our own time, the issue has been joined at a more empirical level than in the past. With the introduction of the subliminal method, largely by psychoanalytic investigators (Fisher, 1954, 1957; Shevrin, 1956; Klein, Spence, Holt, & Gourevitch, 1958; Pine, 1960), there arose a new form of opposition, methodological in nature, claiming that subliminal experiments fell short of adequate experimental rigor. More recently, there has been a veritable explosion of subliminal investigations, which have been comprehensively reviewed by Dixon (1971, 1981). Shevrin has provided two more recent reviews, one on subliminal perception and dreaming (1986), and one on subliminal perception and repression (1990). Contemporary cognitive psychology has gradually and somewhat grudgingly accepted the position that unconscious processes play a significant role in perception and memory, but the line has been drawn against accepting a dynamic unconscious, involving affect, motivation, and conflict.

The research described in this book is an attempt to investigate the revolutionary concept of an unconscious mental life in its full depth, encompassing its narrowly cognitive aspects, which are of increasing interest to cognitive psychologists, as well as its more profoundly disturbing affective, motivational, and conflictual aspects, which have been of enduring interest to psychoanalysts of whatever theoretical persuasion. To accomplish this end, we have developed a new experimental method involving psychoanalytic, cognitive, and neurophysiological dimensions.

Historically, it has not proven easy to investigate dynamic unconscious processes with objective experimental investigative tools. In the past, either the relevant phenomena were oversimplified for controlled laboratory investigation, or, if the richness of the phenomena was retained, it was difficult to establish their objectivity. Therefore, we first had to develop a new approach that allowed for objective investigation of complex, richly detailed phenomena. We developed a method based on convergent operations in which several independent methods are combined so that the strengths of one method compensate for the limitations of another. We have combined psychodynamic, cognitive, and neurophysiological methods into one composite method. The subjective, theory-rich inferences of the psychoanalytic clinician, whose concerns are individual differences, personal meaning, and object relations, have been balanced by the objective cognitive methods of the laboratory. The purely psychological character of both the clinical and cognitive methods have been complemented by a neurophysiological method in which measurements do not depend on any psychological judgment or inference, and, in this sense, are independent of both. In this way, we have put the clinicians' clinical inferences to the test of convergent, independent, cognitive, and neurophysiological evidence. The three methods, working together in the manner described, constitute a powerful new tool for investigating the relationships between conscious and unconscious processes.

The research described in this book has three specific aims: (a) to provide independent, objective evidence for the existence of unconscious conflict in psychopathology, (b) to develop a method capable of allowing this determination, and (c) to explore the relationships between psychological and neurophysiological processes bearing on unconscious conflict and conscious symptom experience.

In thinking about how to best present our research, we recognized the need to meet one important challenge: to communicate to readers in multiple disciplines. Our research requires an understanding of psychoanalysis, cognitive psychology, and psychophysiology. Each discipline has its own phenomena, basic issues, and terminology. The practitioners of these disciplines seldom have occasion to interact with each other or know about each other's work. To describe one method in the technical detail required by one discipline would leave most practitioners in the other two disciplines mystified. Yet, to resort to a nontechnical approach that would make our description equally available to each discipline would result in understandable dissatisfaction among all practitioners because their own technical requirements had not been met. We decided on a two-step approach: first, we describe our investigation in a nontechnical manner so that readers from all disciplines can obtain a general idea of our approach, and then we describe each aspect of our method so that readers with expertise in each area can understand what we have done at a suitable technical level.

Readers might well wonder why we have crafted a method that is so complex and multifaceted. The scientific questions we wanted to investigate require nothing less. As we hope our readers will come to appreciate, our method is no more complex and demanding than the questions we desire to answer. Had we remained within the confines of one or another of the three disciplines, we would not have done justice to a number of crucial questions, the answers to which extend beyond the limited interests of any one discipline. What are these questions?

Our first question derives from a psychoanalytic frame of reference: How can we investigate the nature of dynamic unconscious factors influencing consciously experienced symptoms as objectively as possible, while incorporating the wisdom and experience of psychoanalytic clinicians?

Our second question derives from a cognitive psychological frame of reference: Can the use of subliminal stimulation, a method currently used by cognitive psychologists to investigate preattentive, preconscious aspects of perception, permit us to probe the nature of these dynamic unconscious factors independently of any clinical inferences or judgments?

Our third question derives from a psychophysiological frame of reference: Can physiological measures—specifically, event-related potentials (ERPs)—provide a nonpsychological, nonbehavioral marker for these objectively activated, dynamically unconscious processes that are related to consciously experienced symptoms?

Implicit in these questions are a number of assumptions and hypotheses that need to be made explicit. Each component method and its frame of reference will first be dealt with separately, and then the way in which they fit together in our composite method will be described.

THE PSYCHOANALYTIC METHOD AND FRAME OF REFERENCE

The primary focus of our inquiry is on the relationship between dynamic unconscious and conscious processes. Psychoanalysts claim to be able to determine this relationship on the basis of a clinical method developed and practiced for the past 100 years (Shevrin, 1984, 1991b). At the very least, psychoanalysts claim that their method allows them access to phenomena on the basis of which reasonable inferences about these unconscious influences can be made. Other methods—such as biological interventions and behavioral and cognitive treatments—make no such claim.

No method can stand on its own without the implicit or explicit support of certain assumptions and a theoretical frame of reference. First and foremost, the psychoanalytic method is a *clinical* modality providing a means for treating patients suffering from psychological disorders. Psychoanalysis also lays claim to being an investigative tool, although precisely how and with what limitations remains a matter of controversy. One fundamental assumption, which Rapaport has referred to as "psychological continuity" (Rapaport, 1967), undergirds the psychoanalytic method. Psychological continuity contains two ideas, and each is important in its own right. By assuming that the continuity is "psychological" in nature, the analyst focuses most productively on psychological causes. Specifically, the psychoanalyst conceptualizes the underlying causes as motives, feelings, thoughts, fantasies, or memories—all psychological in nature and, for the most part, concerned with the important people in an individual's past and present life. The other term, "continuity," is of equal importance. Continuity commits the analyst to the belief that a coherent pattern of underlying psychological *causes* determines the apparent discrepancies in conscious experience. These underlying processes are assumed not to be random in nature.

When patients give their accounts of what has led them to treatment, the analysts note that these accounts are seldom manifestly coherent or internally consistent; they usually have striking omissions and apparent irrationalities. Indeed, the complaint or symptom itself is often a clear instance of a discontinuity in the story. One of our patient-subjects described (see Chapter 9) his inability to eat in public without experiencing an intense headache, palpitations, a sudden need to defecate, sweatiness, and shortness of breath. He had no way of understanding why he should be so anxious and distressed when performing so simple an act as eating in public, something he had been doing easily for years. He was willing to concede that his behavior was indeed irrational. He had to either leave the restaurant or suffer an agonizing anticipation that something terrible would happen. After leaving the restaurant, he was miraculously freed of the distressing experiences and was filled with a sense of great relief and enormous puzzlement. The latter, as well as the inconvenience and frustration caused by the symptom, led the man to seek treatment and to become a subject in our experiment. At the heart of the symptomatic experience was something mystifying, troubling, and irrational. The patient was painfully aware that there was really nothing to fear and, indeed, for most of his life, the fear had been totally absent. The analyst's method focuses on this disparity between the patient's rational judgment of the experience and the nature of the symptomatic experience itself.

At this point in the application of the psychoanalytic method, the psychoanalyst departs from other methods, be they behavioral, cognitive, or biological. The psychoanalyst implicitly or explicitly bases further inquiry and understanding on the fundamental assumption of an underlying, broadly defined psychological continuity. The psychoanalyst believes (i.e., assumes) that the disparity between rational judgment and irrational experience would become understandable if the nature of the particular underlying psychological continuity that is currently inaccessible to the patient could be determined.

At first glance, readers might shrug off the special necessity for assuming the existence of nonrandom underlying psychological causes, but it is no small thing: The assumptions of any method may be heuristically necessary, but they stand in constant danger of being undermined by findings from elsewhere. Indeed, as we hope will become apparent, the primary methodological aim of our research is to see whether we can provide sufficient support for this fundamental assumption of psychological continuity on the basis of our composite method, so that other methods that ignore the existence of these unconscious processes do so at their own scientific peril.

From the assumption of psychological continuity, we can deduce a significant corollary—a causative psychological unconscious that is dynamic in nature. The nature of this underlying psychological continuity is unknown to the patient. If it were known, the patient would not experience the discontinuities and irrationalities characterizing the account. The surmise that neither the patient nor the psychoanalyst is aware, at least at the start of treatment, means that the causes are unconscious. The generative cell of psychoanalytic theory, the concept of an *inaccessible causative psychological unconscious,* is thus, from a logical standpoint, an assumption of the clinical psychoanalytic method and not an empirical discovery resulting from the practice of the method. Indeed, the ensuing treatment is aimed at discovering what these unconscious causes are, why they are initially inaccessible to the patient, and how they have affected the patient's life. Without the assumption of a causative psychological unconscious that is inaccessible to consciousness, the psychoanalytic method would be unthinkable and unusable.

Another important assumption concerns the role of free associations. By instructing the patient to say whatever comes to mind, the psychoanalyst assumes that what is revealed thereby will provide linkages to the underlying unconscious causes. The psychoanalyst's attention is especially drawn to anything that seems to impede the patient's flow of free associations. We can now begin to understand why the analyst is especially drawn to discontinuities in the patient's communication. It follows from the psychoanalyst's assumptions that, were the flow of associations unimpeded, the underlying psychological continuity would be revealed directly.

Once we appreciate the nature of these underlying assumptions, we can better understand why the psychoanalyst must encourage the most complete kind of communication on the part of the patient. The psychoanalytic method must favor an unstructured versus a structured interview, and it must allow the patient the freedom to range widely and sample deeply from this inner stream of thoughts. This kind of information constitutes the fundamental data that psychoanalysts then try to understand and explain. Chapter 2 present a fuller exploration of the psychoanalytic method and theory drawn on in the research.

THE COGNITIVE PSYCHOLOGICAL ASSUMPTIONS AND FRAME OF REFERENCE

One could scarcely imagine a method more different from the psychoanalytic method than the cognitive psychological method, which derives entirely from an experimental, not a clinical, tradition. Among the fundamental assumptions of any experimental science are that the investigator (a) must ideally exercise complete control over the means of obtaining the phenomena of interest, and (b) has a clear conception of the relevant variables and has hypotheses about their interrelationships. The experimenter also has in mind alternate hypotheses that are tested by incorporating control conditions into the experimental design. The subject is instructed carefully as to exactly what is required. Responses are designed to be as economical as possible and have been selected with a particular purpose in mind.

Aside from its structured nature, the cognitive theoretical frame of reference also differs from that of the psychoanalytic. The focus is on the nature of cognitive processes, usually meant to include perception, memory, judgment, and thought. Cognitive psychology has been far less interested in affective processes, motivations, fantasies, dreams, and other similar experiences. Experimental cognitive science has neglected pathological phenomena in favor of its traditional concern with normal behavior and a disinterest in individual differences. However, experimental cognitive science shares with psychoanalysis beliefs in psychological causes of behavior and in some unconscious causality, although its range of interest is almost entirely contained within the cognitive sphere and ignores the role of motive and affect.

As cognitive psychology has become more and more interested in preattentive and preconscious processes associated particularly with perception, subliminal stimulation has grown in importance as a tool for investigating these processes (Shevrin & Dickman, 1980; Shevrin, 1992a, 1992b). Long before the interest shown by cognitive psychologists in subliminal stimulation, psychoanalytic experimental researchers had used it to investigate unconscious processes of relevance to psychoanalysts. Thus, subliminal stimulation is a method of interest to both cognitive psychologists and psychoanalytic researchers. From a methodological standpoint, the main advantage of subliminal stimulation is that, for both the cognitive psychologist and the psychoanalytic researcher, it makes it possible to bring unconscious processes into the laboratory and to control the nature of the stimulus and the response, albeit the cognitive psychologist and the psychoanalyst are interested in different aspects of these unconscious processes. By permitting this control, subliminal stimulation allows the investigator to study unconscious processes without resorting to inferences from conscious communication that are relied on by the psychoanalyst. An example might make this distinction clearer. It is certainly possible in clinical medicine to infer from a variety of signs and symptoms what the underlying disease process might be. We might, for instance, infer from a variety of such signs and symptoms that the patient is suffering from a thyroid disorder. We might then introduce radioactive iodine into the patient's system and determine, through a Geiger counter, that the uptake of this radioactive iodine by the thyroid gland is distributed in a manner that suggests serious difficulties in thyroid metabolism. The radioactive iodine is a known probe, as is the nature of its uptake in the thyroid gland. The inference chain is considerably shortened, and the two lines of evidence—the clinical and the laboratory—converge and increase our confidence that our diagnosis is correct. Subliminal stimulation can serve this same methodological function by making it possible to investigate the preconscious phases of perception with stimuli designed to probe these processes. Stimuli might also be designed to investigate the nature of unconscious processes bearing on motivation, affect, and conflict, which are of interest to the psychoanalyst.

PSYCHOPHYSIOLOGICAL ASSUMPTIONS AND FRAME OF REFERENCE

Our interest in neurophysiological indicators originated primarily from the methodological requirement for independent and objective measures and, secondarily, from an interest in the relationships between complex psychological events and brain processes. Specifically, on the basis of previous research (Shevrin, 1973), we were ready to assume that ERPs could serve as a marker for these complex psychological events, both conscious and unconscious. We will discuss in Chapter 4 what we mean by a marker and will compare the concept of a marker to other ways in which the relationship between neurophysiological and psychological processes can be conceptualized. The basic assumption underlying our approach is the widely accepted position that mind and brain are closely related and that processes in the two domains are correlated.

Much research has shown that event-related potentials are associated with psychological events such as attention, response to stimuli varying in response probabilities, and connotative meaning. Additionally, we have shown in previous research that a positive-going amplitude, at approximately 200 msec poststimulus, can differentiate between two subliminal stimuli and varies as a function of stimulus meaning and repression (Shevrin, 1973). In our research, we have developed three main measures of ERP responses to specially selected psychological stimuli:

1. A transinformation method based on the Shannon information-theoretic approach (Williams, Shevrin, & Marshall, 1987; Shevrin, 1988; Kushwaha, Williams, & Shevrin, 1992);
2. A time–frequency feature analysis specially developed to serve our particular research ends (Williams & Jeong, 1992; Shevrin et al., 1992);
3. An adaptive Gabor transform that incorporates three brain parameters in addition to time and frequency (Brown, Williams, & Shevrin, 1995).

But why incorporate a physiological response at all? As indicated earlier, we believe the justifications are both methodological and substantive. Methodologically, a physiological measure such as the ERP provides a nonpsychological, objective method to complement the subjective clinical method and a strictly psychological cognitive subliminal method. If a physiological marker is found for a subliminal stimulus hypothesized by the clinicians to be related to an unconscious conflict, then independent evidence is provided for an unconscious (subliminal) process of a dynamic nature. Thus, the evidence for the existence of a dynamic unconscious is substantially strengthened insofar as the clinician's subjective, highly inferential, and theory-laden hypotheses are supported by objective, independent measures based on a procedure (subliminal exposure) in which unconscious processes are operationally defined outcomes of the procedure itself. Substantively, the incorporation of a physiological method opens the door to discovering relationships between conscious and unconscious processes and brain activity. We believe that we have begun to discover such new relationships (Shevrin et al., 1992).

ORGANIZATION OF THE BOOK

We have organized this book into five parts, titled respectively as Theory, Methods, Results, Clinical Cases, and Conclusions and Future Directions.

In Part One, Chapter 2 is devoted to the underlying psychoanalytic theory, Chapter 3 to cognitive theory, and Chapter 4 to the theory of psychophysiological signal analysis.

In Part Two, the psychoanalytic clinical method as applied to our research is described in full detail for the psychoanalytically oriented clinician in Chapter 5; the cognitive psychological method is described in similar detail in Chapter 6; and the psychophysiological method is set forth for the psychophysiologist in Chapter 7. Each of these technical chapters is introduced by a brief nontechnical outline of the technical detail that follows.

In Part Three, Chapter 8 provides a detailed exposition of the main findings. Part Four, containing Chapters 9 through 11, is devoted to presentation of three cases.

Finally, in Part Five, Chapter 12 discusses the conclusions, implications, and future directions of the research.

THEORY

In keeping with the three perspectives constituting our approach, the chapters in this Part are devoted to presenting our approach to psychoanalytic theory (Chapter 2), cognitive theory (Chapter 3), and psychophysiological theory (Chapter 4). In each instance, the theory necessarily reflects our views, although we believe that the views presented will not be surprising to scientists in each field.

For nonpsychoanalytic readers, we need to note that the psychoanalytic theory described is consistent with one that psychoanalysts would call a structural approach. This approach is best characterized as being based on Freud's original ideas about the organization of the mind into three agencies-the id, ego, and superego. Beyond that, the structural approach accounts for the contents of the mind in normal and abnormal conditions as being made up of so-called compromise formations in which id, ego, and superego influences are accommodated with greater or lesser success. This theoretical approach is to be distinguished from an object relations or self psychological approach, two other important alternative theoretical perspectives within psychoanalysis. However, as we will explore briefly in the introduction to Chapter 2 and comment on more fully in Chapter 12, lines of demarcation among the various theories are not clear-cut and much overlap exists. Although we favor a structural approach, our experimental method can be used in conjunction with the two other approaches. All that would be necessary is a choice of key stimuli according to psychodynamic formulations made on the basis of these other theories. In fact, one can foresee a future possibility of exploring the comparative validity of these different theories by using our method.

In Chapter 3, on cognitive theory, we review the current computational basis for much cognitive theory as well as the broadly accepted distinction between automatic and controlled processes. The latter distinction generally coincides with the difference between unconscious and conscious processes,

respectively. We have tried to point to some of the limitations of the computational view and of the automatic/controlled distinction as they bear on
psychoanalytic theory. We then offer an alternative, based on the quite different approach proposed by the cognitive psychologist Alan Allport
(1989). In our judgment, because Allport's approach is quite consistent with
psychoanalytic theory, it provides a useful bridge.

In Chapter 4, on psychophysiological theory, we undertake to show
how a purely amplitude component approach to the ERP is greatly limited
in reflecting the complexity of brain processes instantiating psychological
processes of the kind in which we are interested. We attempt to show how
this component-based approach assumes that any variability in a brain signal is caused by noise that must be averaged out across many trials. Underlying this approach is the assumption that a given brain response, or signal,
would occur at the same time and in the same way each time, were it not for
the variability introduced by random, non-stimulus related factors. In other
words, the signal is fixed, or stationary in time. Our approach is quite different insofar as it is based on the more likely assumption that brain states
vary from time to time, from one stimulation to the next, not simply randomly, but as a function of repetition itself and other substantive factors.
Thus, true brain signals in response to stimuli are inherently variable and
nonstationary. Methods must be devised to measure this inherent variability. We have set out to measure this variability with the development of the
time–frequency and Gabor logon methods of signal analysis. The implications of these new methods for the study of brain–mind interactions are
discussed.

We hope that, after reading these three chapters, readers who are expert in each of these three different perspectives will have an appreciation
of our overall theoretical frame of reference.

Psychoanalytic Theory

As with most sciences, psychoanalytic explanations have grown and developed over the course of the history of psychoanalysis, giving rise to alternate and competing explanations. In Freud's lifetime alone, psychoanalytic theory evolved through three different stages culminating in the structural theory, familiar as the theory based on the id, ego, and superego. However, this theory has not been without its competitors. Various object relations schools were critical of structural theory for failing to give sufficient emphasis to the role of internalized object representations in explaining neurotic behavior. Self psychological theory has drawn attention to the importance of self-organization and the role of early defects in the self, resulting from unempathic early parenting. More recently, intersubjectivity theory has emphasized the centrality of the actual relationship of the analyst to any understanding of pathology and cure.

Although these different theories diverge in some respects, they overlap in many others. Each theory is complex and multifaceted. For example, identifying crucial hypotheses that, if supported or refuted, would favor one theory over another would be hard. It might be more correct and useful to think of these various psychoanalytic theories as efforts to conceptually *represent* complex phenomena in which different emphases are placed on one aspect or another, that is, early relationship to caregivers, importance of self-organization, and so on. Particular cases may fit better with one theory than another. For example, Mr. A's pathology (Chapter 9) appeared to require emphasis on the early relationship to the mother, involving possible early empathic failure—features compatible with object relations and self psychological theories. On the other hand, the two cases shown in Chapters 10 and 11, in particular Mr. B, seemed readily understandable in structural oedipal terms. Nevertheless, each theory claims to give its own explanation of clinical findings identified as particularly salient to the other frames of reference. Thus, in self psychology, oedipal issues find a place although they are interpreted differently than in structural theory.

It is our belief that *all* psychoanalytic theories share a common assumptive base. We will try to show that these common assumptions underlie the psychoanalytic method. In the psychoanalytic method, the psychoanalyst encourages the analysand to free associate and then listens to these associations with a mental set based on the assumptions described below. (For more detail about these distinctions, see Shevrin, 1984; Brakel, 1991.) Despite sharing the assumptions underlying the method, we believe that *differences* in theoretical perspective emerge in the particular clinical hypotheses used to explain the clinical phenomena brought to light by our common method.

At the same time, we need to make plain that our own theoretical interests derive from the application of a structural frame of reference qualified by the inclusion of topographic considerations that our research makes necessary. We invite *all* psychoanalysts to examine our experimental findings and, in particular, to consider our three case presentations as illustrations of how we have applied structural theory to actual clinical material.

Here, we undertake to present both the shared assumptive base of the method and a careful exegesis of how we have attempted to use structural theory in our research. (The details of our procedure are outlined in Chapter 5.)

To achieve the methodological goals of our research project, it is imperative that the clinical method we use in the research be a true extension of the psychoanalytic method and, as such, share with the psychoanalytic method its basic assumptions. We hold that *four basic assumptions* underlie the psychoanalytic method and are shared by all of the main psychoanalytic schools: Kleinian, self psychology, object relations, and structuralist. These assumptions are (a) psychic continuity, (b) psychic determinism, (c) the existence of a psychological unconscious, and (d) the role of free association. In the section that follows, we briefly describe these four assumptions and discuss how our clinical research method, like the psychoanalytic method, assumes each of them.

Next, we describe *four clinical theories.* We organize the data resulting from the use of the psychoanalytic method (and, by extension, the data from the application of our clinical research method) using these four clinical theories. These four theories concern (a) unconscious conflict, (b) compromise formation, (c) the oedipal complex and associated psychosexual stages, and (d) multi- and overdetermination. We have interpreted our clinical data in terms of these structuralist theories, supplemented by topographic (pertaining to the conscious, preconscious, and unconscious status of mental contents) and developmental considerations. Different psychoanalytic schools (psychoanalytic by virtue of holding the four basic assumptions mentioned above) regard different general clinical theories as best for organizing data from the psychoanalytic material. However, we anticipate that our Kleinian, object relations, and self psychology colleagues will have no trouble in recognizing our clinical material as psychoanalytic, nor in applying our research method using their own general clinical theories. In this way, our method might serve to compare the validity of these different theories—a task that has thus far proven elusive.

Later in this chapter, we show how we have utilized the theories of unconscious conflict, compromise formation, the Oedipus complex, and multi- and overdetermination in our actual clinical work, demonstrating their explanatory capacity.

Finally, we address two questions often raised by nonanalysts acquainted with our research. These questions and their answers reveal further facets of psychoanalytic clinical theory.

THE FOUR BASIC ASSUMPTIONS

Psychoanalysis, as a discrete branch of science, has its own method. Like any method, the psychoanalytic method has a number of built-in assumptions that are necessary in order for the method to function. Assumptions of the psychoanalytic method, like those of any method, are taken for granted; thus, they can neither be discovered nor proven from data generated by use of the method (Freud, 1915/1957; Edelson, 1984; Shevrin, 1984; Brakel, 1991).

The psychoanalytic method is based on four major assumptions (Rapaport, 1967; Shevrin, 1984; Brakel, 1991). The first two assumptions, psychic continuity and psychic determinism, are special versions of two assumptions of scientific endeavors in general—continuity and determinism. To assume continuity is to presume lawfulness (though not necessarily regularity); to assume determinism is to take for granted cause and effect. *Psychic* continuity, then, is the assumption that all psychological events—including those that seem inconsistent, such as symptoms, gaps, slips of the tongue, and other parapraxes—are not only lawful but can be rendered psychologically meaningful. *Psychic* determinism holds that even such apparent psychic discontinuities as symptoms, parapraxes, and gaps are not only caused in general, but often have primary psychological causes in particular and are capable of being explained, at least in part, on a psychological basis. We should make clear here that we are intending the broadest possible interpretation of "psychological" when we speak of psychological meaningfulness and psychological causation. There is no restriction at the level of assumptions of the method. Erroneous beliefs and other cognitive distortions would be included, as would faulty memories, defects resulting from early failures in empathy, and conflictual wishes. In other words, anything properly described as psychological can potentially provide psychological explanations and causes.

Before Freud, scientists favored organic causal explanations (certainly an improvement over positing demonic and supernatural causes) as primary for *all* mental symptomatology. Constitutional brain defects, viral illness, physical traumas, or heredity were thought to account for hysterical symptoms, obsessions and compulsions, anxiety, and phobias, no less than delusions, hallucinations, and frank cases of delirium. Indeed, an urgent task for all modern mental health clinicians is to determine whether the primary etiology of a particular problem is psychological or organic. In this connection, it should be stressed that the assumption of primary psychological causation, for many cases, denies neither cases where mental symptoms are caused primarily biologically (e.g., organic brain syndrome, psychoses, or some cases of major depressive illness), nor the necessary brain mediation of all mental events, including neurotic symptoms, although these are usefully considered primarily psychologically caused.

The third assumption, that of a psychological unconscious,[1] follows from the first two assumptions. A psychological unconscious is posited,[2] such that if unconscious contents and processes were taken into account, the apparent discontinuity would resolve. The fourth assumption tells us that it is through the use of free association that the significant unconscious elements will be revealed or inferred in order to resolve seeming psychic discontinuities.

A brief clinical example demonstrates how the four methodological assumptions operate. A woman patient is upset and angry about a vacation her analyst will take in two weeks. She is even more concerned that her analyst will soon get pregnant and ultimately abandon her. This is what she felt happened when she was two years old and her brother was born. She has been in psychoanalysis for several years and it isn't hard for her to say how much she hates her psychoanalyst for "cancering" [sic] her sessions. This slip of the tongue is a seeming discontinuity in her associations (we assume psychic continuity). Psychic determinism and the positing of a

---

[1] Rapaport (1944) considers this a corollary rather than a separate assumption.

[2] In the clinical portion of our research, which is an extension of the psychoanalytic method, the unconscious is again assumed or posited. A primary goal of the research reported in this book is to show that, with the use of methods where the unconscious is not assumed (i.e., the subliminal method and the ERP method), independent evidence for the unconscious can be gained.

psychological unconscious hold that psychologically unconscious causative content can be found, which, when known, would restore continuity. Indeed, positing that the patient's wish that what might grow inside of her analyst will be a cancer, not a baby—something that would cause the analyst as much pain as she believes her analyst's pregnancy would cause her—allows us to understand the slip of the tongue.

Free associative material can sometimes directly fill in gaps or clarify inconsistencies (e.g., a momentarily repressed memory can return). However, as in the case of the "cancering" slip, the contents produced by free association can themselves be different from ordinary waking thoughts and/or can be seen to relate to the gaps and inconsistencies only if further inferences are made, based on certain hypothesized principles of transformation. These hypothesized principles of transformation posit certain mental mechanisms—condensation, displacement, part for whole, symbolic representation—that account for the discontinuities in free associations (Freud, 1900/1953; Edelson, 1984; Brakel, 1994).[3] Thus, free associative connections need not be thematic or logical; instead, there can be clang associations, or associations contiguous or tangential along any dimension or mixed dimensions (e.g., a patient who was a chemist talked on and on about a routine chemical extraction, only later realizing he was anxious about an upcoming dental extraction). We are, of course, describing what Freud (1900/1953, 1911/1958) termed the primary process mode of organization that is prominent in dreams and symptoms as well as free associations. From the vantage point of this methodological analysis, the primary process is an explanatory theory that follows from the four assumptions previously described.

The "cancering" slip illustrates another important aspect of the free association assumption of the psychoanalytic method: Unconscious causes influence and affect conscious processes in both direct and indirect ways. For example, a previously repressed memory may appear quite *directly* in consciousness, as when Elizabeth von R suddenly remembered, in the course of her treatment with Freud, that at her sister's deathbed she had thought that now she could marry her brother-in-law (Freud, 1893/1955). However, the unconscious cause is revealed *indirectly* in the slip "cancering." The conscious intent is to say "canceling." The discontinuity takes the form of an additional meaning (cancer), appearing discontinuously on the basis of the

---

[3] Wherever there is an inconsistency, a truly explanatory unconscious cause is posited as necessary. Some set of principles of transformation therefore becomes a necessary entailment of the four assumptions as soon as the method generates primary process, or seemingly irrational types of free associations. The particular principles of transformation—condensation, displacement, part for whole, symbolic representation—are not necessarily the only (or even the best) such principles. They are the ones analysts have found useful to make sense of the data generated.

unconscious intent. The hypothesized unconscious cause has to do with anxiety and fear that the analyst, once pregnant, will abandon the patient.[4]

That unconscious causes are revealed through indirect manifestations is a significant corollary of the free association assumption of the psychoanalytic method that poses weighty and difficult problems. For example, establishing the validity of this theory requires independent empirical support not thus far available. All we wish to claim here is that the assumption and its corollary are necessary for the method.

Edelson (1988) addresses himself to this issue as he discusses Freud's (1900/1953) positing of "two theorems, the 'basic pillars' of his technique: 'when conscious, purposive ideas are abandoned, concealed purposive ideas assume control of the current ideas, and . . . superficial associations are only substitutes by displacement for suppressed deeper ones' (Freud, 1900/1953, p. 531). He [Freud] indicates also . . . that he appreciates the necessity for providing evidence independent of the method and its use in the psychoanalytic situation to warrant acceptance of these theorems" (p. 270).

Free association, within the psychoanalytic method, entails two other conditions:

1. The analyst's explicit role is primarily devoted to exploring the patient's free associations, wherever they lead (i.e., including about the analyst), in order to learn about the patient and to help the patient learn about himself or herself (in other words, toward analyzing the patient);
2. The patient, among diverse motives for freely associating, necessarily has a conscious intention of learning about himself or herself and getting psychoanalyzed. Although within an analysis this motivation is often far from uppermost, it is implied to exist throughout (Brakel, 1993).

As will be clear from the description of the clinical team's operations in Chapter 5, the first three assumptions of the psychoanalytic method are identically assumed in our clinical research application. After all, our subjects are basically undergoing the same sort of evaluation as would patients being evaluated for psychoanalysis, and our clinical evaluation team members are operating much as they would in evaluating patients for psychoanalysis in their consulting rooms. There are, of course, some differences.

---

[4] This hypothesis does not rule out other possible causes that might influence why the slip took the linguistic form that it did. For example, the form of this slip obeys the rules of morpheme structure—it is a syllable that is replaced ("cel" by "cer"). For an extended discussion of this and other issues in the experimental investigation of slips, the reader is referred to Baars (1992).

Most psychoanalysts do not emphasize DSM-III-R diagnostic labels, and most do not administer a battery of psychological tests (see below for more discussion of the differences). However, noting symptoms, learning of the major unconscious conflicts, and formulating psychodynamic assessments—all through a number of open-ended, nonstructured interviews—constitute the essentials of evaluations for psychoanalysis *and* evaluations using our clinical research method. In both types of evaluation, psychic continuity, psychic determinism, and a psychological unconscious are assumed.

But what about free association, the fourth assumption of the psychoanalytic method? We contend that our clinical research method assumes free association, and this is not merely on the grounds of our use of open-ended rather than structured interviews. Rather, as is true for psychoanalytic patients and psychoanalytic clinicians, in our clinical research method, free association is embarked on by our subjects in the context of a motivation to understand their problems, with the (correct) expectation that we are also attending to these associations to likewise understand their problems. Such patients (or subjects) need not be consciously free associating; perhaps they are not giving up conscious control of their thoughts. Nonetheless, in the clinical context (and in our research extension), sequences of ideas and nonverbal behaviors, no less than contents, constitute free associative material.[5]

FOUR GENERAL CLINICAL THEORIES

The psychoanalytic method—and our clinical research extension of the method, when applied—yields data and discoveries. These data are then organized according to various general clinical theories. In this section, we offer detailed definitions of four fundamental clinical theories that we have found helpful in explaining data and discoveries arising from application of the psychoanalytic method and/or our clinical research extension. Like the assumptions themselves, these clinical theories cannot give any evidential warrant to what the method has assumed because the theories have embedded within them various assumptions of the method. For example, the clinical theory concerning causative unconscious conflicts assumes psychic determinism and continuity and tautologically assumes a psychological unconscious. These four theories also entail other constructs and explanatory

---

[5] An example of a method related to psychoanalysis that does not assume free association may prove useful. Psychobiography is such an example. Although it is sometimes claimed that a writer's journal entries, for instance, can be considered equivalent to free associations, they, in our view, cannot be the same because, in such productions, there is no reason to impute any motivation to get analyzed.

concepts needed to organize the findings. These constructs and concepts are discussed in the following sections (boldface type indicates their occurrence).

Unconscious Conflict

We, like most analysts, hold as a clinical theory that unconscious conflicts are important causative contributors to all varieties of psychological events, including much of what is consciously experienced—for example, symptoms. (Symptoms, which we discuss below, are particularly important for our research purposes.) Our claim for causative unconscious conflicts provides organization to the data yielded when the psychoanalytic method is used; along with other clinical theories, the theory of causative unconscious conflicts allows us to explain these data. However, in order to understand just what the theory of causative unconscious conflicts specifies, we must ask what these unconscious conflicts are; how, why, and under what circumstances do they occur?

Unconscious conflicts are extremely common. We can gain an idea of the extent of their occurrence by examining the simplest type of unconscious conflict—any and all instances of even partly unconscious wishful fantasies that are felt to be either unacceptable or ungratifiable. (Note that these "judgments" about the fantasies can also be unconscious in whole or in part.) A fantasy is felt to be unacceptable or ungratifiable insofar as the subject holds it to be a consequence of, or to lead to, one of several **childhood situations of danger** initially identified by Freud (1926/1959)—loss of object, loss of object's love, castration anxiety, or loss of one's own self-regard. Thus, if a boy wishes to kill his father in order to have a more intimate and exclusive relationship with his mother, this is unacceptable on several counts: he loves his father, killing is bad, his father may retaliate during an attack, and so on. If this same boy envies his mother's capacity to give birth and wishes to do so himself, this wish is ungratifiable owing to its impossibility, and humiliation may result from having had such an impossible wish.

Consistent with the **pleasure principle,** it is in attempting to avoid these dangers and their attendant unpleasurable affects (the anxiety and/or depression associated with unacceptable or ungratifiable wishful fantasies) in accord with one's **psychic-reality**-bound view of best adaptations, that the unconscious conflicts result in various **compromise formations** among the familiar **tripartite psychic structural systems—constructs termed id, ego, and superego** (Freud, 1923/1961), where each represents different functional aspects of mental life. In referring to the id, ego, and superego as constructs, we are indicating that there is no material id, ego, or superego, despite the fact that they are misleadingly called psychic structures. Further, there is no pure manifestation of id, ego or superego. Each is a convenient label for a number of interrelated psychological functions (Beres, 1965). Each, owing to its differing characteristics, is thought of as a necessary contributor to every **compromise formation.**

The id, according to Moore and Fine's *Psychoanalytic Glossary* (1990), "is a concept that encompasses the mental representations of the instinctual drives" (p. 90). The ego has been considered to be a collection of functions—those serving perception as well as those that are "object and reality related, defensive, regulative, synthetic and integrating, autonomous and executive" (p. 62). Finally, these same authors characterize the superego as the agency that "sets up and maintains an intricate system of ideals and values, prohibitions and commands (the conscience); it observes and evaluates the self, compares it with the ideal, and either criticizes, reproaches and punishes, leading to a variety of painful affects, or praises and rewards, thereby raising self-esteem" (p. 189).

Compromise Formations

By definition, compromise formations are composite wholes resulting from the interaction of the id, ego, and superego functions. Unlike the strictly construct status of these three psychic systems, and different too from the necessarily nonconscious operations in their formation, particular instances of resultant compromise formations, by virtue of consisting of observable contents, do have a different ontologic standing. To these content-rich instantiations, which are recognizable as any psychological event (dream, fantasy, parapraxis, transference manifestation, object or career choice, symptom or character trait), we can apply the general construct "compromise formation" with its three components entailed.

To understand further the nature of compromise formations, it is necessary to distinguish between the process of *compromise forming* and the content or product of that forming process. The process that results in compromise formations is always a nonconscious, nonrepresentational process of which we cannot become aware, just as we cannot become aware of the firing of neurons. The content of the compromise formation produced, on the other hand, is representational and can be conscious, preconscious, or unconscious (Shevrin, 1991a).

We note here that the process of compromise forming, in relation to the resultant content, has much in common with the production process versus the content aspect of free associations. The conscious contents that are the products in both cases can demonstrate primary process characteristics. We claim that these primary process characteristics can be considered indicative of: (a) unconscious contents requiring disguise in order to be consciously acceptable (and thereby accessible) and (b) processing necessarily outside of consciousness (i.e., nonconscious operations affecting the disguise of content via displacement and condensation distortion).

In our formulation of psychoanalytic theory, these topographic considerations are central. It is our hope that, in future work related to our research, independent evidence can begin to be provided for the assertion that primary process contents indicate nonconscious processes and unconscious causes influencing conscious contents. Positive findings would go a long way toward reintegrating a new topography into psychoanalytic theory—one where conscious, preconscious, and unconscious designations are not merely descriptive but signify different modes of mental organization (Snodgrass, Shevrin, Brakel, & Medin, 1995).

Immediately, certain problems with the clinical concept of compromise formation arise:

1. Are simple perceptions, single ideas, and fleeting desires really compromise formations? Is each an outcome of an interaction among id, ego, and superego functions?
2. Must a conflict (unconscious and conscious) among these three systems necessarily be a part of each compromise formation, as some theorists have held (Brenner, 1982)?
3. Are Heinz Hartmann's concepts of "autonomous ego functions," "conflict-free sphere of ego functioning," "change of function," and "secondary autonomy" meaningful and useful (Hartmann, 1958)?

These questions have no definitive answers. We will, however, offer what we consider to be the most coherent hypotheses.

Taking question 3 first, we think Hartmann's concepts do remain useful, even if we find that a conflict is necessarily a part of every compromise formation (question 2). Any seeming contradiction is indeed only apparent, for the existence of a conflict among the three agencies in no way precludes various unconflicted functions that are operating smoothly at the same time and even within the same psychological event. Here is a constructed example. Carol accurately registers the perception of her father's smiling face. She then is outraged and walks quickly away because she believes (and construes) a leer to lurk behind his manifest smile. Remembering that we know his smile looked just as she perceived it, let us make a further assumption. We know that his smile, to any neutral outside observer, would look like (and be construed as) the smile of a proud father. Thus, although Carol's visual perceptual registration is itself not interfered with by the conflict, there is obviously a conflict. Further, Carol's conflict can and should be differentiated from another constructed case, Diane's, in which the father's smile is not properly perceived at all, but is seen as a grimace instead—the registration itself is caught up in the conflict.

With regard to question 1, we believe it is most consistent to regard simple perceptions, single ideas, and fleeting desires as compromise formations, that is, as composites of id, ego, and superego components. We take this position insofar as even the simplest perception can be seen to have a motivational (id) and a value (superego) aspect, and the most fleeting desire cannot be felt without a number of quietly operating ego and superego functions. (For example, if the desire is knowable and articulable, even to oneself, or involves a memory or sensation, various ego functions are required. If the desire concerns one's self-regard or something forbidden or morally "incorrect" with regard to another, superego aspects must play a role.)

Question 2 is the most difficult. Even granting that there can be non-conflicted areas of some (and perhaps all) compromise formations, our problem regarding the necessity of a conflict in each and every compromise formation has not been addressed. From a logical point of view, the question is insoluble; those positing necessary conflict can always "posit" one in disagreement with their colleagues who "demonstrate" psychological events without conflict. Thus, all we can frankly claim for our position, which follows, is that it is surely tenable: The set of compromise formations is a large set encompassing two subsets—compromise formations necessarily associated with conflict and compromise formations not necessarily so associated (i.e., those where id, ego, and superego work in harmony toward a cooperative composite).[6,7]

Fortunately, for the purposes of our research, question 2 need not be answered. The compromise formations we have worked with are symptoms; and symptoms are the compromise formations most uncontestedly associated with conscious and unconscious conflict.

Symptoms

A symptom is a particular type of compromise formation; it expresses yet distorts aspects of underlying unconscious conflict(s). Like other such compromise formations, a symptom is taken to consist of conflict and compromise among id, ego, and superego functions in an attempt to maximize gratification and adaptation while minimizing pain with respect to the classic danger situations. So, how are symptoms different? Although

---

[6] This last subset could be further subdivided: (a) compromise formations arising out of conflict; now with "change of function" no longer in conflict; and (b) compromise formations where id, ego, and superego interact and compromise, without even a history of conflict.

[7] Perhaps a term less connected with conflict than "compromise" would help here—"composite" or "combination" formation might more accurately describe the largest, most general category.

symptoms arise no differently than, say, the psychological aspects of dreams or parapraxes, out of the anxiety and/or depression associated with unconscious conflicts, symptoms are, by definition, maladaptive. Some symptoms, although they relieve an immediate sense of danger or hopelessness, are harmful, particularly in the long run. For example, an inhibition of capacities may take place in order to avoid a phobic stimulus. Other symptoms may not even be effective with respect to unpleasurable affect, as anxiety or depression, can concern the symptom itself. In still other cases, a piece of reality may be involuntarily given up.

To demonstrate this process, let's take the case of Bob, a little boy suffering from both anxiety and depression over a wish that, in his view, is both unacceptable and ungratifible. He wishes to be preferred by his mother over his brother, John. Suppose that various compromise formations could be made, each of which consisted in an unconscious connection (in fact, a displacement) between John and the family dog, Spot. If Bob then wished to be preferred to the dog, if he even wished to deprive the dog of his mother's love forever, this couldn't possibly cause him to lose his mother's love—as might an effort to displace John in his mother's affection. Further, Bob could easily believe himself already far preferred to the dog. Thus, in compromise formations with this displacement, both anxiety and depression could potentially be reduced while Bob remains quite unaware of the elements that are hostile and degrading toward John.

Let's consider this displacement with these wishful contents, first, as part of a compromise formation of one sort, a parapraxis. We find Bob calling the dog John, or putting John's favorite cereal into the dog's bowl. At worst, Bob might feel silly or get criticized; at best, everyone might laugh. The unconscious conflict that caused the parapraxis remains, but unpleasurable affects, both anxiety and depression, are lowered.

Suppose, instead of this parapraxis, the best compromise formation now available to Bob is a symptom. There are many reasons one could offer as to why, at a given time, the best compromise formation possible is a less than good one. In this case, for example, John might have recently been taken ill, heightening Bob's sense that his wish is unacceptable; or, Bob might have just been overpowered physically by John, increasing the urgency of his wish. However, this is only a partly satisfactory answer. Even with these new circumstances, we can still ask: Why is a symptom the best compromise formation possible now? Why can't a less harmful parapraxis or dream result? Questions like these are problematic for our theory and, unfortunately, are seldom raised and less often answered. Nonetheless, the same displaced wish, the same hostile elements, the same consideration of conscience could result in Bob's symptomatic fear of dogs. As with the parapraxis, the relationship with his brother is spared although the causative unconscious conflict remains. However, anxiety and perhaps depression have not been reduced; in fact, they have increased. Although some, including Bob himself, might try to explain the heightened anxiety largely as new anxiety about dogs, we feel that the psychoanalytic explanation is more complete and compelling. Bob's new fear of dogs, as a resultant compromise formation, has incorporated, not decreased, his initial anxiety associated with the unacceptable wish to be preferred. (Also, Bob's hostility toward his brother has now been projected as well as displaced, again increasing, not diminishing, his anxiety.) Regarding depression, although one might claim that Bob now feels bad because he's too big a boy to fear dogs, the psychoanalytic understanding offers a more encompassing explanation. Secondarily, Bob may feel bad about fearing dogs; however, the increased depressive affect indicates that his symptom, the compromise formation, has included and not diminished the depression associated with Bob's belief that his wish to be preferred to John is ungratifiable.

Transference Manifestations

No account of psychoanalytic theory can be complete without including transference. Transference manifestations are among the most important discoveries of the psychoanalytic method. No matter which group of general clinical theories psychoanalysts from different schools have used to organize the data, transference manifestations are, in every case, central findings to be explained. Transference manifestations can be considered to belong to the class of compromise formations, because each transference manifestation consists of id, ego, and superego components.

Transference manifestations are a specific type of compromise formation. Transference is understood as a repetition of aspects of the experienced past—including one's unconscious conflicts, unconscious (wishful) fantasies, character traits, identifications, and various components of one's original object relations—in a new and often distorted version, with a new object (e.g., the psychoanalyst).

Following Brenner (1976, 1982), we agree that transferences are ubiquitous; they are not restricted to the psychoanalytic situation. However, the psychoanalytic situation does bear a special relationship to transference manifestations in two ways. First, application of the psychoanalytic method yields transference manifestations as data. In other words, when a patient freely associates, material that can be understood as transference manifestations arises spontaneously. Second, the psychoanalytic technique recommends that analysts handle transference in a special way. Brenner (1976) states: "It is an analyst's attitude toward the transference and the use he makes of it that are the hallmarks of analysis, not the presence of the transference. . . . In analysis the transference is to be analyzed . . . —it is to be understood and interpreted" (p. 131).

As we hope will be evident in the clinical case chapters of this book (Chapters 9 through 11), we handled the transference manifestations of our subjects as we would our psychoanalytic patients: we attempted to understand these manifestations in an analytic fashion.

The Oedipus Complex

The oedipus complex is a central concept in our view of psychoanalytic theory;[8] further, it is both complex and central as an organizer of human development and experience. Nagera (1966, p. 54), who surveyed Freud's vast writings on this subject, says: "He [Freud] stated explicitly on several occasions that the [O]edipus complex is the 'nuclear complex' of neuroses. Thus, he said: 'It is to be suspected that, together with its extensions, it constitutes the *nuclear complex* of every neurosis, and we may expect to find it no less actively at work in other regions of mental life' (1910, p. 47)."

Grossman and Kaplan (1988) explain that there are tasks special to this phase, that only the oedipal-age child, possessing increased cognitive and emotional maturation, can negotiate. For example, the oedipal child must begin to acknowledge and contend with the consequences of generational differences. Unlike oral- and anal-phase instincts, which the child can satisfy no less than the parents despite the constraints parents place on the maturing child (e.g., you may eat that later; you can urinate, but do it in the toilet), oedipal longings, from the child's viewpoint, are not fulfilled equally—the big parents always go to bed together, but the child is small and always alone. Positive and negative oedipal longings alike are frustrated, and narcissistic injuries can be aroused.

Grossman and Kaplan (1988) state that "the optimal direction for development of the oedipal stage is assimilation of defeat without a sense of alienation, vulnerability, damage, inferiority" (p. 329). Yet they point out how elusive an ideal resolution is "in part from the issues of the stage itself. The problem of the oedipal period involves a set of identities and roles, namely masculinity and femininity, father and mother, child and adult, which are achievable only at different times in future development" (p. 329). No wonder this phase, in all its complications, is so universally formative. The fact that a multitude of different unconscious fantasies and unconscious conflicts derive from the multifaceted oedipal phase of life should come as no surprise. This is not to say that various unconscious conflicts and fantasies

---

[8] Although the oedipus complex may not be a central clinical theory in every psychoanalytic school, it is important in every such school.

from earlier stages are less alive. Recast during the oedipal phase (and used to disguise oedipal concerns), preoedipal conflicts, contents, and modes contribute to the nature of an individual's Oedipus complex and beyond.

What concepts have been implied in our statements regarding the Oedipus complex? The following **developmental concepts** derive from data obtained from applying the psychoanalytic method, organized to yield the discoveries that are now givens.[9]

1. An epigenetic (necessary sequential) unfolding of **psychosexual phases** occurs in human development. These phases have been called oral/tactile, anal, phallic, oedipal (both negative-phase oedipal, in which same-sex parents are the desired object, and the more familiar positive-phase oedipal triangle), latency, and adolescence.

2. Individuals, owing to their **psychic reality construal** of aspects of their external and internal situation (i.e., their age-influenced experience of their parents as people and as objects of wishes; various traumas; and so on), suffer **fixation points** (and, in extreme cases, some areas of arrest) along the course of development. **Regressions** to such problem areas are typical, both to fend off the dangers and the attendant unpleasurable affects that are associated with more advanced phases, and to attempt to gain gratification of earlier longings. Hence, notwithstanding the centrality of the Oedipus complex, the psychodynamic assessment of any individual will include preoedipal as well as oedipal elements.

Multidetermination and Overdetermination

We make use of one additional overarching clinical theory in understanding psychoanalytic data. We have left this theory for last, hoping that the earlier pages will have provided some familiarity with each of the composite parts of this concept—a concept that is essentially an extension of our thinking about compromise formations. We are claiming here that compromise formations should indeed be considered **multi- and overdetermined compromises** on several levels—among the conscious, preconscious, and unconscious aspects of the tripartite functional systems; with conflictual and nonconflictual aspects; yielding conscious contents, often in primary process mode; frequently representing various transference manifestations

---

[9] By considering these concepts givens, we in no way diminish the vast number of confirming instances that psychoanalysts and people involved with child development accrue empirically every day.

with elements from preoedipal, oedipal, and adult phases—all contributing
to the content of resultant compromise formations.[10]

CLINICAL APPLICATION

Having set forth the basic assumptions of the psychoanalytic method (as we
see them) and the four major clinical theories (and other entailed concepts)
used to understand data and discoveries generated by the method, let us now
proceed to demonstrate how, in our clinical method—one that we regard as a
research extension of the clinical psychoanalytic method—we utilize the aspects of psychoanalytic theory discussed in the previous section.

The clinicians in our study undertake four tasks or steps, in the following order (for a more detailed account, see Chapter 5).

1. Diagnosing the subject
2. Describing the conscious symptom
3. Formulating the unconscious conflict
4. Selecting words

Diagnosing the Subject

The fact that we chose subjects who empirically fit a particular diagnostic
entity in no way reflects our regard for this descriptive/manifest labeling as
a classification of interest to psychoanalysts. Rather, the diagnostic entities
of "social phobia" and "pathological grief reaction" were chosen because of
the research nature of our work. Both diagnostic categories are associated
with a variety of manifest symptoms. For us, symptoms are compromise formations and, in this general formal respect, are not different from character traits, dreams, daydreams, and all sorts of waking, nonsymptomatic

---

[10] The psychoanalytic theory of conflict and compromise formation has been
championed most articulately by Arlow and Brenner (1964) and Brenner (1976,
1982). As should be evident, we owe much of our own formulations to Arlow and
Brenner and to other structuralists (Abend, 1989, 1990a, 1990b; Boesky, 1982, 1983,
1988). However, especially owing to the findings we are presenting in this book, we
are proponents of a new reintegration of topographical concepts. Unlike Arlow
(1975), we do not view the structural theory as indicative of a Kuhnian (1962) paradigm shift in psychoanalysis; in fact, we hold that, far from being incompatible, the
data of the psychoanalytic method can best be organized and understood only when
topographic, developmental, and structural considerations are simultaneously applied.
For us, these three theories are at the same level of abstraction. We feel that the structuralists are mistaken in considering structural theory overarching.

behavior classified as normal behavior (i.e., other compromise formations). However, we do recognize certain advantages in working with the particular type of compromise formation classified as a symptom.

First, the presence of a diagnostic classification of particular symptoms allows reasonable homogeneity, at least at the level at which each of these labels can be applied. A group of subjects with such tangible complaints allows ready identifiability of subject population and potentially reduces uncontrolled variation. Second, the efficacy of different treatment modalities can be compared. Third, from a practical standpoint for our research, symptoms bring our subjects to us. Patients/subjects seek our services, and participate by associating, with the hope of understanding and relieving their symptoms.

Fourth, and most significantly, symptoms are advantageous to use with our particular research paradigm. We are attempting to test the hypothesis that words representing a subject's conscious experience of a symptom will, on ERP measures, be reacted to differently (thereby forming a separate category) from words representing the unconscious conflict(s). A symptom, more than any other type of compromise formation, provides us an enduring, discernible, compact, single entity about which conscious aspects can be elucidated and underlying unconscious conflict(s) can be reasonably inferred coterminously and contemporaneously.

Describing the Conscious Symptom

In this step of our work, the subjects' own awareness of their symptoms and their explanatory ideas regarding the symptoms' causes are taken at face value. Thus, there is a good deal of agreement among the four judges regarding this phase of our assessment. By inquiring about a conscious symptom and learning a subject's causal explanations regarding the symptom, we are provided with a detailed, specific, and unique expression of the subject's experience of the symptom.

Mr. C, for example, has a social phobia. He is symptomatic in his avoidance of eating in public places. He is aware that a specific fear involved in his symptom concerns eating in front of people, despite the fact that he wants to eat with his friends. Mr. C then offers some causal explanations.

1. He remembers almost choking on some steak at age seven. He wonders: Has he not gotten over that event?
2. His current symptoms began after some rotten fish had been served at his table. He feels this incident must have made him sick.
3. He believed that some organic problem might have caused the problem and went to a doctor.

The symptoms and the conscious explanations that provide specificity are all, in our view, manifest though displaced and distorted versions of unconscious conflicts associated with the unconscious content comprising fantasies. Although the congruence is imperfect, having a social phobic symptom is like having had a particular type of dream (say a "typical" dream—like an examination anxiety dream). Here, the conscious symptom and the explanations the patient/subject believes to be causal are like the recounting of the particular manifest dream, along with glosses and associations. As is true for manifest dreams (and glosses and associations) in relation to the latent dream thoughts they simultaneously disguise and represent, we must remember that symptoms (and conscious explanations) are displacements; thus, they are more consciously acceptable versions of the underlying conflicts, contents, and fantasies that have remained largely unconscious.

Formulating the Unconscious Conflict

The third step of our clinical task is to "figure out" these displacements, aiming at inferring the underlying unconscious conflicts and fantasies comprising the symptom. Already, some can argue that four interviews and a battery of psychological test responses are insufficient data on which to base such inferences; that only long-term analytic data would potentially suffice. We acknowledge this argument. We proceed, however, with the same spirit and in much the same fashion as we do when working with a dream (or any other compromise formation) when sitting behind the couch. We believe even our best interpretive efforts can lead only to an approximate understanding of the underlying unconscious conflict(s)—at every stage of an analysis! Thus, continuing with the dream analogy, just as we take the entire content and form of an analytic hour (including the transference)—not just direct associations—to be associative to a dream recounted in that hour, we utilize all the data of the four interviews and tests (including the transference), not just those that are directly symptom-related, as relevant associative material toward our best approximation of the most relevant unconscious fantasies and conflicts.

Despite the limited data, we nonetheless found a surprising degree of independent agreement concerning two matters that are important for the clinical theory.

1. Regularly, in different subjects, the same symptom was fueled by very different unconscious conflicts and fantasies, even when the conscious experience of the symptom seemed quite similar. This point is of some importance, for it addresses a potential criticism—namely that, for

psychoanalysts, particular symptoms have only a small finite set of potentially causative unconscious conflicts, so that agreement among analysts is not only probable but trivial. Actually, we hold that the same manifest symptom can be caused by a great variety of unconscious conflicts. As an example, one social phobic subject, whose conscious symptom involved a fear of going to places where men and women mix, was thought by all four clinical team members to have a significant (significant for his general psychodynamic picture as well as in relation to his symptom) unconscious conflict concerning exhibitionistic wishes and their prohibition. Another social phobic, Mr. A (described in Chapter 10), identified his main symptom as an inability to be in any situation where people meet socially and/or professionally. Yet, all four judges agreed that exhibitionism had no more than a peripheral significance in the case of Mr. A. Instead, we eventually understood Mr. A's phobia as a means to remove himself from situations in which he felt dangerously enraged; any gathering of more than two people in which he felt he was not being given his due produced great hostility.

2. We regularly agreed that even subjects thought to have similar unconscious conflicts underlying their symptoms were not similar in terms of an overall psychodynamic formulation that included an assessment of ego functions and general developmental phase considerations. We found, for example, that two of our subjects, both with exhibitionistic conflicts, demonstrated very different dynamics. One subject's unconscious conflict over exhibitionism arose from primal-scene fantasies differently elaborated at successive developmental phases, with particular preoedipal regressive positions more manifestly significant than the centrally organizing oedipal phase (from which the regressions took place). Traumatic events (traumatic because of their occurrence at key developmental periods) could account for such a picture of fixation and regression. In contrast, the other subject's phallic–Oedipal wishes to be "the star," outshining a rival, was felt to be the most salient exhibitionistic conflict. Here, we agreed that there did not seem to be much preoedipal regressive contribution.

Areas of Agreement and Disagreement among Us at the Level of Actual Clinical Data

We will take up very schematically, for the purpose of this chapter, the clinical data themselves, contrasting areas in which we agreed with areas in which we did not concur, in order to highlight our use of the particular aspects of clinical psychoanalytic theory described above.

Whereas, almost by definition, the four clinical evaluation team (CET) members and the subject would describe the same "conscious experience of the symptom" (step 2), the task requiring the formulation of an unconscious conflict (step 3) is both more inferential and much more complicated. What has surprised us is that, for each subject, we have *always* had a high degree of agreement regarding the central importance of a particular component of his or her unconscious conflict(s); this component, necessarily described in general, was deemed central to that subject's symptom and to his or her psychodynamics by all! Here are two examples, in an attempt to capture the general, yet highly particular, level of our agreement. For one of our phobic subjects, we were all impressed with the centrality of unconscious conflict(s) over exhibitionism. With Mr. A, we again all agreed that projection of conflicts concerning his destructive aggression was the most significant element. Sometimes, each CET member cited the same bit of clinical manifest data (with similar inferences as to its unconscious content) as evidence. However, we had no such clear consensus regarding answers to questions such as: Which exhibitionism? Which projected destructive aggression? Owing to what? Each CET member characterized the origin and nature of the basic constitution of the central conflict somewhat differently. With Mr. A (see Chapter 10 for fuller details), each judge emphasized a different psychosexual developmental phase as most significant, and/or a different degree of ego function interference was noted. One judge believed a developmental arrest accounted best for the findings; another cited a massive fixation and regression; a third felt that ego defects were causative and contributory (not just resultants); and the final judge felt that a trauma during the consolidating oedipal phase made any of the three options possible, although obscuring any possibility of now knowing which option (or which combination).

To recap, by the end of the third step, we *always* had a consensus about important unconscious contents and a significant component of the unconscious conflict(s) thought both to underlie the symptom and to comprise a major component of unconscious fantasies central to our subject's psychic life. However, we sometimes also had two or more competing views about other particulars of the unconscious conflict.

Selecting Words

The fourth step, selecting words, will be taken up in great detail and depth in Chapter 5. Hence, only a brief outline of the mechanics of our task is given here, and a few comments are offered on how selecting words is related to our use of aspects of psychoanalytic theory.

The word-selection criteria for conscious symptom words and unconscious conflict words are the same. They are:

1. The words must have been uttered by the subject in the course of the evaluation protocol.
2. The number of letters (and spaces) in the word (or phrase) must be less than or equal to 16. (This is a practical constraint imposed by the tachistoscopic side of the experiment. See Chapter 8 for experimental details.)
3. The words must be judged to capture and represent either the conscious symptom or the salient unconscious conflict(s) with as little overlap as possible between conscious and unconscious conflicts. (We do not want to obscure whatever experimental effects are obtained—i.e., brain responses distinguishing between unconscious and conscious words). Thus, although it is desirable to choose words that we regard as nodal—words that capture the different conflictual aspects of the unconscious conflict—for our selections of unconscious conflict words, those words should have little to do with the words representing the conscious symptom experiences.

We must determine which theoretical considerations underlie our word choices. In important respects, the word selection process itself derives from the same clinical and technical theories[11] that form the basis for formulating any interpretation. If we regard an interpretation as a clinician's utterance conveying a partial understanding of the patient, derived (partly intuitively) from an enormous wealth of available material (all of the communications up to that point), word selection can be seen as an even more highly condensed version of the same process. (Interestingly, clinicians often use the exact words uttered by their patients, both in interpretations and in case reports, to capture and convey essential features.) Choosing conscious symptom words can be seen as analogous to the clarification type of interpretation. Selecting unconscious conflict words more closely resembles interpreting aspects of the unconscious conflicts of which the patient was not yet aware; the interpretation, if successful, then facilitates awareness.

Although we as clinical experimenters are not subject to the requirements of timing and tact that are ever present in interpretations within the analytic situation, we do labor under significant constraints when we choose words. One constraint is the number of letters. More importantly, in the analytic situation, there is no need to separate interpretations pertaining to those elements of which the patient is consciously aware from interpretations concerning still unconscious material. In fact,

---

[11] Technical theories are those that pertain to how best to apply the method.

in an analysis, such a separation would not only be artificial but would detract from the patient's sense of conviction, which can grow from adding that which was not in awareness to that which was.

Finally, we must confine our word choices to those words that are actually spoken by the subject in the course of the interviews and diagnostic tests. Because countless numbers of words are uttered, this does not at first seem a serious hindrance. However, consider the clinical setting for comparison. Here, the analyst is allowed truly free verbal expression, not just in terms of vocal qualifiers—intonation, tone, pitch, loudness or softness of voice, and other contributors to interpretation—but also in an unrestricted selection of words. The analyst can at times use the *analyst's* words, stimulated by the patient's productions, to enhance the patient's self-understanding. This type of word selection is vital to the analytic process and is, in part, what makes the analytic process vital.

Conclusions Regarding the Clinical Evaluation Team's Contribution

As clinical experimenters through all four steps in our process, we are aware that ours is a situation derived from, but not identical to, the clinical psychoanalytic situation. Assumptions of the psychoanalytic method (along with psychoanalytic clinical theories and concepts) underlie and inform the conduct of our evaluations, our diagnoses, our assessment of conscious symptoms and unconscious conflicts, and our word selections. Although in significant ways the particular requirements of our experimental protocol necessitate constraints on the application of the psychoanalytic method (sometimes, constraints that are frustrating for psychoanalytic clinicians), we hope to have shown that our clinical research method is indeed a true extension of the psychoanalytic method and that this different perspective, in the context of our research as a whole, will ultimately prove enlarging and enlivening for psychoanalytic theory itself.

TWO FURTHER QUESTIONS

Two questions have been raised by nonpsychoanalytic readers of our research—questions that we feel psychoanalytic theory can help explain and that demonstrate some additional features of psychoanalytic clinical theory. The questions showcase the robustness of psychoanalytic theory; as a theory, it is remarkably comprehensive and flexible. We do not claim, however, that these psychoanalytic explanations rule out the possibility of other competing explanatory concepts.

Question 1

If, as we hold to be true, specific unconscious conflict(s) are the primary causes of a large group of psychological symptoms,[12] how can we explain instances of improvement in such symptoms, even symptomatic abatement, without significant resolution of the unconscious conflict(s) involved? In other words, can we account for symptoms disappearing over time or for a symptom stopping with a change in external environmental circumstances?

We believe that we can explain these outcomes. First, although we hold that specific unconscious conflict(s) are causally related to and indeed cause symptoms, and we further hold that these unconscious conflicts are *necessary causes* of symptoms, we do not hold that such unconscious conflicts are *sufficient causes* for symptoms. Simply stated, other conditions must obtain and contribute for a particular symptom to form and to be maintained.

One of these "other conditions" can be strictly environmental, in the following way. Suppose a man who swims in the ocean for an hour each day develops a shark phobia. Further suppose it is agreed that the most significant underlying conflicts have to do with castration anxiety over phallic sadism. If the man decides to do his swimming in a pool and never has occasion to enter the ocean again, he may properly describe a disappearance of his symptom. No one could claim a resolution of the unconscious conflicts felt to be causal; we may even say the man now suffers from an inhibition. Yet, it is not in a trivial sense that this symptom is gone. This particular symptom requires not just the described set of unconscious conflicts, but also a specific environmental factor. The external environmental factor is analogous here to the day residue and other manifest features in a dream. Indeed, in an analysis, the very same unconscious conflict(s) can be expressed in one manifest dream on one day, with that day's residue, and again the next day, or next week, or next month, in very different manifest dreams with different day residues.

What about a symptom's disappearance over time? This we believe can happen because of "development." In this context, let us define development in terms of the myriad of life factors (not strictly environmental, as above) that, independent of analyzing, can effect shifts in compromise formations, including symptoms. Thus, to claim, as we do, that analysis of unconscious conflicts and compromises, mainly in the transference reexperience of them, constitutes the most efficacious method for producing shifts in compromise formations, in no way implies that less predictable changes in compromise formations cannot spontaneously occur. A man who has felt too small all of his life, owing to perceptions of childhood, can suddenly or

---

[12] The psychological symptoms associated with the psychoses might best be understood as primarily biologically caused.

gradually realize that he is big enough for what he, as an adult, wants to do. For instance, this could happen after a successful job-related incident, after realizing that he has been a big man to his kids, or in conjunction with a feeling that he can satisfy his wife!

Finally, we want to take up the special case in which a neurotic symptom remits just when an external life problem arises—for example, the onset of a physical illness. We believe different instances of this phenomenon have different causes, including aspects involving environmental changes and development. However, we should also keep in mind something more dynamic: the causative unconscious conflict has been partially touched on in such a way that the symptom no longer is the compromise formation that best expresses the multidetermined factors. In many of these cases, for example, the self-punitive aspect of the symptom has received such abundant reinforcement from "reality" that the symptom itself can be dropped.

Question 2

This question, almost a reciprocal of question 1, is: Why and how do symptoms remain, sometimes even after considerable analytic work involving the (seemingly) causative unconscious conflicts? Our two answers are variations of each other, with each predicated on the condensation and the over- or multidetermination concepts alluded to earlier in this chapter.

One symptom can simultaneously express several different causative unconscious conflicts in disguised form. A symptom considered nodal would certainly be highly condensed, fueled by an over- or multidetermined complex network of unconscious conflicts, with many psychosexual levels of different instinctual, ego, and superego components represented. Closely related to the condensation and over- or multidetermination in our mental functioning is its essentially conservative nature.[13] Thus, if 52 important unconscious conflicts exist, why make 52 different symptoms, if one symptom can express all 52 unconscious conflicts simultaneously? Then, even after much analytic work, it certainly is plausible that some important unconscious conflicts could remain.

Let us take up the same problem from a slightly different angle. Suppose we could be sure that all of a symptom's underlying causative unconscious conflicts had been experienced, addressed, worked through, and understood, and the symptom still remained. How could we account for this? Again, let us assume conservation with regard to certain psychic contents and

---

[13] This in no way precludes the equally essential repetitive/redundant nature of psychic operations, such that the same single unconscious conflict could contribute to many compromise formations.

processes. Could it not be that an as-yet-unanalyzed unconscious conflict (different from the 52), only now coming to the forefront owing to the progress of the analysis, would use the preexisting symptom, rather than forming a different symptom. An everyday example might prove useful. As any analytic treatment progresses, it is expected that various unconscious conflicts underlying symptoms will be increasingly understood. But might not the symptom take on new meaning for the patient, owing precisely to its continued existence? The symptom could now represent to the patient, for example, the analyst's helplessness, a way to defeat the analyst, or a way to remain inferior to the analyst—or any or all of these! Thus, something not at issue in the symptom's formation becomes an issue in its maintenance.

One might reasonably conclude, from the questions raised, that the fate of unconscious conflicts must remain forever unknowable. After all, arguing as psychoanalytic theoreticians, we have claimed that a symptom can disappear, although a significant causative unconscious conflict remains, *and* that a particular symptom can endure, notwithstanding good analytic resolution of important causative unconscious conflicts. Psychoanalytic data will not prove illuminating on this issue, nor (we believe) will outcome research data. Independent evidence regarding the fate of unconscious conflicts could, however, be obtained through a follow-up design of the research method we describe in this book.

Thus, a subject's brain (specifically, ERP) responses to the selected words would be compared before and after a psychoanalytic treatment. Would responses to the unconscious conflict words be different after a successful treatment? Would the ERP responses indicate that these words no longer form a cohesive category? Follow-up results with subjects undergoing other treatments could also be obtained. Likewise, subjects choosing no treatment could serve as controls by being retested at intervals matched to treated cases. In short, we could begin not only to track these indicators of unconscious conflict, but to get preliminary data on what treatments (if any) affect them.

Cognitive Theory

In this chapter, we first present a review of theoretical positions characterizing cognitive psychology at this time. We then explore the relationships between these cognitive science views and psychoanalytic theory, as presented in Chapter 2. The chapter concludes with a consideration of our main findings in the light of this theoretical discussion.

Contemporary cognitive theory is based primarily on an analogy with the computer. To those who maintain a strict equivalence point of view between cognitive processes and the computer, the latter, far from being simply an analogy, is considered to be a case in point. According to this point of view, we can directly learn how the mind works from how computers work. The mind is viewed as simply another kind of computer. A less extreme position holds that computers can greatly assist the cognitive theoretician in simulating various hypothesized cognitive processes and can greatly help in figuring out the complex steps involved in any cognitive process.

In either case, resorting to the computer as a fundamental metaphor for cognitive processes has made it possible for cognitive science in the 1950s and, gathering speed, in the 1960s and 1970s, to advance beyond the limitations of behaviorism. By considering the mind to be equivalent to a computer, cognitive psychologists could allow themselves to look into the "black box" abjured by behaviorists. More importantly, the interest stimulated by computers and the sequences of steps involved in complex processes of computation made it possible for cognitive psychologists to free themselves of behaviorists' preoccupation with behavior and to turn their attention to underlying *mental* processes modeled on sequential steps similar to those in a computer.

Perhaps the single most important parallel derived from comparing the mind to a computer is the central importance ascribed by most cognitive theorists to a "computational" view of the mind; the various stages of cognitive processes constituting a mental event are describable in terms of a set of numbers and mathematical operations on them. If "computation" is the quantitative account of a cognitive process, "information processing" is the qualitative step-by-step analysis of what happens to a mental content (i.e., perception, memory, judgment, and so on) as it takes shape and influences other mental contents and processes. This step-by-step cognitive process, in psychological terms, is explained quantitatively on the basis of a series of computations. "Information" refers to the specific mental contents; "processing" refers to a computational account of what happens to the information. At the foundation of this computational view of information processing is a basic "cognitive architecture" or frame within which information is processed. The cognitive architecture imposes certain constraints on what information can be processed and how.

There are at least two different points of view concerning the nature of this cognitive architecture: symbol-based architecture versus connectionist architecture.

SYMBOL-BASED ARCHITECTURES

Illustrative of the symbol-based architecture viewpoint is the theory of Pylyshyn (1989). According to Pylyshyn, three levels constitute the classical computational cognitive architecture:

1. *The semantic or knowledge level.* At this level we explain why people, or appropriately programmed computers do certain things by saying what they know and what their goals are and by showing that these are connected in certain meaningful or even rational ways" (1989, p. 57).
2. *The symbol level.* "The semantic content of knowledge and goals is assumed to be encoded by symbolic expressions . . . the codes and their structure, as well as the regularities by which they are manipulated, constitute another level of organization of the system" (1989, p. 57).
3. *The physical (or biological) level.* "For the entire system to run, it has to be realized in some physical form; the structure and the principles by which the physical object functions correspond to the physical or biological level" (1989, p. 57).

The fundamental problem that the particular cognitive architecture and its three constituent levels explain is how "a physical system, like a human being, behaves in ways that correspond to the knowledge-level principles, which at the same time are governed by physical laws" (1989, p. 61). According to Pylyshyn, there is only one explanation for how knowledge-level principles can be causally realized: by encoding in a system of symbolic codes, themselves physically realized, the physical properties of the codes that cause the behaviors in question. This approach raises two critical questions: (a) How is knowledge encoded in a system of symbolic codes? and (b) How does the manipulation of symbolic codes lead to action? The latter problem is identified as a question of *cognitive control*, referring to the principles that govern how knowledge at the semantic level is transformed into behavior on the level of action by way of internal representational symbolic coded processes. More simply put, how does what one thinks result in what one does (and when doesn't it?)?

We will see later that there is a parallel between Pylyshyn's distinction between the symbolic and coding level and the next level, which involves the *cognitive control* necessary to transform, in some way, the symbolic code into action or behavior. One form this has taken in cognitive theory is to conceptualize the encoding process as "automatic" and the translation of these codes into action as "controlled" processes. One can draw a further parallel. For Pylyshyn, the symbolic encoding is a rule-following process and, in that sense, is "automatic." Cognitive control has to be selective, goal-oriented, and sensitive to context if the resultant action is to be adaptive.

The cognitive architecture organized in terms of the three levels defined above provides the framework and the machinery through which the various cognitive algorithms are realized. A problem of considerable importance is how the function of cognitive architecture imposes limitations on which algorithms can be carried out. This problem is further underscored by a more basic issue that Plyshyn believes to be at the assumptive base of all cognitive architectures modeled on computers: All computers have built-in primitive arithmetic operations and numerical expressions for their different constituents. Quite specifically, the computer operates on the basis of a numerical code. When the output of one operation is zero, a second operation receiving that output (as a result of the computer hardwiring) will output one, zero, or some combination of ones and zeros, depending on the program coding. Literally then, numbers activate the hard-wired on–off electrical signals that are the physical instantiation of the numerical codes. Pylyshyn carefully points out that these arithmetic operations and numerical expressions may or may not be inherent in *cognitive* architectures. In other words, the mind may not, in fact, work that way. Yet, computer-based cognitive architectures are built on this conventional assumption. Pylyshyn notes somewhat cautiously that this is "an assumption that clearly needs to be independently motivated and justified" (1989, p. 77). He further comments that little attention has been paid to this requirement for independent support of this fundamental assumption. (See Chapter 2 on the similar states of psychoanalytic assumption.)

Pylyshyn concludes his theoretical presentation of a symbol-based cognitive architecture with a statement imposing severe potential limitations on any such view:

> It would . . . not be entirely surprising if some of our favorite candidate cognitive phenomena got left out. For example, it could turn out that consciousness is not something that can be given a computational account. Similarly, certain kinds of statistical learning, aspects of ontogenetic development, the effect of moods and emotions, and many other important and interesting phenomena could simply end up not being amenable to a computational account. Substantial components of such phenomena could, for example, require a non-computational explanation, say in terms of biochemistry or some other science. (1989, p. 86)

One could argue that Pylyshyn has quite seriously qualified or even compromised his position insofar as only the narrowest notion of mental process would appear to be securely computational in nature. As with our presentation of psychoanalytic theory, in which we identified certain basic assumptions and presuppositions for which independent evidence is required, we can see that Pylyshyn is well aware of at least one crucial presupposition—mental processes, like computer operations, are based on arithmetic operations and numerical expressions. This assumption is at the heart of the computational approach; it is what is meant by a *computation*. Pylyshyn takes care to say that there is little independent evidence to support this claim, and he adds that little attention is being given to the necessity to obtain such evidence. In the light of our approach, we can only sympathize with his concern. Too little attention has been paid in psychoanalysis to *its* underlying assumptions.

When Pylyshyn speculates that many cognitive phenomena may require explanation based on other sciences, like biochemistry, he appears expressly to distinguish computational explanations from explanations based, for example, on chemical reactions in which it is not numbers that are "sent" but specific chemical "messengers" or neurotransmitters having particular chemical properties. The same considerations apply to purely psychological explanations as to chemical explanations. We may choose to *model* in computational terms and to use the computer as an efficient "logic machine" (i.e., as an almost error-free rule-following apparatus unaffected by mood, bias, or inattention—unlike human operators) to explore various implications or further consequences of these presumed properties, but that is not the same thing as asserting that in the brain or mind such numbers are sent—it would be to confound the model and how it is instantiated in the computer with how the brain or mind actually works.

Another underlying assumption is not made as explicit by Pylyshyn. As he states, computer architecture places limitations on what algorithms will work. For example, compare serial and parallel computers with respect to the kinds of algorithms that each can accommodate. This notion of some structurally determined, limited capacity has found its way into cognitive theory, particularly in theories of attention, and bears on the concepts of automatic and controlled processes previously discussed. The latter are limited in capacity but they determine what emerges in behavior, just as the final step in a program determines what will emerge as the result of its previous operations. Not all cognitive psychologists or attention theorists share this view of the significant role of a limited-capacity system. Even this narrower view of the place of a computational approach has been challenged as inadequate to account for the nature of any mental process.

A CONNECTIONIST VIEW

The main departure distinguishing connectionists from advocates of a symbol-based cognitive architecture involves the replacement of symbols with networks. For Rumelhart (1989), a leading exponent of a connectionist view, a network is an organization of nodes and the links connecting them. Each node is a particular feature (i.e., of a perception), and the links between nodes constitute the relationship among these features. A symbol is a particular pattern of network activation. As a result, a separate level of cognitive architecture to represent symbols is rendered unnecessary.

Underlying the connectionist views is a weaker artificial intelligence (AI) assumption than is true for the symbol-based views: The computer is seen as a helpful means for simulating "systems whose operations are very different from the computer in which they are run" (Rumelhart, 1989, p. 133). We have previously discussed how Pylyshyn himself raises concerns as to how far a computational view can be extended and looks on it as an untested assumption. Rumelhart appears to agree and, in fact, assumes that systems such as the brain operate on quite different principles from computers. In large measure, the computer metaphor is replaced with a brain metaphor. Computer architecture is replaced with "neuronally inspired" brain models based on some abstract conception of what a neuron might be. In effect, the reticulation of neurons, axons, dendrites, and synapses is modeled in the form of nodes (neurons) and their interconnections (axons, dendrites, and synapses). Properties are assigned to these elements that may or may not accord with actual physiology. However, any computer simulation will be relevant and meaningful only to the extent that (a) actual brain properties and their effects on each other are modeled computationally and (b) computational operations have the capacity to model brain operations. Suppose one were to assume that brain processes can be modeled like a language such as English; the subsequent modeling would be constrained by the rules of English, which may or may not allow for modeling certain neural properties. The same problem exists when one language is translated into another; it is often difficult for the second language to "model" (i.e., to translate exactly) the first language because of differences in rule structures, unique meanings, and so on. We do not fully know how constraints intrinsic to a computational approach limit what we can model or simulate in the brain because we do not fully understand how the brain works—that is, what its rules are. Thus, the connectionist view is based on the same computational assumption as symbol-based views, but it takes a different form: All brain processes can, in principle, be modeled computationally. As Pylyshyn points out, there is as yet no independent evidence for either form of the computational assumption. Besides working on different, noncomputational principles, brain processes may not lend themselves to computational modeling. These important considerations should be kept in mind as we proceed with a brief account of connectionist theory.

Activation is the means through which a network becomes functional. When a network is activated, a series of complex computations is occurring in the network. As with symbol-based views, computations involve "sending numbers" throughout the network that serve to activate its nodes (i.e., send numbers to other nodes) and their interconnections. A particular node is activated or inhibited depending on what summation of numbers reaches it from other nodes; links have different numerical weights, so the pattern of activation at any particular node will be the numerical summation of the weights of all the links connecting to it. When modeling networks on brain anatomy and physiology, connectionist theorists attempt to include in their conceptualizations everything that is known about the brain. For example, scientists know that real neurons, as compared to computer elements, are relatively slow by a factor of 1 million milliseconds for neurons versus nanoseconds for computers. Most cognitive processes studied so far take about one second. Thus, at most, a hundred processes are possible within one second. Because cognitive processes appear to involve many more steps within the given time frame, it becomes necessary to posit parallel and distributed processing agencies. Many slow processes acting simultaneously in different parts of the brain can compensate for the slowness of neuronal activity relative to computers.

In computers, knowledge is stored in certain units or files. In the connectionist model of the brain, knowledge is located, as already mentioned, in the patterns of postulated connectivity. No additional symbol-level process is necessary to access knowledge.

There are seven fundamental working elements in any connectionist network.

1. A set of processing units (nodes and links).
2. A state of activation defined over the processing units.
3. An output function for each unit that maps its state of activation into an output.
4. A pattern of activation among units.
5. An activation rule for combining inputs impinging on a unit in its current activation state to produce a new level of unit activation.
6. A learning rule whereby patterns of activation are modified by experience.
7. An environment within which the system operates.

In addition to these postulated working elements and the fundamental computational assumption, there is the further representational assumption that the units constituting a particular system of connections represent (stand for) certain aspects of the environment or inputs from the environment. A good example would be a perceptual microfeature detector activated by perceiving a diagonal line.

Several problems arise with this connectionist model of how the brain works and, by implication, how cognition occurs. Connection theory requires that the network be "taught" how to represent a given input (i.e., a letter or a word). This learning takes place by a process of successive corrective iterations in which it is essential that the model letter or word be known so that it can act as a reference for these corrective iterations. Although much learning takes place with a worked-out model in mind (e.g., learning a new language), it is also the case that much learning takes place in the absence of a known model (e.g., early perceptual learning).

Even if it were possible to "teach" a network without a model, a problem remains. In connection theory, identifying the *boundary* of the network system does not seem to be possible. The assumption of parallel and distributed systems all connected to each other by links of varying strengths makes it logically impossible to draw a boundary around any one particular network because all networks are connected to all other networks. As a result, connection theory requires that we *know in advance*, for example, that the letter "k" is being learned, because simply by observing the network activity there is no rule by which one would know where the network for "k" ends and the network for other letters or other activity begins. This problem is finessed when an isolated, closed network is constructed and targeted for a particular task. However, in the brain, this is not the case at all, especially as it is assumed that the brain is intensively parallel and that many subsystems are simultaneously active.

As a result of this boundary problem, connection theory is caught in an endless regressus. We need to know that we see the letter "k" before we can teach the network "k," but we cannot, independently of the report, know what network "represents" "k." Therefore, on what basis in connection theory do we know "k"? At best, we can say that somewhere in the brain a pattern of excitation exists that represents "k," but in connection theory terms, we cannot identify exactly where it is, no matter how many simulations we might run.

In contemporary cognitive psychology and cognitive neuroscience, connection theory plays an important role. The nature of what is "automatic" in the information processing is often defined in terms of "spreading activation" in a network in which the activation is constrained only by the particular nodes and their connecting links. A cognitive process is considered "controlled" when activation is constrained by a task determining how the network is activated. In effect, the controlled processes play the role of the "teacher" by providing the reference point or model for what is known, setting boundaries to network activation, and selecting task-relevant information from an undifferentiated spreading activation. The concept of parallel and distributed processes intrinsic to connection theory is also a central feature of cognitive theorizing. Yet, it is clear that connection theory is limited by the basic computational assumption and by its inability to provide an independent model for knowledge acquisition. Instead it needs to rely on what is already known in the form of a teacher.

ALLPORT'S SELECTION-FOR-ACTION THEORY FOR AN ATTENTION MOTIVATION SYSTEM

When we shift our interest from broadly based computer models to more specific cognitive theories that have more immediate relevance to our purpose, we find, as already indicated, that the computational assumption and the connectionist model are widely drawn on. Thus, in the joint concepts of controlled and automatic processes, the notion of spreading activation in a network is central to an understanding of automaticity, and limiting or guiding that activation is central to an understanding of controlled processes. To put it differently, controlled processes establish the boundaries that, as we have seen, cannot logically be drawn from within connectionist theory itself. Another metaphor might make this important distinction even clearer: Water spills in all directions, limited only by the natural obstacles in its way, unless channeled by dams, levees, and retaining walls. The water spilling in all directions is equivalent to spreading activation, and the natural obstacles in its way are the network nodes and their varying strength of connections; together, they constitute automaticity. The dams, levees, and retaining walls constitute the controlled processes. In older psychological language, automatic processes are habits, and controlled processes are voluntary actions. In more contemporary terms, automatic processes are defined as involuntary, effortless (i.e., not drawing on attentional resources), autonomous, outside of awareness, and unintentional. Controlled processes, by contrast, are voluntary, requiring effort (i.e., drawing on attentional resources), contingent, conscious, and intentional. There is no place in this framework for unconscious intentional processes, such as is called for in psychoanalytic theory or as our results strongly suggest is the case. The controlled/automatic distinction would rule out unconscious defenses (because these are also motivated) and unconscious conflict. In more general terms, unconscious processes ("automatic," in cognitive theory terms) cannot be shaped in any way by unconscious intentions or motives. Control can only be exercised from the direction of consciousness, a traditional position derived from the prevailing 19th-century view that psychology was primarily the study of consciousness.

The close linking of intention to consciousness in cognitive psychology also derives from the cognitive experimental paradigm itself, in which a task or instruction given by the experimenter is accepted and acted on by the subject as his or her intention and goal in the experiment. In the conventions operating in experiments, the subject is to have no other intention or goal than the one defined by the task given by the experimenter. The controlled processes are the inner counterpart of this external arrangement. The controlled processes define a task or goal shaping the automatic processes. The automatic processes can have no intention of their own; in this respect, they are parallel to the passive role of the experimental subject who is to have no private or personal intention (as well he or she might!). To the extent that the controlled/automatic explanation of cognition holds sway, there is little basis for believing that cognitive theory could be compatible with psychoanalytic theory. Fortunately, the controlled/automatic explanation is much criticized within cognitive psychology, and considerable contradictory evidence exists. A viable alternative is available that enables us to explore the suggestive ways in which cognitive and dynamic explanations can be related.

Allport (1989) has provided perhaps the most telling critique of theories based on a controlled/automatic dichotomy; he has also suggested an interesting alternative. His critique not only cites contrary evidence, but it delves into the assumptive foundations of the theory and reveals their weaknesses. According to Allport, two basic assumptions underlie the controlled/automatic dichotomy: (a) the notion of limited capacity and (b) the serial organization of early/late selection. The former assumption applies to controlled processes; the latter applies to automatic processes. In visual perception, the basic cognitive paradigm used by Allport, early/late selection, posits that sensory (i.e., feature analysis) and spatial information processing occurs initially, followed by object identification and categorization. Controlled/automatic theories differ with respect to the point in early/late selection when controlled processing takes over. In early selection theories, controlled processes take over prior to object identification and categorization; in late selection theories, controlled processes take over after object identification and categorization, which can take place automatically (i.e., without intention or consciousness).

Allport points out that recent findings in the neurophysiology of visual perception demonstrate that feature analysis, spatial location, and object identification occur in parallel systems. Object identification may, in fact, occur before knowledge of location. Tellingly, in lateral neglect (in which the person cannot experience any sense of possessing half of his or her body), distorted representations of whole objects enter into this bodily spatial disorder, indicating that object representations are present along with the disorder in spatial attention. There is good reason to believe that any prevailing serial order is a function of task rather than of any hard-wired sequence.

Allport also points out a further corollary of the previously cited assumptions: Once controlled processing supervenes, automatic processing ceases. After a task determines what stimulus properties will be assigned to controlled processing, processing of all other stimulus properties ends. Allport argues, with some validity, that in this approach, selective cueing (by the task) and selective processing are confounded. Selective attention can be directed to one set of stimuli by particular instruction or cue; at the same time, selective *processing* may continue for uncued stimuli.

In place of a limited-capacity, early/late hierarchical model, Allport argues that recent evidence requires postulating a multiplicity of attentional functions, none of which needs to be central, as in one fixed, dominant control process to the exclusion of any other processing. Instead, multiple and simultaneous adaptive tasks require a constant prioritization of functions related to adaptive actions in the real world. Efficient adaptation also requires that a currently lower-priority task be instantaneously capable of assuming top priority so that concurrent processing of lower-priority tasks is adaptively useful. For a time, an animal may be devoting top-priority attention to devouring its prey, but at the same time, it needs to process cues that could immediately alert it to the presence of enemies. To place the theory in a clinical setting, a patient may be consciously attending (giving top priority) to the manifest content of a particular therapeutic exchange, but he or she may, at the same time, be unconsciously processing cues related to underlying transference feelings bearing on some unconsciously expected danger (i.e., loss of parental love). Or, as in our experimental setting, the subject may be alertly attending to the fixation point and the blank field, while at the same time the subliminal stimulus registers and is simultaneously processed out of awareness.

Of equal importance, for our purposes, is Allport's linking of complex attentional acts to motivation, which is rare among cognitive theorists.

Adaptive prioritization can only occur on the basis of some hierarchy of intentions related to a given environment. As Allport states, adaptive prioritization depends on "some means of evaluating, or at least estimating, the relative *motivational importance* [italics added] and temporal urgency of the potential threats and affordances *outside* the current attentional engagement, relative to the estimated importance of urgency of the *current* [italics added] activity or activities" (1989, p. 653). He continues, "I should . . . add, as a further indispensable attentional function, continuous (parallel) monitoring of the environment (internal as well as external) for changes relevant to current and long-term goals" (1989, p. 653).

We note that Allport carefully includes internal as well as external monitoring as indispensable to adaptive attentional functioning. By linking attention to motivation and including internal as well as external monitoring, Allport provides a basis for relating cognitive theory to a psychodynamic conception of conscious and unconscious processes. Allport does not himself discuss the relationship of his conception of a multifunctional attentional motivational system to awareness or its absence, although his views are not incompatible with those concepts. When, for example, Allport talks about the "relative motivational importance . . . of potential . . . affordances *outside* the current intentional engagement," one can see that he is postulating that motives other than the immediate central motive in the "current attentional engagement" can result in simultaneous processing of environmental stimuli. These motives can thus shape processes beyond those defined by the momentarily central task. As a consequence, the notions of automatic and controlled lose their distinctness: Controlled processes, in the sense of being affected by motives, can go on outside of the focus of current attention. Moreover, the source of these motives can be external (i.e., environmental threat) or internal (i.e., needs such as hunger, thirst, or sex). The picture one can draw from Allport's model begins to approximate a psychoanalytic model in which internal and unconscious motives that are related to basic needs or drives shape cognitive processes both within and outside consciousness, once we link consciousness with the current attentional engagement. As we shall see when we next consider recent research and theory in social cognition, once contradictory evidence forces the controlled/automatic distinction to be abandoned, the role of intention, so closely tied to controlled processes, causes difficulty.

A SOCIAL COGNITIVE PERSPECTIVE

In an opening chapter of the aptly titled book *Unintended Thought*, edited by Uleman and Bargh (1989), Bargh presents a complex view of the role of automaticity in social perception and cognition. The book title unambiguously conveys the central thesis of this collection of papers on unconscious processes as seen from a social cognitive perspective: Intention (motivation) is conscious, while unconscious processes are unintentional (unmotivated). Automaticity is defined entirely in terms of one property: "not requiring conscious guidance to run to completion" (Bargh, 1989, p. 24).

Much as Allport does, Bargh takes the distinction between automatic and controlled to task, citing evidence from a variety of social perception and cognitive research to demonstrate that autonomic processes are conditional and that circumstances dictate which properties of automaticity are operative. Thus, research has shown that automatic processes are not effortless, requiring no attention; attentional resources are required (Kahneman & Henik, 1981). Also, motor habits that are considered automatic, such as typing, driving, and walking, insofar as they are readily stoppable and clearly intentional, share properties with controlled processes. The effort to distinguish controlled and automatic processes on the basis of multiple-related properties does not appear to stand up under close conceptual and empirical scrutiny.

Whereas Allport is clear in linking motivation at all levels, internal as well as external, to attentional processes (those in focal attention and those at the periphery), Bargh links intention solely to conscious processes but then encounters some difficulty in maintaining this position. Instead of unconscious intention, Bargh resorts to a dispositional view of the forces "running" automatic processes. One such set of dispositions is made up of "chronically accessible social constructs," (Bargh, 1989, p. 12) such as honesty, selfishness, and aggression, assessed on the basis of paper and pencil tests. Research is cited to show that these social constructs can be activated by "relevant proximal stimulus information . . . without the need for conscious intentions or goals or attention, or any awareness that the information has been thus categorized" (Bargh, 1989, p. 12). These social constructs are nonmotivational causes of behavior—in particular, of preconscious, automatic processing highly influential in producing social stereotypes and misattribution of personal attitudes to external stimuli. Feeling states are other nonmotivational causes. People who were interviewed after seeing various films were more positive or negative in their judgments on a variety of unrelated matters, depending on the emotional tone of the movie they had just seen (Forgas & Moylan, 1987). These social constructs and feeling states are not movitational in nature. But could, for example, the importance of honesty to a person be based on fear of personal dishonesty or the need to placate authority? Could the influence of a feeling state be related to powerful wishes that might result in negative attributions to seemingly unrelated matters because of sado-masochistic wishes that have been aroused? Questions of this nature are not raised; the existence of one type of social construct or another, or the presence of individual variability in such attitudes, is attributed to "life experiences" or the "long-term social environment" (Bargh, 1989, p. 12).

Nevertheless, some problems emerge in attempting to link intention to consciousness, and nonmotivational causes to unconscious or automatic processes. Bargh himself reports experimental evidence that goal-directed thought can continue after conscious attention has been shifted elsewhere. A good example is the "tip-of-the-tongue" phenomenon. After an initial conscious effort fails, the attempt to retrieve an elusive name may be dropped and other matters attended to; then, at some later point, the lost name suddenly pops into consciousness. As Bargh notes, "the search for the answer goes on in these cases autonomously without conscious awareness or control to achieve the desired goal after all" (1989, p. 26). Bargh also cites the work of Ghiselin (1952), who has identified many examples of unconscious problem solving achieved by scientists, poets, and artists, where "goal-oriented" and therefore apparently intentional unconscious thinking occurs. Bargh finally does concede that "it is possible that chronic motivations may manifest themselves in a totally automatic way beginning with preconscious activation by triggering situational features of the overarching goal structure" (1989, p. 26). However, Bargh wishes to distinguish this kind of unconscious motivation from the "Freudian notion of 'unconscious' goals and motivations in which the person is never aware of having such goals in the first place" (1989, p. 26).

Let us briefly examine Bargh's notion of a goal-directed autonomic process. He does appear to concede that there can be an intention guiding an automatic process, but the origin of this goal or intention is within consciousness itself and, in fact, occurs after "a great deal of conscious thought and effort" (1989, p. 26). The unconscious intention is, as it were, borrowed from consciousness, and it retains its importance because of its relevance to some conscious task. Yet, Bargh cites other evidence that "intrusive and uncontrollable conscious thinking may in fact be attributable, at least in part, to the operation of unsatisfied goals of long-standing importance to the person" (1989, p. 26). He is referring to research on uncontrollable ruminations and obsessive thinking caused by traumatic events. Presumably, these "goals of long-standing importance" are entirely conscious in origin. At the very least, then, there are unconscious intentions associated with automaticity, albeit ones borrowed from consciousness.

How different is this from the psychoanalytic conception of repression according to which certain unacceptable desires may appear consciously and then are quickly banished from consciousness? When Elizabeth Von R, a patient described by Freud (1893/1955) in his Studies on Hysteria, entertained the wish, at her sister's deathbed, that she could now marry her sister's husband, it was an entirely conscious thought. However, the thought was then immediately repressed, causing "automatic" mayhem in the form of various symptoms, all of which kept her from achieving the goal of finding any husband, let alone her widowed brother-in-law. Psychoanalysts might further infer that lying behind the wish for her dead sister's husband was an earlier childhood wish for winning her father away from her mother, but this might well have been conscious in childhood and later repressed. There is no real contradiction between Bargh's position and psychoanalysis. The extensive evidence he cites can equally support the psychoanalytic view of the role of intention in unconscious processes: that automatic (unconscious) processes not guided by ongoing conscious intentions can be guided by unconscious intentions having their origin at one time or another in consciousness. One is, however, left with the thought that the notion of automatic has lost all specificity and conceptual force; it would simply be less confusing to re-place it with the concept of the unconscious.

SUMMARY AND CONCLUSIONS

What can we learn from this examination of cognitive theory with refer-ence to our presentation of psychoanalytic theory in Chapter 2 and its bearing on our findings? These implications are organized here under three headings: (a) the concept of computation, (b) the controlled/automatic distinction, and (c) conscious and unconscious processes.

The Concept of Computation

Much cognitive theory is linked to the computer in at least two different ways: (a) the computer as, in effect, a form of mind from which one can learn how the mind and even the brain work—the so-called strong artificial intelligence (AI) position as developed by Pylyshyn, and (b) the computer as a model for, rather than an instance of, the mind and the brain, the so-called weak AI position developed by Rumelhart. For either position, the computa-tional operations of the computer are basic to most views of how cognitive processes work. Computation refers to the numerical code on the basis of which information is relayed from one point to another in the computer. As Pylyshyn points out, it is an unproven assumption as to whether actual cog-nitive processes work on this basis; totally different processes might be in-volved, based on entirely different kinds of codes that might be biochemical, electrophysiological, or purely psychological in nature. Rumelhart, on the other hand, sees the computer and its computational numerical codes as use-ful tools for simulating models of brain functioning. The permissive assump-tion he must make is that the constraints posed by these numerical codes and their instantiation in a particular hardware do not seriously limit what can be modeled of how brain processes actually work.

The computer turns out to be a seductive siren who makes us talk her language, no matter what meanings we employ. Not surprisingly, cognitive scientists like Allport appear to depart significantly from a strictly literal

use of the term "computation." Allport, citing Marr, a cognitive neurosci-
entist, approvingly states:

> Understanding any complex mental function no doubt requires explana-
> tion at many different levels. David Marr, particularly, emphasized the
> importance of clear explicit formulation at the level of what he called
> the *computational theory*, that is, the level at which the overall *purposes*
> or goals of a given category of cognitive processes are to be specified and
> at which the internal and environmental *constraints* under which they
> must operate, and that make those processes possible, are formulated.
> (1989, p. 631, italics in original)

This formulation contains little about numbers and much about purposes, goals, functions, and levels of organization—all terms that could be biological or psychological in nature—yet these terms appear to be subsumed
under "computational theory." As often happens in scientific usage, a term
with a clear and delimited reference becomes much more general and ambiguous over time. At best, what is left is a vague allusion to something quantitative whose exact character is determined by the specific subject matter
(i.e., vision, attention, and so on) rather than by the way computers operate.
It is instructive to recall Pylyshyn's admonition that the extent to which
true computation explains the full range of cognitive processes remains an
untested assumption.

The Controlled/Automatic Distinction

A similar fate appears to have overtaken the controlled/automatic distinction, in the sense that the two concepts have undergone considerable modification, if not outright dismantling, as described by Allport in cognitive
psychology and by Bargh in social psychology. In place of the controlled/
automatic distinction, Allport offers a theory emphasizing a complex hierarchy of attention-motivational systems capable of rapid shifts in priorities.
Control is determined by the interaction of external environmental demands with internal motivational requirements. Attention, and presumably
consciousness, is directed at the combination of environmental demands and
motivational requirements that receives the highest adaptational priority.
What were formerly designated as automatic processes are simply those of
lower priority, which are momentarily capable of shifting into the focus of
high-priority attention as adaptational requirements change. A fluid hierarchy of this kind necessitates that processing of lower-priority systems continue simultaneously with high-priority systems; otherwise, rapid priority
shifts could not take place with optimum adaptational success. As a result,

controlled processes (high-priority systems) cannot preempt automatic processes as stipulated in the usual form of controlled/automatic theory.

Although Bargh appears to share much of Allport's misgivings about the controlled/automatic distinction, unlike Allport, he wishes to save the concept of automaticity by defining its essential character in terms of an absence of intention. According to Bargh, motivation is always conscious. Even when the evidence suggests that unconscious, goal-directed, automatic processes exist, Bargh wants to save intention for consciousness by insisting that the origin of these automatic intentions is always conscious. We have argued that, much as Bargh would like to distinguish this position from Freud's, there is no contradiction between psychoanalytic theory and Bargh's theory on this score. Dynamic repressed contents have their original source in consciousness (Freud, 1915/1957). If there is a significant difference between Freud and Bargh, it has more to do with the different fate of the originally conscious intentions than with their origin. Bargh's automatic intentions can readily be brought back to consciousness and thus would be viewed psychoanalytically as preconscious; Freud's repressed intentions cannot readily be brought back to consciousness and thus are viewed as dynamically unconscious.

Interestingly, what appear not to be so readily available to consciousness in Bargh's theory are the "chronic social constructs" that are dispositional in nature and act as nonmotivational causes of automatic influences on consciousness. These chronic social constructs are inherently nonmotivational; they are defined as personality traits or characteristics of the individual, like intelligence or temperament, that can exercise enormous influence on behavior but are not themselves intentions or motivations. In psychoanalytic theory, dispositional traits of this nature are also to be found in what are termed "ego factors." These ego factors exist as nonconscious constraints on behavior, similar to procedural memory—a repository of rules, perhaps most prominent of which are the rules of language.

However, in psychoanalytic theory, any goal-directed activity that has some gratification as its aim has to involve a motive, either conscious or unconscious and often both at the same time. Unconscious motives are not dispositional influences on behavior like innate intelligence; they are active organizers providing the impetus for behavior. Innate intelligence is dispositional because it is a characteristic of an individual, independent of any particular motive. Similarly, the fragility of glass is an inherent characteristic of glass as a material and, in that sense, is dispositional, but it takes the force of gravity to cause the glass to break when dropped. Gravitational force is functionally analogous to a motive. Another analogy might serve to make this important distinction clearer. The engine of a car literally provides its motive power, while the wheels and other body parts exercise constraints as to how this motive power is transformed into motion. A car without an engine would not move; *how* the car moves depends on the wheels and other body parts. When, in our research, we posited the existence of certain unconscious conflicts, we hypothesized that quite specific unconscious motives were at work; otherwise, our formulations would not qualify as psychoanalytic in nature. These motives were not dispositional constraints but active motors setting the psychic apparatus in motion.

Conscious and Unconscious Processes

Are there qualitative differences between conscious and unconscious processes that are not caught up in the spurious distinctions between controlled and automatic processes? Allport does not address this question. He simply posits a shifting hierarchy of attention-motivational systems without specifying any qualitative differences in modus operandi between those attention-motivational systems of high priority and those of low priority still undergoing processing. Bargh, on the other hand, draws attention to an interesting difference: When automatic processes influence consciousness, they are experienced as noninferential givens, even though an inferential process may have occurred unconsciously. For example, a person characterized as having honesty as a chronic social construct will be especially sensitive to issues of honesty and will judge faces on that basis, but will experience these judgments as inherent in the stimulus rather than as a personal bias. A psychoanalyst might say that these judgments, just like the effects of unconscious motives, are peremptory in nature and are not open to conscious critical appraisal. In this respect, Bargh's theory and psychoanalytic theory concur that unconscious processes can be qualitatively different from conscious processes, and they concur even as to the nature of some of the differences.

In what other ways might conscious and unconscious processes differ qualitatively, given the cognitive theories thus far reviewed? One other way derives from network connectionist theories and their application to controlled and automatic processes. Several examples might clarify the nature of this distinction. Posner and Boies (1971), when talking about "preattentive" processes or those processes preceding consciousness of a stimulus, have demonstrated that the stimulus initially activates a wide variety of codes in addition to the code that is related to the immediate conscious task. Thus, if a subject is told to press a button only when lowercase letters appear, the experimenter could demonstrate through subsequent savings effects that uppercase letters were also activated. Marcel (1983) demonstrated that a pattern-masked word, such as bank, would activate its multiple meanings, although it would only activate its contextually relevant meaning when presented unmasked and, thus, in consciousness. Apparently, preattentive or unconscious processing results in spreading activation throughout a connectionist network that is not limited to the meanings related to a conscious task, but is constrained only by the structure of the network itself. For Bargh, spreading activation would qualify as automatic; he would claim that it is not guided by a conscious intention, or any intention, because, for Bargh, there are no unconscious intentions.

Interestingly, in psychoanalytic theory, there is a set of concepts comparable to spreading activation: the notion of mobile or unbound cathexes that characterize primary (as opposed to secondary) processes. First, it should be noted that the concept of cathexis is similar in its conceptual function to the connectionist concept of activation: It refers to that which sets processes in motion. *Bound* cathexis would be comparable to controlled processes; *unbound* or *mobile* cathexis would be comparable to spreading activation. Whereas the *spread* of activation in automatic processes is determined only by the structure of the network and could, in principle, spread throughout all networks because all networks are connected, mobile cathexis appears to be constrained by certain rules of organization referred to as a primary process level of organization. According to psychoanalytic theory, this level of organization is primary in the sense of being developmentally early, so that childhood cognition is marked by primary process organization. Just as much of conscious childhood content is superseded and soon repressed, so these childhood cognitive modes function unconsciously. Although the nature of primary process organization is by no means fully worked out in psychoanalytic theory, there are certain telltale indicators of its operation: alogical thinking, a tolerance for contradiction, a part standing for the whole, and something tangential or unimportant taking on the burden of reference for quite important and psychologically threatening desires and thoughts. These primary process indicators are frequently noted in dream reports and, when looked for, are not uncommon in everyday waking thought. Primary process indicators can be summarized under the headings of condensation, displacement, and symbolism, the main mechanisms hypothesized by Freud to be at work during primary process ideation. These mechanisms characterize infantile wishes that fuel motivations and are also used in the service of significant defensive activity related to repressing these motivations.

Thus, the psychoanalytic concept of the primary process differs from the connectionist theory of automatic spreading activation in two important respects:

1. Rather than being constrained solely by the structure of a network, as in spreading activation, the primary process activates a network on the basis of these different principles of organization. Networks are *reorganized* in accord with primary process principles rather than simply activated randomly and infinitely.

2. Motives—wishful and defensive—influence the course of this reor-
ganizing activation to meet defensive needs.

Insofar as activation is *controlled*, both by principles of organization and
motivation in the operation of the primary process, we can see how unconscious processes can be both controlled and intentional, the former at
variance with the usual distinction between controlled and automatic
processes, the latter at variance with Bargh's contention that unconscious
processes are unintentional.

IMPLICATIONS FOR OUR RESEARCH

We consider here the implications of this theoretical analysis for our method
and findings. As described in Chapter 2, the clinical method is based on the
assumption that unconscious motives exist. In our examination of Allport's
theory, we have seen how he closely links motivation to attention; how,
through the interaction of environment and motivation, adaptive requirements are determined and priorities for attention are set. Moreover, the existence of a given high-priority attention-motivational system does not
preclude the simultaneous processing relevant to other nonpriority systems
that are not the focus of attention at the moment. Although Allport does not
address concepts such as conscious and unconscious, it would do no violence
to his theory to maintain that it is highly likely that high-priority attention-
motivational systems are conscious and that all of the other systems are unconscious and are no less motivational in nature.

Bargh would like to deny the existence of unconscious motives. We
have seen, however, that the evidence he cites creates problems for this
view. He, in fact, ends up talking about unconscious intentions, but tries to
explain them away by ascribing their origin to consciousness. We have
pointed out that this ascription does not contradict psychoanalytic theory.

On the basis of our theoretical analysis, we can conclude that our assumption of unconscious motives is consistent with the findings cited by
Allport and Bargh. The assumption of unconscious motivation can fit well
with current research in cognitive and social psychology.

When we next turn our attention to the subliminal/supraliminal laboratory method, we can again benefit from Allport's analysis. We can recast
what our subjects are doing as follows: Their conscious task is to fixate a
dot, look as alertly as possible into the surrounding visual field, and report
whatever they see. The high-priority attention-motivational task is to
alertly pick up whatever stimulus is presented. A word may be flashed too
quickly for conscious perception, but it registers and is processed by other

systems that are not, at that moment, of high priority but are nevertheless important with respect to other motivational requirements.

We next consider the role played by brain responses. Their important function is to detect the unconscious processing of the stimuli and to allow us to compare this unconscious processing with the processing that occurs in consciousness when the same words are presented supraliminally. Our findings then tell us that there are qualitative differences between conscious and unconscious processing, depending on whether the words are related to unconscious conflict or to conscious symptom experience. The electrophysiology of the brain is different when unconscious conflict is involved. On the basis of our current method, we cannot say whether the psychological processes occurring during unconscious processing obey the rules of primary process organization. We can say, however, that the unconscious conflict words constitute a category only when presented subliminally; thus, some unifying organization is present unconsciously. For the unconscious conflict words that are presented subliminally, activation is not spreading solely as a function of network nodes and connecting weights; if that were the case, diverse categories would be activated. However, this does appear to happen supraliminally for the unconscious conflict words—the opposite of what would be expected on the basis of controlled/automatic theory but quite consistent with psychoanalytic theory (see Chapter 8 for a full presentation of findings).

Psychophysiological Theory

An initial question needs to be answered: Why use brain responses at all? We can safely say that most psychoanalytic and cognitive research relies entirely on psychological measures of various kinds. Many researchers are loath to involve brain responses because new measurement and methodological complexities are encountered, as are potential philosophical questions bearing on the seemingly intractable mind–body problem. Moreover, it is argued that satisfactory explanations can be worked out entirely at a psychological level. At the same time, cognitive psychology has recently developed in an interdisciplinary direction, giving rise to the new field of cognitive neuroscience. Nothing quite comparable has happened within psychoanalysis, although there have always been some purely theoretical attempts to incorporate neurophysiological concepts. Indeed, Freud himself was the first such theorizer and we will consider his views on the subject next, after which we will also consider other views.

First, as Nagel (1994) has recently pointed out, psychoanalysis from the start has been based on a materialistic metaphysics, in which a real, knowable world is taken for granted. When Freud first tried his hand at a comprehensive theory, in *Project for a Scientific Psychology* (1895/1950), he cast it in neurophysiological terms. Presciently, he posited the existence of a basic nervous system unit comparable to the neuron, and "contact barriers" between these units comparable to synapses. Freud's neurophysiological theory was not published in his lifetime and only came to light years later. Opinion has been divided on its importance and relevance to contemporary psychoanalysis. Some believe (as they surmise Freud did, because he never published his *Project*) that it was an early, premature, and failed effort to found psychoanalysis as a "hard" science. Others believe that whatever meritorious ideas the effort possessed were incorporated into Freud's later theorizing in *The Interpretation of Dreams* (1900/1953) and in his metapsychological papers.

Pribram and Gill (1976) have taken a quite different position, asserting in their careful reassessment of the *Project* that it should be taken seriously as a pioneering effort to ground psychoanalysis in neurophysiology and contains Freud's basic conceptualizations of the mechanisms explaining psychoanalytic phenomena. For Pribram and Gill, the *Project* is also a forerunner of modern cognitive control theory and, as such, they believe it can provide cognitive psychology with clinical applicability, something it currently lacks. For readers interested in a provocative exploration of the relationships among cognitive psychology, neurophysiology, and psychoanalysis, the Pribram and Gill volume will be rewarding. For our present purposes, we need only note that Freud, as early as the *Project*, desired to root psychoanalysis in biology and to consider the mechanisms of the mind to be instantiated in brain processes. Pribram and Gill draw forth from this early effort many suggestive parallels between Freud's theorizing and contemporary cognitive psychology and neurophysiology.

If, as Freud supposed, conscious experience is in some way associated with brain processes, unconscious processes must be similarly associated. This conclusion must follow from the fundamental assumption of a materialistic metaphysics. Thus, it should be possible to detect brain responses associated with unconscious processes—and, indeed, our research provides empirical support for this position. Among psychoanalytic theoreticians since Freud, perhaps the most extreme position on the importance of brain processes to psychoanalysis has been taken by Rubenstein. Following Freud, Rubenstein (1976) pointed out that, in a psychoanalysis, the psychoanalyst does not directly know the unconscious; the nature of the unconscious is always inferred from experiences consciously reported by the patient or from behavioral enactments that the analyst takes to be evidence of unconscious influences. Moreover, the analytic relationship is between two persons experienced entirely in a psychological mode. However, Rubenstein argued, neurophysiology offers a way in which the unconscious could be known directly without inference. He referred to this neurophysiological approach as being on the level of the organism rather than the person. From Rubenstein's viewpoint, the event-related potentials (ERP) measures we have relied on, associated with subliminal (unconscious) processes, are measures of the unconscious that do not require any inference from conscious experience. The words we have selected from the patient protocols are inferences on the level of person, but the ERP responses to those words are measures on the level of the organism and do not require such inferences. But are ERPs such noninferential measures? Can we, for example, "discover" from the ERPs the psychological nature of these unconscious processes? The answer has to be rather, that the ERPs become meaningful on the basis of our prior knowledge that the words flashed subliminally have been inferentially selected by clinicians from the patients' conscious experiences and are thus contingent on this prior knowledge. In these important respects, an understanding of the ERPs requires inferences that refer back to the person level of experience.

Our own position is different from Rubenstein's. Brain responses are vitally important, not as noninferential measures of the unconscious but as a convergent set of operations based on "harder," more objective measures than clinical judgments that are, at the same time, independent of these clinical judgments. Our justification is primarily methodological rather than theoretical. However, it may be possible to discover suggestive differences in the brain responses associated with unconscious processes, and these differences might lead to new hypotheses on the nature of the *brain processes* associated with the unconscious. As discussed in more detail in Chapter 12, we believe our results point the way to a new understanding of the neurophysiological character of unconscious processes.

In our research, brain responses serve a methodological function similar to that of laboratory tests in physical medicine, with one important difference: Brain responses cannot be considered the final arbiter, as is the case with some laboratory tests, because the underlying theory relating the brain response findings and the clinical inferences has not been worked out. For example, we do not know why a high-frequency feature, discussed at great length in Chapter 8, occurs early subliminally and later supraliminally for unconscious conflict words. We have no theory relating the ERP parameters to unconscious conflict, but we can say that these ERP parameters are associated with, or are markers for, unconscious conflict. When we call them markers, we mean that these ERP parameters are statistically significant indicators of unconscious conflict, but we do not know whether they are an intrinsic part of the cause-and-effect chain involved in the neurophysiology of unconscious processes or are simply a noncausal concomitant. The term "markers" is used in this latter sense in genetics. A particular gene might be discovered that has a strong association with a given phenotypic characteristic, but it may or may not be causally involved in the production of that characteristic. When we next turn to consider why we have selected ERPs as our brain measure, we will see that ERP researchers have paid considerable attention to these methodological issues.

Within the field of ERP research, a certain dialectic has prevailed between those who approach the psychological interpretation of ERPs with considerable caution, calling attention to the known limitations of ERPs, and those who, although aware of these limitations, believe that ERPs have much to offer in the study of psychological processes and cite considerable research to buttress their position.

The fact that there are limitations to ERPs should not surprise us. Our multimethod approach is based on the realization that no method is free of limitations; but, by relying on a model of convergent operations that is made up of different methods, our aim is to compensate for the weakness of one method with the strengths of another. Thus, the rich but necessarily subjective nature of the psychoanalytic clinical method is compensated for by the objective nature of brain responses. However, what limitations do we need to be aware of when using the ERP method?

ERPs are produced by synchronous activity within large neuronal populations. For this reason, ERPs might more readily reflect the integrated neuronal activity involved in complex psychological processes distributed over wide regions of the brain. By the same token, it becomes impossible to identify specific localized regions of the brain and to know how each might be contributing to the complex, integrated activity accompanying psychological processes. As Allison, Wood, and McCarthy have pointed out, the identification is impossible because of the "aggregate, incomplete, and biased character of surface ERPs" (1986, p. 18). By aggregate, they are referring to the fact that activity from many different areas and levels of the brain is superimposed so that the resultant ERP signal is a composite rather than a partitioned representation of these different areas and levels. Or, as they put it, "the contribution of each neuron (and each gross anatomical structure) can lose its identity in the summation. Just as there is no way of answering the question 'How many different values were added to yield the sum 43, and what are they?', there is no way to determine from the instantaneous potential difference between two electrodes the number of distinct sources that have contributed to that potential difference and their relative contributions" (1986, pp. 17–18).

The ERP is incomplete because there is no way of knowing from the signal itself whether all of the brain regions and levels related to a given psychological event have been reflected in the ERP. Lastly, the ERP is biased because one brain process or another may be more or less fully represented in the ERP, not as a function of its important role in the given psychological event, but because of some favorable location with respect to the recording electrodes.

Perhaps it would be helpful to compare the ERP method to a space camera orbiting the planet Venus. What the camera records is subject to the conditions prevailing in the atmosphere surrounding Venus, the properties of the planet surface, the time of the planetary day, the planetary season, the distance of the camera from the planet surface, and so on. Many of these conditions will not be known in advance (e.g., the nature of the planetary surface), and they may have an aggregate effect on the camera film. Images filtered through an unknown atmosphere may cause difficulty in sorting out the planet's surface features. The photo record would be incomplete because the camera can scan only a certain portion of the planet surface, and it would be biased insofar as we would have no way of knowing what features are truly characteristic and central to understanding the nature of the planet (i.e., volcanoes, deserts, and so on). Nevertheless, reception of pictures of Venus is an exciting scientific event. Why? Because the pictures contain information that was not previously available in any other way, albeit they yield confusing, incomplete, and biased information. Then the hard work of reducing confusion and of completing and removing bias from the information must begin. The same holds true for ERPs.

Although Allison, Wood, and McCarthy (1986) are thorough in pointing out the limitations of ERPs, they also believe that the ERP method can make important contributions when its limitations are kept in mind. They refer to the use of ERPs as "purely psychological tools . . . designed to determine the mapping between psychological processes and ERPs, no matter how complex that mapping might be" (p. 24). At the same time, they warn against expecting that any one-to-one mapping exists or that any particular component, voltage direction, or latency is unequivocally related to a particular psychological event. They leave open the question as to what new mapping rules will prove useful. However, they also believe that ERPs might assist in the discovery of "patterns of organization in the CNS not evident in, or not yet discovered with, other experimental methods" (p. 24).

Although acknowledging the limitations spelled out by Allison, Wood and McCarthy (1986), the position taken by Donchin (1986) affirms, on the basis of extensive empirical work, that "ERPs provide a rich class of responses that may, within the appropriate research paradigm, allow the study of processes that are not *readily accessible* [italics added] to experimental psychologists by other means" (p. 245). For Donchin, what are not readily accessible and are of interest to experimental psychologists are the "subroutines" of information processing that constitute a given psychological event such as remembering. For us, what are not readily accessible and are of great interest are the unconscious psychological processes. At the same time, Donchin is careful to point out that he does not relate specific ERP parameters to "specific neuroanatomical entities, but rather to specific functional processors" (p. 245). In effect, he advocates the position we have taken: ERPs are markers whose cause-and-effect relationship to the underlying neurophysiological entities and to the psychological events is at present unknown but is ultimately knowable.

Once these important caveats are borne in mind, several specific facts about ERPs are generally accepted: (a) the distinction between *exogenous* and *endogenous* components of the ERP, (b) gross localizations of sensory systems with respect to known brain regions, and (c) the real time character of ERPs.

Exogenous components are found earlier than 100 msec poststimulus and, as defined by Donchin, "reflect early neural processing of the features of the stimuli presented. They are obligatory responses to stimuli whose amplitude and latency are responsive to changes in the physical characteristics of the stimulus, and whose scalp distribution is determined by the sensory system activated" (1986, p. 245). Examples of exogenous components would be early amplitude increases as a function of increased loudness or brightness of a stimulus. These changes would be measurable at the occipital region for visual stimuli and at the temporal region for auditory stimuli. Endogenous components, on the other hand, occur later and are responsive, not to physical parameters of the stimulus, but to task-related processing of the stimulus. Thus, an amplitude component somewhere between 250 and 450 msec, the so-called P300, might be greater in response to a rare stimulus as compared to a frequently occurring stimulus in an "oddball" experimental design. Or, as Wong, Shevrin, and Williams (1994) have found, the P300 is greater for a stimulus conditioned to a mild shock than to an unshocked control stimulus. Wong, Shevrin, and Williams (1994) also found a negative voltage shift occurring subliminally at approximately 2500 msec, the time just before the shock had been previously administered to the same stimulus supraliminally. Although the subject was unaware of the stimulus, the ERP contained evidence that an unconscious expectation of a shock was present. In the research reported in this book, the time–frequency features of interest occur between approximately 200 and 600 msec, in the range associated with endogenous ERP activity.

Readers may have noted that the actual latencies of ERP events of interest are relatively fast, being measured in milliseconds or, at most, in seconds. Quite complex psychological events occur with great rapidity, very likely as a function of the many parallel distributed processes associated with a given psychological event. Visual perception involves, at latest count, approximately 30 different brain regions that need to be integrated to produce the perception of a unitary object. ERPs reflect the speed with which these processes occur.

REVIEW OF RELEVANT ERP STUDIES

Insofar as our research is concerned with the subliminal and supraliminal processing of word meanings, research that deals with either word meaning or subliminal processes is reviewed here. With respect to word meaning, the most relevant studies are those by Chapman (1979), who demonstrated that words drawn from the extremes of the Osgood (Osgood, May, & Miron, 1975) connotative dimensions of pleasant–unpleasant, active–passive, and weak–strong could be differentiated on the basis of a principal component analysis of ERPs. In our own research, we have used words drawn from the extremes of the pleasant–unpleasant (evaluative) dimension. Brown, Lehmann, and Marsh (1980) have demonstrated that verbs and nouns can be differentiated on the basis of different scalp distributions of ERP components. They have shown this to be the case for verbs and nouns in English and Romansh, the indigenous language of Switzerland. By showing that the same linguistic distinction can be reflected in ERPs in two different languages, it cannot be argued that the distinction is limited to certain words contained only in one language. Apparently, an underlying differentiation exists between verbs and nouns that cuts across at least these two representatives of Indo-European languages. Words representing action and those representing objects must be processed differently in the brain. In this research, we go beyond connotative word meaning into the realm of deeper structural characteristics of language organization. Interestingly, ERPs appear to be able to reflect this underlying organization.

Kutas and Hillyard, in a series of studies, have discovered a late ERP component, the N400, which appears to index distance in associative strength between words, as well as categorical differences (Kutas & Hillyard, 1989). In a typical experiment, sentences composed of seven words, where the seventh word completes the meaning of the sentence either sensibly or with a non sequitur, are presented to subjects. The ERP is obtained to the seventh word. When the word is totally unrelated to the meaning of the sentence, the N400 is increased in amplitude as compared to when the word is related to the sentence meaning.

The Chapman, Brown, and Kutas studies amply demonstrate that the endogenous parameters of ERPs can reflect complex semantic and linguistic meanings. Our research adds further to this body of work by showing that *individual* word meanings having significance only to one person can also be measured by ERPs.

RESEARCH ON ERPs AND SUBLIMINAL PROCESSES

In previous research, Shevrin and colleagues have identified ERP parameters associated with subliminal stimuli. They have shown that a positive-going component in the P200 range discriminates between two closely matched stimuli different only to the extent that the experimental stimulus was made up of meaningful objects while the control stimulus was a dummy version of these objects. The P200 component is larger for the meaningful stimulus. An interpretation has been offered in terms of unconscious attentional processing (Shevrin & Rennick, 1967; Shevrin & Fritzler, 1967; Shevrin, 1973).

Libet, Alberts, Wright, and Feinstein (1967) demonstrated that a below-threshold somatosensory stimulus gives rise to an early (P100) ERP component. They argued that later components should be associated with consciousness. Their P100 differentiating component qualifies as an exogenous rather than an endogenous component, and, as such, it is more closely related to the physical characteristics of the stimulus. Our own P200 would more likely be related to endogenous aspects of the stimulus associated with the meaning for which our results provided evidence. Words related to the meaningful, experimental stimulus were associated by subjects after subliminal exposure of the experimental stimulus and not after the dummy control.

Kostandov and Arzumanov (1977) have also reported ERP findings for subliminal stimuli. In fact, their model is quite close to our own insofar as they used emotionally loaded words that were related to the alleged crimes of criminal suspects. These words referred to objects or other incidentals of the crime that could only be known to the actual perpetrator. When they compared supraliminal and subliminal ERPs to these emotionally loaded words and to neutral control words, they found that subliminally the P300 was greater for the emotionally loaded words than for the neutral words, and that the latency for the former was earlier. A P300 component is endogenous and thus is related to stimulus meaning. Others, however, like Libet, Alberts, Wright, and Feinstein (1967) and Posner (1982), have hypothesized that later components such as the P300 are associated with consciousness. One might then argue that either their subjects were conscious of the purported subliminal stimuli or that P300, under the given conditions of stimulus presentation, is not associated with consciousness. Unfortunately, the Kostandov and Arsumanov report is not clear on exactly how they established subliminality. In our own work, we have paid careful attention to these conditions and have, in fact, found that endogenous ERP components are associated with subliminal stimulation. However, the matter must remain equivocal insofar as we have not identified a P300 component in our subliminal ERPs. A P300 component, unlike other endogenous components, may be associated with consciousness.

Another line of ERP subliminal research was initiated by Libet, Wright, and Gleason (1982). They discovered a readiness potential occurring some 500 msec prior to a conscious decision to perform a spontaneous movement. Apparently, the conscious experience of making a decision to perform an action is preceded by a brain activity occurring prior to consciousness. This readiness potential is a negative-going, ramplike ERP taking anywhere from 500 to 200 msec to occur. Wong, Shevrin, Williams, and Marshall (1988) have demonstrated that obsessive subjects have a longer, more ramplike readiness potential than nonobsessive subjects, suggesting qualitative differences in preconscious brain processes.

In a study referred to previously, Wong, Shevrin, and Williams (1994) have shown that a negative-going voltage shift occurs in subliminal ERPs obtained to stimuli previously conditioned to a mild shock supraliminally. This voltage shift occurs just prior to the time at which the shock had been administered supraliminally. Because other ERP research has associated this negative-going voltage shift to the expectation of a stimulus, some have referred to it as an expectancy wave. If this interpretation is correct, then what Wong, Shevrin, and Williams have found may be related to the cognitive aspect of signal anxiety, a vitally important concept in psychoanalytic theory.

Two other subliminal researches have been published by Barkoczi, Sera, and Komlosi (1983) and Brandeis and Lehmann (1986). Both deal with lateralized subliminal visual stimuli and demonstrate that subliminal stimuli appear to follow known principles of lateralization.

Conclusions

We can conclude from this overview of the nature and role of event-related potentials that there are important substantive and methodological roles for ERPs in psychological research. The ERP emerges as a prime marker for connotative word meaning, parts of speech, associative strength, and category membership, as well as of subliminal processes related to preconscious decision making, emotional significance, unconscious expectation, and unconscious conflict. With respect to unconscious processes, ERPs constitute the only way (other than inference from conscious communications) to investigate them. ERPs have the further advantage of being based on operations that are totally independent of clinical judgments, and they are classically objective in nature insofar as no judgment is involved in their measurement.

METHODS

Having given our readers some idea of the overall theoretical frame of reference within which our research has been conceived, we turn next to a detailed consideration of the three interrelated methods drawn from this frame of reference.

The first chapter in this Part (Chapter 5) describes in detail the clinical method on the basis of which our patient-subjects were evaluated, our understanding of the underlying unconscious conflict that developed, and the key words selected. In Chapter 2, we showed how our clinical method was, in our judgment, entirely consistent with psychoanalytic theory and practice. In Chapter 5, each step in the method is described carefully and completely so that the psychoanalytic reader, in particular, can judge how successfully we have achieved our objective. Our hope is that the nonanalytic reader, although not fully appreciating the implications for psychoanalytic theory and method, will nevertheless obtain a clear picture of our clinical method and how it contributed to the research.

The chapter on the subliminal cognitive method (Chapter 6) reviews the history of research on subliminal perception as it bears mainly on our own research, stressing research that has incorporated questions concerning the dynamic as well as cognitive unconscious. Chapter 6 also deals with the history of the criticism of subliminal research from within cognitive psychology as well as the efforts to deal with these criticisms. On the whole, readers will learn that criticisms have been constructive, as reflected in the growing consensus within cognitive psychology as to how to perform methodologically acceptable subliminal experiments. Further underscoring this largely successful response is the increasing number of cognitive studies of unconscious processes appearing in cognitive science journals.

The chapter on the psychophysiological method (Chapter 7) will appear to psychoanalytic and cognitive science readers as being heavily technical. This level of technical detail is necessary if we are to adequately present the nature of the method and the innovative methods of signal analysis that we have developed, which are unique to the field but of great methodological utility to us. Without these innovations, our main research objectives could not have been achieved. Conventional methods did not work, for good reason. As already described in Chapter 4, conventional ERP approaches are largely based on an assumption of stationarity in brain signals. From this standpoint, nonstationarity or latency variability is produced by noise, rather than by meaningful, systematic changes in brain processing from time to time. Our methods are based instead on the latter understanding of brain process variability. In particular, the time–frequency and adaptive Gabor logon methods described in Chapter 7 attempt to capitalize on this inherent, meaningful variability. The psychoanalytic clinician might liken our approach to the way in which clinical phenomena are understood. In different contexts, the same content might have different meanings and different content might have the same meaning. The psychoanalytic clinician is prepared for a great deal of both intra- and interindividual differences. The psychophysiologist, on the other hand, much like the cognitive psychologist, looks on such variation as the "noise" that must be eliminated in a good experiment. We invite the psychophysiologist and the cognitive psychologist to consider an alternative strategy in which such variability is part of what needs to be understood and is intrinsically related to the phenomena under study.

The Psychodynamic
Clinical Method and
Word Selection Procedure

The word selection process is of critical importance to our research because the words and phrases selected are none other than the experimental stimuli. These word stimuli are later presented tachistoscopically to research subjects in the laboratory while ERPs are collected. Let us place the word selection process in the chronological sequence of the research as a whole (see Table 5.1 for the sequence of steps). Each subject was given a thorough psychodynamic evaluation, including at least three exploratory interviews aimed at clarifying the symptom and exploring the related unconscious conflict(s); a psychological testing, including WAIS-R, Rorschach, and TAT, aimed at revealing the deeper characterological and defensive structures as well as underlying conflictual themes; and a medical–psychiatric interview, aimed at clarifying the DSM-III-R diagnosis and uncovering any other symptoms or problems that would make the subject unacceptable for research purposes. All interviews and the testing were audio-recorded and transcribed. Each of four clinical judges carefully read the transcripts and independently wrote a psychodynamic formulation that included: (a) the patient's conscious description of his or her symptom and (b) the judge's own understanding of the unconscious conflict hypothesized to underlie and, at least in part, cause the conscious symptom. On the basis of these formulations, each judge selected words and short phrases used by the subject during the interviews and testing. These word selections represented two categories: (a) words that best reflected the patient's conscious experience of the symptom and (b) words that best reflected the putative unconscious conflict. After a series of word ratings made by all four judges, 8 words best reflecting the conscious symptom and 8 words best reflecting

TABLE 5.1. Sequence of Research Steps

Step	Procedure
Step 1: First psychodynamic interview	Consists of an unstructured interview aimed at eliciting a description of the symptom and exploration of dynamic or developmental themes that might reveal unconscious conflict related to the symptom.
Step 2: Psychological testing	Wechsler Adult Intelligence Scale, Revised Rorschach (Rapaport–Schafer method of administration; i.e., Inquiry comes immediately after Free Association for each card and the card is not seen by the subject during Inquiry)
	10 Thematic Apperception Test cards
Step 3: Medical–psychiatric interview	It aims to clarify whether patient meets DSM-III-R criteria for social phobia, has some other diagnosis, or has problems that exclude him or her from the research (e.g., current substance abuse, evidence of brain insult).
Step 4: Second psychodynamic interview	Continues step 1.
Step 5: Psychodynamic formulation	Transcripts of interviews and testing are sent to judges who study them and submit a written psychodynamic formulation and nominate words used by the subject that best represent the conscious symptom and unconscious conflict.
Step 6: First word ratings	Words selected by the judges in step 5 and 36 Osgood control words (see Table 5.2) are alphabetized and submitted to each judge for initial independent ratings.
Step 7: First clinical evaluation team (CET) meeting	Consists of comparison of formulations and identification of areas of consensus and disagreement, with focus on the unconscious conflict; collection of written psychodynamic formulations, and distribution of quantitative results of first word ratings.
Step 8: Second word ratings	Word lists are submitted to judges for a second rating after feedback consisting of (1) discussions during first CET meeting; (2) results of first word ratings.
Step 9: Data summary	First psychodynamic consensus is summarized and submitted to all judges for emendations or approval. Results of second word ratings are distributed to judges.

TABLE 5.1. (Continued)

Step	Procedure
Step 10: Third psychodynamic interview	Its aim is to elicit from the subject associations that may allow a decision for one formulation of the unconscious conflict as against another raised by CET members during the first CET meeting.
Step 11: Third interview transcripts	Transcripts are submitted to judges, who revise their psychodynamic formulation if necessary and nominate new words from third interview.
Step 12: Third word ratings	Word nominations from third interview are added to the first word list. The composite list is submitted to judges for third rating.
Step 13: Second CET meeting	Its aims are to develop a final consensus and define remaining areas of significant disagreement. As time permits, some discussion of word selections and third word ratings may take place. Second written psychodynamic formulations are collected, and quantitative results of third word ratings are distributed.
Step 14: Final consensus	Final psychodynamic consensus is summarized and submitted to judges for emendations or approval.
Step 15: Fourth word ratings	Composite word list is resubmitted to judges for fourth rating, after discussions of first and second CET meetings have occurred and results of third word rating have been distributed for perusal.
Step 16: Final word selection	Eight words or short phrases best representing the conscious symptom, and eight representing the unconscious conflict are selected along with eight pleasant and eight unpleasant words to serve as controls. Additional criteria of word length and frequency of usage are applied when final selection is made.
Step 17: ERP laboratory session	Conscious, unconscious, pleasant, and unpleasant words chosen for each subject are presented tachistoscopically in both subliminal and supraliminal conditions while ERP data are collected. Subject fills out paper-and-pencil rating scales, tries to group the words consciously into categories, and has a short debriefing interview following the laboratory session.

Note. Psychodynamic clinical procedures include interviews and tests.

the unconscious conflict were finally selected. In addition to these 16 "pathological" words, 16 control words were selected. The control words (8 pleasant and 8 unpleasant) were drawn from the evaluative dimension of Osgood's research (Osgood, May, & Miron, 1975) on connotative meaning (see Table 5.2 for the full list of Osgood words from which our controls were chosen). Finally, the 16 pathological words and the 16 control words were presented both subliminally and supraliminally to the subject in a tachistoscope while ERPs were recorded. The most fundamental hypothesis of our research was that the different categories of words (i.e., conscious symptom,

TABLE 5.2. Osgood Evaluative Words

Ordinary unpleasant words (E−)	Ordinary positive words (E+)
Air pollution	Apple
Atomic bomb	Bath
Cancer	Bread
Cheating	Care
Criminal	Cleanliness
Crying	Flower
Debt	Fresh
Devil	Friendship
Earthquake	Kindness
Envy	Peace
Evil	Pleasant
Failure	Pocket radios
Filth	Quality
Hunger	Right hand
Lying	Space travel
Noise	Spring
Nonbeliever	
Poison	
Poor people	
Sickness	
Sin	
Trouble	

Note. The Osgood ordinary unpleasant and ordinary pleasant words were selected from the endpoints of the Osgood evaluative scale: E− = unpleasant, E+ = pleasant. All these words were added to the conscious symptom and unconscious conflict words selected by the judges, and made up the full list rated by the judges. How these ratings were done and taken into account is described in the text.

unconscious conflict, and pleasant–unpleasant) were likely to be associated with distinguishable features of the ERP.

One of our primary aims has been to lean entirely on clinical expertise in this word selection process (further discussion of our emphasis on clinical expertise occurs in the Introduction). That is, the judges on the clinical evaluation team (CET) had been selected precisely because they were experts in making psychodynamic diagnostic judgments. The judging task was designed to allow them to function as closely as possible to their usual clinical practices. Following a study of the transcripts, each judge was asked to produce independently a written account of his or her formulations of the conscious symptom and the unconscious conflict. Further each judge was to select words or short phrases used spontaneously by the subject that, in the judge's mind appeared closely associated with either the subject's conscious experience of the target symptom or the unconscious conflict the judge believed to be related to that symptom.

Our reliance on clinical judgment for selection of the experimental stimuli that were later presented to subjects in the laboratory is one feature that makes this research approach a *convergent* one (Shevrin, 1988). On one hand, the process of clinical judgment includes intuitive and subjective components and thus is not open to an entirely objective description. On the other hand, the laboratory process is an entirely objective procedure: The methods by which the words were presented to the subjects tachistoscopically, by which the ERP data were collected via EEG electrodes, and by which these data were analyzed, can be stated with specificity and are open to careful examination. Of central importance is the fact that the laboratory data were collected by methods entirely independent of clinical judgment. Thus, the convergence hoped for was one between the results of expert, albeit subjective, clinical judgment (i.e., the stimulus words) and the results of a relatively objective laboratory procedure involving data produced by methods quite independent of the clinic (i.e., subliminal/supraliminal presentations, ERP data, and subsequent statistical analysis).

Our dependence on the clinician's expertise in this fundamental way was based on the assumption that such expertise, even if not of the same objective character as the laboratory method, nonetheless exists. A significant corollary is that scientific experiment is not the only, nor the most usual, method of knowledge accumulation. Expert knowledge as contributed by our clinicians would likely be part of what scientist and philosopher Michael Polanyi (1958, 1967) called "personal knowledge" or "the tacit dimension." This expert knowledge is embedded in an uncertain mix with erroneous beliefs, and we cannot with assurance separate the knowledge from the error at this time. Yet, it continues to be an important fact of life that knowledge of this kind is accumulated through experience and study in a wide variety of careers and occupations. Most of this knowledge, however, is not accumulated by means of scientific experiment or controlled empirical research.

We believe this reliance on expert judgment is a strength. Poorly understood expert judgments cannot be fully formularized, and when researchers attempt to substitute an operational procedure for such judgments (i.e., to "empiricize" them), they usually lose what was valuable in the original judgments (Bond, Hansell, & Shevrin, 1987). As Polanyi (1967) wrote "It is impossible to account for the nature and justification of knowledge by a series of strictly explicit operations" (p. x).

However, this question might be asked: What are the fundamental assumptions on which these expert clinical judgments were based? Our word selections were based on our assumption of a psychoanalytic point of view for understanding the individual and his or her symptoms. (See Chapter 2 for a fuller exposition of these assumptions.) We assumed that the individual's verbal and nonverbal communications to us were unconsciously organized and unconsciously, as well as consciously, meaningful. That is, within the subject's speech as well as his or her nonverbal behavior, an expert can find clues (Arlow, 1979) or "unintended giveaways" of central conflicts around which the subject has, usually unwittingly, organized thoughts, feelings, and behavior in relation to highly significant other persons (e.g., parents or siblings). When such psychic conflicts give rise to distressing problems or symptoms, the individual sometimes comes to a professional for treatment. When the psychodynamic clinician listens to a patient, certain portions of the patient's presentation often appear to have an especially close connection with the patient's significant conflicts. These elements might include certain vivid descriptive phrases or images, notable nonverbal behaviors, images, and so on. Often, the clinician finds particular phrases or accounts of events that seem to epitomize the patient's central conflicts. The clinician often uses such examples in interpretations to the patient as well as in conveying a sense of the patient in clinical summaries. Our word selections were only extensions or refinements of this usual method of psychodynamic listening and clinical inference. Ordinary clinicians do not *have to* select specific verbalizations as representatives of central unconscious conflicts, though they *may* do this in an intuitive fashion. However, we required of ourselves a selection of small units of the subject's unconsciously organized verbal communication for research purposes. These units were the words or short phrases we believed to best represent the subject's conscious symptom and inferred unconscious conflict.

THE PSYCHODYNAMIC FORMULATION

Since the psychodynamic formulation attempted to capture the essentials of the clinicians' thinking concerning the unconscious conflict and exercised an influence over their selections and ratings of the words, we now describe the process by which the CET arrived at a consensus psychodynamic formulation and provide an example of one such consensus. (Table 5.1 will again likely be helpful in keeping an overview of the research steps in mind.)

After reading the transcripts of the first two evaluation interviews, the psychological testing, and the medical–psychiatric interview, each clinician was asked to formulate in his or her own words (a) a description of the subject's conscious experience of the symptom, (b) an account of the subject's own understanding and explanation of the symptom, and (c) an account of the clinician's understanding of the unconscious conflict believed to, at least in part, cause the conscious symptom. During the first CET meeting, each clinician read aloud his or her psychodynamic formulations. Discrepancies and disagreements were then discussed in an attempt to reach a consensus. Topics were also suggested that the interviewer might discuss with the subject in the third exploratory clinical interview, in order to resolve differences among the clinicians. After the third interview was conducted and the judges had read its transcription, each clinician made revisions as deemed necessary in his or her psychodynamic formulation, resulting from any new information obtained in the third interview. During the second CET meeting, these changes were read aloud, and discussion again was aimed at reaching a consensus psychodynamic formulation.

The following is an example of a consensus psychodynamic formulation. (This consensus is for Mr. X, the same subject who is used as an example in Table 5.3 and from whose interview an example is reproduced and discussed later in this chapter. We drew examples from the same subject to facilitate the reader's understanding of our procedure.)

There appears to be broad agreement that [Mr. X's] focal conflict had to do with phallic competitive wishes, but that it was unclear concerning the extent to which these phallic competitive conflicts were regressive primarily from a later oedipal struggle or the extent to which they were a fragile transition point toward a more powerful regression toward primarily sadistic, likely anal, impulses. In other words, it isn't clear whether his difficulty with phallic competitive feelings toward males is because he fears seeing them as rivals for a prize (e.g., an admired and loved woman), or whether the anxiety of the phallic competitive impulses comes from their admixture with powerful earlier sadistic impulses. Some of the evidence as we read it suggests that he has great anxiety over strong affects and impulses of any kind which would favor the earlier origin of his current difficulty with competitive strivings. There seems to be agreement that the symptomatic compromise in the phobia saves him from a more wholesale regression into a passive homoerotic position with respect to a powerful authority figure so that he experiences anxiety under those circumstances but performs nevertheless.

TABLE 5.3. Partial List of Alphabetized Word Selections for Mr. X

Rater's Name: Judge 1   Subject: Mr. X
Date: November 15, 1994

No.	Word	Cons. rating	Uncons. rating
1	A little worm	−9	6
2	Achieve heights	−6	4
3	Agitation	6	−4
4	Air pollution	−9	−9
5	Alice	−6	2
6	Appendage	−9	5
7	Appendages	−9	3
8	Apple	−9	−9
9	Ask a woman out	9	−3
10	Ask out	6	−5
11	Athletic	−7	1
12	Atomic bomb	−9	1
13	Attack	−3	3
14	Authoritarian	−7	2
15	Baby sitter	−9	0
16	Back end	−9	0
17	Bath	−9	−9
18	Batting slump	−9	3
19	Belt	−9	−3
20	Big commotion	−9	6
21	Bitter	−7	0
22	Bomb	−7	1
23	Boss	−1	1
24	Bread	−9	9
25	Broke it off	−5	5
26	Cancer	−9	−9
27	Care	−9	−9
28	Challenging	4	5
29	Cheating	−6	−5
30	Cristized	0	0
31	Cleanliness	−9	−9
32	Competition	−2	7
33	Competitive	−5	5
34	Confrontations	−2	2
35	Control	3	5

Note. Partial list of alphabetized words and one judge's ratings. Note that there are four ordinary unpleasant (E−) words and five ordinary pleasant (E+) words included here. Of these, all E+ words are rated as not belonging to either the conscious (Cons.) or unconscious (Uncons.) conflict categories. Of the four E− words, one (atomic bomb) is rated a 1 on belongingness for the unconscious conflict category. This word would not be used. We can also see a beginning theme emerging for the unconscious conflict in the choices of "a little worm" (−9/6), "appendage" (−9/5), "broke it off" (−5/5), all putatively related to castration anxiety, as well as the countertheme of ambition and competition in "achieve heights" (−6/4), "big commotion" (−9/6), competitive (−5/5).

OUR USE OF THE DELPHI METHOD
FOR WORD SELECTION

While wishing to utilize the strengths inherent in expert clinical judgment when selecting the word stimuli for the subsequent laboratory experiment, we also chose to strengthen the expert judgment process through use of the Delphi method (Linstone & Turoff, 1975). Dalkey (1975, p. 236) described the Delphi method as follows:

> (1) the exercise involves a group; (2) the goal of the exercise is informa-tion, i.e., the exercise is an inquiry; (3) the information being sought is uncertain in the minds of the group; (4) some preformulated systematic procedure is followed in obtaining the group output.

Dalkey (1975, p. 239–240) also stated the two basic assumptions underly-ing the use of the Dephi method:

> "(a) In situations of uncertainty (incomplete information or inadequate theories) expert judgment can be used as a surrogate for direct knowl-edge. . . . (b) In a wide variety of situations of uncertainty, a group judg-ment (amalgamating the judgments of a group of experts) is preferable to the judgment of a typical member of the group, the "*n* heads are bet-ter than one" rule.

Thus, our aims in using the Delphi method were to select word stimuli on the basis of "corporate" or group expert judgments, as opposed to merely de-pending on the judgments of a single expert, and to use a "preformulated systematic procedure" in obtaining the corporate judgments, one that could be readily understood and replicated by others.

The Delphi method was incorporated into the word selection process in the following manner.

1. Each expert nominated words from the transcripts.
2. All of the judges' word nominations were put together in a compos-ite list and arranged alphabetically (see Table 5.3 for an example, again taken from Mr. X's case).
3. Each judge rated each word nomination in terms of how represen-tative it was of the conscious symptom and/or the unconscious con-flict using the scale in Figure 5.1.
4. The judges met as a group to discuss their views of the patient and of the reasons for at least some of their word ratings. These discus-sions represented feedback that judges could later use in their sub-sequent word ratings.

+9 +8 +7 +6 +5 +4 +3 +2 +1 0 −1 −2 −3 −4 −5 −6 −7 −8 −9

Definitely belongs   I don't know   Definitely does *not*
to the category being judged(i.e., if this word   belong to the category
conscious symptom   belongs to   being judged (i.e.,
or unconscious conflict)   either category   conscious symptom *or*
                                                            unconscious conflict)

FIGURE 5.1. Nineteen-point belongingness rating scale. (See Appendix A for full background for deriving this scale and the accompanying formula in Figure 5.2.)

5. In addition to discussion in a group, each judge was provided with the complete rating results from the immediately prior ratings so that these too could be used as feedback and could inform subsequent word ratings.

Thus, words were rated on four occasions, and, on the second through fourth ratings, judges received feedback from discussion and/or prior ratings to feed forward into their subsequent ratings. The mathematical formula used to rank words (see Figure 5.2) in terms of how well they reflected the conscious symptom and unconscious conflict *combined* all four judges' ratings to determine each word's rank. Thus, the ranking represented the results of the *corporate* expert after each step of rating. The eight words best reflecting the conscious symptom and the eight words best reflecting the unconscious conflict were always chosen from among those words that were at the extremes of the fourth and final ranking. Selection of the final eight words in each category was also governed by two more considerations: (a) balancing for frequency of usage for English-speaking persons in psychotherapy (Dahl, 1979) and (b) length of word or phrase.[1]

THE WORD SELECTION PROCEDURE

In what follows, we describe the word selection procedure as we have applied it up to the present (see Table 5.1 for an overview of the research steps). The expert judges initially received the transcripts of the first two psychodynamic evaluation interviews, the separate medical–psychiatric interview, and the psychological testing. Two of the four judges were asked to read the *interview*

---

[1] For the stimuli to be within the fovea during tachistoscopic presentation, the combined number of letters and spaces was limited to 17. The details of these considerations are described in Chapter 8.

$$D_c - D_u$$

where

$$D_c = 1 + \sqrt{(9 - \text{Conscious Mean})^2 + (9 + \text{Unconscious Mean})^2}$$

and

$$D_u = 1 + \sqrt{(9 + \text{Conscious Mean})^2 + (9 - \text{Unconscious Mean})^2}$$

and

Conscious Mean = average of ratings across all judges in the conscious symptom category for the particular word in question.

Unconscious Mean = average of ratings across all judges in the unconscious conflict category for the particular word in question.

The reader can better understand the formula by examining a limiting case: Let us imagine a "perfect" conscious word, for example, one where every judge rated it +9 in the conscious symptom category *and* −9 in the unconscious conflict category. Thus, the conscious *mean* would be +9 and the unconscious *mean* would be −9. In this case $D_c = 1$ and $D_u = 25.46$. Finally, this "perfect" conscious word's $D_c - D_u$ score would be −24.46. In the other limiting case of a "perfect" unconscious word, $D_c = 25.46$, $D_u = 1$, and $D_c - D_u = 24.46$. Thus, better conscious words receive higher *negative* scores and better unconscious words receive higher *positive* scores (with −24.46 at one extreme and +24.46 at the other).

FIGURE 5.2. Formula for ranking word nominations. (See Appendix A for the mathematical derivation of this formula.)

materials first and to write psychodynamic formulations of symptom and unconscious conflict based on interview materials alone, prior to reading the psychological test transcript. The same two judges were also asked to nominate words or short phrases used by the subject that they believed reflected either the symptom or the conflict. The other two judges were asked to do the same with the *psychological test* transcript prior to reading the interview transcripts. (Usually, on the basis of the tests alone, judges cannot make a formulation about the consciously experienced symptom because the subject normally does not discuss the symptom when responding to tests. The symptom is, of course, explored in detail in the interview format.) When each judge had made formulations and nominated words based on either interviews or tests, this process was repeated for the other set of materials not examined initially. During this process, there was no discussion between judges about any of these materials, about their formulations, or about the words they were nominating. All judges brought their word nominations in at a designated time. Duplicates were removed and then the full list of possible Osgood pleasant–unpleasant words was added (see Table 5.2 for this list). The whole list of words and short phrases was alphabetized. This alphabetical list was quickly returned to the judges, who then rated each word on a 19-point scale of "belongingness" (explained below) in relation to the conscious symptom category and the unconscious conflict category (Figure 5.1 shows the rating scale). In other words, each nominated word and each Osgood word was rated by each judge twice—once for its belongingness to the conscious symptom category as it was understood by the judge, and once for its belongingness to the unconscious conflict category as it was understood by the judge. These first ratings were entirely independent because no discussion between judges had yet occurred.

The 19-point rating scale runs from +9 through 0 to −9. A positive rating is a judgment of the degree to which a word belongs to the category under consideration. A rating of +9 indicates the strongest possible belief that the word *does* belong and a +1 rating indicates the weakest. The 0 point is used to indicate that the judge does not know whether the word belongs. A negative rating indicates the degree to which the judge believes the word does *not* belong to the category under consideration. A rating of −9 is the strongest degree of belief that the word does *not* belong, whereas a −1 rating is the weakest.

Table 5.3 shows an example of a partial list of words and phrases as they are alphabetized and sent to each judge. Note that the judge merely makes two separate ratings for each nominated word or phrase. First, the judge must determine the degree to which the word or phrase (e.g., "a little worm") is associated with the subject's conscious symptom: +9 if it's very closely related to the symptom, 0 if the judge does not know, or −9 if the word seems extremely unrelated to the symptom. The judge then repeats the same process for the same word or phrase, only asking how associated the word or phrase appears to be with the unconscious conflict, as the judge understands this conflict.

During the first CET meeting, each judge read his or her psychodynamic formulation and a discussion followed. The aim was to reach a consensus among the judges on the nature of (a) the subject's conscious experience of symptom and (b) the unconscious conflict inferred to underlie the symptom. Typically, most of this meeting has been occupied with discussion about the psychodynamic formulations because the interviewer needed to develop questions about what issues required further exploration with the patient in the next interview. Relatively little of the time has been spent in discussion of the word selections.

All judges' initial word ratings were fed into the formula in Figure 5.2. This formula produces a number reflecting how unanimously the judges agreed that the word was a more "pure" representative of the conscious symptom or of the unconscious conflict. All words were then ranked; those voted most purely representative of the conscious symptom were ranked at the top, and those most representative of the unconscious conflict were ranked at the bottom. This ranked list was given to each judge as feedback to use in making the next judgments; that is, each judge could see the degree of consensus concerning each word and could use this in the next word ratings.

Immediately following the first meeting, judges again rated each word in the list twice—once for its belongingness to the conscious symptom category and once for its belongingness to the unconscious conflict category—as they understood these now on the basis of their own formulations, their discussion of the other judges' formulations, and the feedback concerning the previous word-rating results. Then, a third psychodynamic interview took place and was transcribed. Each judge received a copy of this transcript and was thereby given an opportunity to revise his or her formulations based on new information and to nominate new words from the third interview. Again duplicate word nominations were removed and new words were added to the list, which was again alphabetized and submitted to the judges for their third rating just prior to the second CET meeting. During the second CET meeting, the third interview was discussed. Feedback about the results of the second word ratings was also distributed prior to the second CET meeting. The second CET meeting usually focused most attention on the formulations, particularly of the unconscious conflict, which is far more subject to disagreement and controversy. Some time may have been spent on discussion of the judges' rationale for selecting a word as being a particularly significant reflection of either conscious symptom or unconscious conflict. A fourth (and usually final) word rating took place after the second CET meeting. This word rating, too, was preceded by feedback to judges about the results of the third ratings.

The Formula Used for Ranking Words

A formula was developed by Robert Marshall for ranking the words in terms of their representativeness of each of the two categories (see Figure 5.2), based on the MYCIN approach developed by Shortliffe (1976) for medical diagnosis. The assumptions underlying this formula suggest that the *best* conscious symptom word would have an average rating across judges in the conscious symptom category of +9, and an average rating across judges of −9 in the unconscious conflict category. The formula assumes that the *best* unconscious conflict word would receive an average rating across judges of −9 in the conscious symptom category, and an average of +9 in the unconscious conflict category. However, in the case of the Osgood control words, the ideal average rating across judges would be −9 in both categories. Here, the idea is that whatever control words are selected from among the pleasant–unpleasant word nominees, they should have no relationship at all to either the conscious symptom or the unconscious conflict as judged by experts. A scatterplot reflecting the ideal clustering of conscious symptom, unconscious conflict, and Osgood words in the two-dimensional space implied by our belongingness rating scales is shown in Figure 5.3.

The judges have had considerable discussion regarding the appropriateness of the assumption that the ideal conscious symptom word or phrase would have no relation at all to the unconscious conflict. The discussion arose because the assumption that an ideal conscious symptom word should be unrelated to the unconscious conflict appeared to contradict the theoretical belief that symptoms are compromises reflecting both the proscribed impulses and the defenses against these impulses, and thus *must* be significantly related to the unconscious conflict (Brenner, 1982; Shevrin, 1988; also see Chapter 2). The resolution of this issue seems to lie in recognizing that, although the psychodynamic theory of compromise formation does assert that *a symptom* is a compromise reflecting the unconscious conflict, this theory

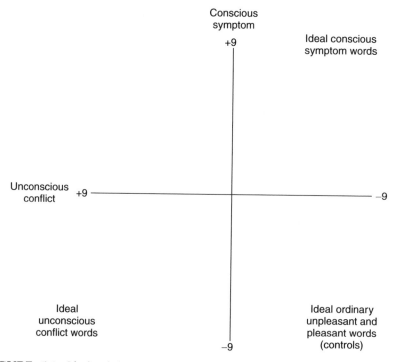

FIGURE 5.3. Idealized locations of conscious symptom, unconscious conflict, ordinary unpleasant, and ordinary pleasant control words. As exemplified in Table 5.3, the control words should receive −9 for belongingness on the conscious symptom and unconscious conflict belongingness scales. An ideal conscious symptom word should receive a +9 on the conscious symptom scale and a −9 on the unconscious conflict scale. An ideal unconscious conflict word should receive a +9 on the unconscious conflict scale and a −9 on the conscious symptom scale.

does *not* require that each and every *word* used by a patient to talk about his or her symptom must *also* reflect the same compromise formation and to the same degree. In fact, when selecting among nominations for best conscious symptom words we *tried* to select those we judged to be more distant from the unconscious conflict. The symptom itself is not *identical* with the words used by the patient to talk about the symptom. Psychodynamic judges might determine that *some* words the patient uses to talk about the symptom *are* associated with the putative unconscious conflict; however, the theory of symptoms as compromise formations in no way requires that *all words* used to talk about the symptom must themselves be compromise formations *of the same kind and to the same degree* as the symptom itself.

WHAT PRINCIPLES MIGHT UNDERLIE JUDGES' UNCONSCIOUS WORD NOMINATIONS AND WORD RATINGS?

Each of our judges nominates only a few words, from among the thousands of words used by a subject throughout interviews and testing. These few words are those that seem to be most evocatively related to the subject's conscious experience of symptom and the judge's inferential and intuitive sense of the subject's unconscious conflict. In relation to the conscious symptom, there is little disagreement among judges that the subject has, in fact, used a particular word to vividly describe the symptom experience or to refer to the context within which the symptom usually takes place. Most of the *disagreement* concerning words occurs because the judges differ as to the degree to which a particular word reflects the *unconscious conflict*. For this reason, this section focuses solely on attempting to articulate at least some principles that might be involved in this quintessentially clinical, inferential, and intuitive judgment.

Edelson (1975, 1988) noted that "we have no adequate theory . . . of the psychoanalyst's act of understanding" (Edelson, 1988, p. 78). Arlow (1979) has certainly also referred to some of the mystery surrounding psychoanalytic clinical inference. We have ideas about clinical inference, clinical intuition, and clinical empathy, which are certainly beginning steps toward a theory; yet, a great deal is left to be explained and articulated. The principles underlying our judges' assessments that a particular word or phrase reflects, represents, or is evocatively related to the subject's unconscious conflict are likely to be the same principles underlying other acts of psychoanalytic interpretive understanding. A fundamental assumption of psychoanalytic understanding is that patients frequently convey, through their words, gestures, and the totality of their self-presentation, meanings that are active and dynamic in their minds but of which they are unconscious. In other words, unconscious conflicts are *dynamic* in the following sense: They continue to exert a selective and formative influence on thoughts, feelings, and behaviors that *are* available to consciousness (Arlow, 1969; Edelson, 1988, pp. 218–221), although this influence itself and its effects on behavior are *not* usually reflected in consciousness. This assumption has a corollary that is crucial to the psychodynamic enterprise, including our judges' unconscious conflict word selections and ratings: At least a portion of an individual's behavioral output—thoughts, feelings, and verbal and nonverbal behaviors—serves functions and carries meanings that can be interpreted, although fallibly, by a psychodynamically knowledgeable observer, even when the acting individual is unaware of these meanings. This is such a basic assumption that Edelson contends that accounting for how unconscious processes cause psychologically important effects is "*the* central question psychoanalytic theory must answer" (1988, p. 218).

For the purpose of this chapter, our focus is on how psychodynamically knowledgeable observers interpret, even though fallibly, unconscious meanings. Perhaps the best way to approach this process of clinical judgment is by way of a vivid example (other examples are to be found in the three case presentations in Chapters 9, 10, and 11). One of our subjects, Mr. X, was a 31-year-old single male who presented for the first time to a mental health professional with a social phobia of moderate severity. He had recently obtained his Ph.D. in the natural sciences and had been hired in his first professional position. Upon assuming this job, he was also selected as a member of a prestigious government-appointed policy committee. The other members of the committee were older, more experienced experts, mostly males, who had substantial reputations throughout the community. Mr. X found, to his chagrin, that he experienced surges of anxiety and intensely distressing physiological arousal when called on to state to the group his name and affiliation, as members took turns introducing themselves. These same symptoms had occurred once when he recently had tried to ask a woman out for a date. In Mr. X's case, these intense performance anxiety experiences were his consciously experienced and reported symptoms, the reasons he sought treatment.

From among the thousands of words of interview and testing transcripts from Mr. X's evaluation, in retrospect we found that the four CET judges unanimously and independently emphasized a two-page segment from the third psychodynamic interview as highly related to what they inferred to be Mr. X's unconscious conflict. Indeed, although only eight words or short phrases are ultimately selected as unconscious conflict stimuli (UCS), two of the eight came from this segment ("internal flame" and "soft story"). A closer examination of this segment of dialogue between the interviewer and Mr. X may help in identifying some of the principles guiding the interpretation of unconscious meanings.

I: Have you had any other recollections about you and your family, since we last talked? We covered a lot of ground.

Mr. X: Yeah . . .

I: Sometimes covering the ground opens up some new ideas . . .

Mr. X: Yeah . . . sure . . . yeah . . . one interesting one [patient himself was struck by something "interesting" about this recollection], and . . . obviously I've put, since we started this, quite a bit of thought . . .

I: Yeah, it sounds like you really have.

Mr. X: Yeah, well, it's a problem that I need very badly to deal with and want very badly to deal with . . . I'll be honest with you, becoming almost . . . with this process . . . somewhat impatient [i.e., the lengthy evaluation process of interviews and testing!] . . . in terms of . . . not feeling like I'm getting results and I . . . I think I'll remain patient for the time being, understanding that there is an end to this and . . . ah . . . hopefully a result as well. Ah . . . there was an incident actually came to mind, I think just a couple of days ago, that . . . ah . . . far be it for me to be the psychiatrist, but . . . and . . . I put emphasis on it, whether emphasis should be put on it or not I don't know, but it did come to mind . . . that was a . . . I guess I must have been in grade school . . . ah . . . and I recall sitting in the living room of the house one evening and . . . writing a story . . . I guess what brought this to mind is that you had asked, had anything happened, interactions I guess of some sort between the parents and myself that I . . . deemed traumatic [patient's word not interviewer's!], or that left a firm impression on my mind and . . . it . . . this did come to mind. And I was writing a story, and it was a fairly elaborate story if I recall and . . . this story had to do with a . . . fairly good memory of a . . . of someone reporting a house being on fire, calling a fire department, the fire department coming and I came up with the end of the story by saying, attempting to say, it was eternal flame and [inaudible]. Well I used the word internal flame, and drew some laughs from my parents and I . . . that . . . as I recall . . . and pretty significant . . . I was very embarrassed about the situation, significant impression on me. Now, to draw the next step . . . and think . . . is that . . . does that incident in my life . . . has that incident in my life had an influence on my interactions in the situation that I'm in now [i.e., the symptom which brought him for treatment] . . . far be for me to decide that, but . . . one did come to mind . . .

I: Like one little word really brought the house down?

Mr. X: Well, it . . . I . . . not so much bring the house down, I think it..the reaction was very subtle, but the impact is very significant. . . .

I: Any thoughts as to why the impact would have been so . . . significant for you?

MR. X: Ah . . . yeah, a couple I had, to me they're fairly obvious. One is that the story I think was probably . . . could . . . by myself be construed, and even at that time, as fairly soft, not something typical of a male . . . to write. [Note that there is nothing "obvious" about this particular construal of the story's import.] Ah . . . the other is that . . . ah . . . I've lost my line of thought [cognitive interference or "momentary forgetting" (Luborsky, 1988)]. Well, the other one I assume was . . . the fact that I used the wrong word or something like this . . . and the embarrassment again of being cristized [slip of the tongue] . . . criticized in that situation by my parents and when I say criticized, it was . . . it was really very subtle . . . umm . . . and yet . . . I think I recall being laughed at . . . ah . . . although not outwardly criticized or outwardly laughing . . . I detected I suppose a . . . a . . . criticism or a . . . a gibe . . . or a sneer . . . whatever [inaudible].

I: Uhhuh . . . what comes to mind when you think about it now, why you might have made a slip like that, "internal flame"?

MR. X: I have no idea, lack of knowledge of the word I suppose, I think that could be it.

I: When you think of houses and fire and eternal flame, what were you meaning? You said it was "soft."

MR. X: Well, I . . . I don't think I drew the story out. I'm not sure I could draw the story out . . . umm . . . if I remember it correctly it was something about having someone report a fire . . . in a house . . . and having the fire department come and a big commotion made and then finding out it wasn't really a fire, it was . . . an eternal flame . . . umm . . . what, what . . . and even, I'll be honest with you, telling that story right now I find somewhat embarrassing [spontaneous report of distress] Now . . . again . . . not typical . . . as I would classify it, a typical male . . . macho . . . type of story that one would tell . . . that a male would tell I guess. And I suspect, again . . . in that type of situation, again make a mistake . . . [inaudible]

In this excerpt the subject *consciously* remembers an embarrassing incident with his parents. Moreover, he does not merely remember silently in the privacy of his own thoughts, he verbally describes the incident to the interviewer in detail. As clinician-observers our task was to search the transcribed *conscious* verbal productions of the subject for clues suggesting that emotionally-charged *unconscious* meanings may have also become active and influential through their association in the subject's mind with what he was discussing consciously. We hypothesize that Mr. X's conscious recollection and verbal description of this incident with his parents activated a whole network of *unconscious* meanings and emotional significances. The conscious talk and conscious experience Mr. X had while speaking during this excerpt are hypothesized to be heavily influenced by these activated unconscious meanings.

What clues may have caught the attention of psychodynamic clinicians seeking evidence that unconscious conflict may have been activated?

1. The recollection was elicited by a relatively unstructured question from the interviewer, and thus was a relatively spontaneous production of the patient's.
2. The segment illustrates several phenomena that psychodynamic theory associates with unconscious conflict. There is a slip of the tongue ("cristized" for criticized—a possible unconscious reference to Christ, a male authority figure who was violently killed), a salient aspect of the recollection itself is a slip (internal flame for eternal flame), the patient loses his train of thought once (a momentary forgetting; Luborsky, 1988), and there is a report of spontaneous emotional arousal (embarrassment) as he retells the recollection to the interviewer.
3. The content of the recollection itself closely parallels the presenting symptom, that is, it involves a surge of very distressing feelings—embarrassment or humiliation—in connection with verbally presenting something to an audience (in this case his parents) and somehow feeling imperfect or incompetent in front of that audience.
4. A primary conflict is illustrated in this segment, that is, an alternation between a competitive challenging of the older male interviewer on the one hand ("far be it for me to be the psychiatrist"; "becoming almost, . . . with this process . . . somewhat impatient"), and reluctantly submitting on the other ("I'll remain patient for the time being"). This parallels a key aspect of the unconscious conflict our CET judges had already identified as central *before this third interview took place* (for evidence of how the clinicians saw Mr. X's unconscious conflict before the above interview took place see the consensus formulation for Mr. X reproduced earlier in this chapter, see p. 75).

The psychodynamic formulations based on the first two psychodynamic interviews, the medical-psychiatric interview, and the psychological testing of this subject emphasized conflicts over competitiveness with his father.

What sort of rough theory sketch might be advanced to give an account of the relationship between the unconscious meanings conjectured to be activated and the just-described clues that we allege to be effects of that activation? We provisionally propose that any conscious experience is part of a network of both conscious and unconscious mental associations. The conscious experience activates these associations in the sense that they begin to exercise a larger influence over the subsequent contents of conscious and unconscious processes. If the activated associations are conflictual, that is, if they are implicated with intense negative emotions and elicit unconscious attempts to avoid distress by warding off conscious experience of unpleasant mental contents, a knowledgeable observer can often detect clues that this is occurring.

Such clues often include those seen in the above excerpt: cognitive interferences such as slips of the tongue and momentary forgetting are more likely to occur. Experiences of distressing emotion may occur (e.g., Mr. X's report that he felt embarrassed while merely recounting the recollection to the interviewer). Mental and behavioral "metaphors" (Arlow, 1979) are often produced unconsciously which parallel key aspects of what has been activated in the subject's mind. For example, the content of Mr. X's symptom paralleled the content of the recollection, and the experience of being embarrassed telling the interviewer the recollection was yet another repetition of this same parallel. (The parallel referred to is the sequence: (a) Mr. X "performs" in some manner for an audience; (b) Mr. X perceives and/or anticipates that the audience's response is/will be derisive; (c) Mr. X experiences a surge of very unpleasant emotion such as embarrassment; (d) Mr. X experiences a powerful urge to escape this unpleasant feeling by escaping its perceived causes.) Associated with the activation of conflictual unconscious contents, it is not unusual to see evidence of what psychoanalytic theory conceives as transference (i.e., behavior based on repetitively occurring, maladaptive interpretations of interpersonal relationships which are emotionally charged and usually include misconstruals of the other person's motives and behavior). For example, Mr. X prefaced his embarrassing recollection with remarks which we see as examples of a key conflict: he first expresses impatient challenges to the older male interviewer and yet follows these with the assurance that he will continue to cooperate and submit "for the time being." We conjecture that all these are evidence that conflictual unconscious meanings were activated in the subject's mind in association with the telling of his childhood recollection, and that it was these clues which drew our psychoanalytic observers' attention to this small transcript segment.

In turn, these clues likely draw attention to key phrases in this segment which the judges believed reflected the unconscious and conflictual meanings activated. "Internal flame" is obviously at the heart of the embarrassing recollection and could be conjectured by the judges to be associated with ideas and feelings of hostile competitiveness, that is, anger and aggression can be likened to an "internal flame." Another speculation would associate the phrase he meant to use with his parents, "eternal flame," with President Kennedy's assassination. The latter event could be construed as a horrifying example of a male subordinate's aggression against an authority figure. "Soft story" refers to the subject's somewhat puzzling construal of his own story as "soft." He associates the term "soft" with the meaning "not . . . a typical male . . . macho . . . type of story." This could be associated again with conflict over hostile competitive impulses in relation to his father: he wants to be "macho" but his conflict makes him go "soft" and fail. This may connote the submissive side of him that was also judged to be expressed when he assured the interviewer he would "remain patient for the time being."

SOME ANALYSES OF THE RELIABILITY OF WORD RATINGS

We present below some results of interjudge reliability analyses of our word ratings, but we believe some substantial caveats regarding such reliability analyses are in order. Although these reliability coefficients give a numerical idea of the degree of interjudge agreement, there are three important reasons for refraining from attaching undue significance to them.

1. These coefficients reflect the degree of agreement over the *entire list* of nominated words, a list including from 159 to 245 words. However, because only 16 words are finally selected from the extremes of each list and those words are selected based on relative unanimity of agreement (see the formula in Figure 5.2), the degrees of disagreement on the majority of words that are not at the extremes are of little relevance to the experiment.
2. Since the laboratory experiment yielded significant results, this in itself would be evidence that the word selection process (i.e., the process by which the laboratory stimuli were collected) was not likely to have been entirely unreliable or random.
3. There is currently no acceptable method of evaluating the *adequacy* of reliability coefficients anyway; that is, there is no acceptable method for determining whether 0.60 is adequate or 0.80 is necessary, especially when the fact that different judgment tasks have different degrees of difficulty is taken into account.[2]

Thus, the value of interjudge reliability coefficients like those presented below is moot. Nonetheless, they give a numerical representation of the fact

---

[2] The difference between the average reliability of our conscious symptom word ratings versus that of our unconscious conflict word ratings is a case in point. The judgment of belongingness to the unconscious word category is much more difficult than that for the conscious word category. It is reasonable to expect both judgments to achieve the *same* reliability standard, say .80? We think not. See Bond, Hansell, and Shevrin (1987, pp. 743–747) for a full discussion.

TABLE 5.4. Intraclass Correlations for Five Subjects for Conscious Symptom Words and Unconscious Conflict Words

Subjects	Number of words selected	Reliability of conscious symptom words	Reliability of unconscious conflict words
Mr. C	159	0.86	0.50
Ms. Y	168	0.77	0.57
Mr. X	179	0.76	0.58
Mr. B	219	0.78	0.51
Mr. A	245	0.72	0.41

that judges agreed substantially better on the conscious words than on the unconscious words.

For five of the subjects, for whom the word-rating data were easily manipulable because they were already on computer disks, interjudge reliability coefficients were computed. Intraclass correlations (Winer, 1971, pp. 283–289) were used to estimate the degree of reliability across all four judges and all of the words that were independently rated during the first rating. Recall that these first ratings are independent because no discussion between judges has occurred. The results are ranked in Table 5.4.

The reliability coefficients are ranked in order of the number of words rated because this was not a constant. Subjects with fewer words (and thus, fewer ratings) tended to have higher reliability coefficients. Moreover, the subject with the largest number of words had the lowest reliabilities in both categories. However, the number of words may be confounded with degree of disagreement among the judges. For example, although there was agreement among the judges on the central aspect of Mr. A's unconscious conflict, there was also considerable disagreement about other aspects (see Chapter 9 for details). Mr. A's case had even more than the usual controversy over how to view the conscious symptom (see Chapter 9).

Agreement among the judges is easier for the words reflecting the conscious symptom than for these reflecting the unconscious conflict. This outcome makes sense because, ordinarily, the subject is quite clear about his or her symptom and uses certain words to describe the conscious experience of it. On the other hand, because the unconscious conflict is very much a matter of clinical inference on the part of each judge, it is a more subjective and controversial matter. However, it is important to bear in mind that the research did not rely on these ratings, submitted to reliability analysis and made prior to the first CET meeting but, in accord with the Delphi method, relied on only those few words that were most agreed-on after the judges reached final consensus.

The Subliminal
Cognitive Method

Before we describe and discuss the nature of the subliminal method as currently employed in cognitive psychology, and the history of the method, a few general observations are in order.

Traditionally, psychology has been divided into three main subject areas: (a) cognition, (b) affect, and (c) conation. This age-old tripartite division traces its origins to Plato. Cognition includes such functions as perceiving, learning, judging, remembering, and thinking. The cognitive functions of the mind might be summarized as all those relating to how knowledge is acquired, maintained, and used.

The affective aspect of psychology refers to the experiencing and expressing of emotion or feeling in reaction to some external or internal event. Emotional reactions can be defined along a number of dimensions, such as good–bad, pleasant–unpleasant, threatening–nonthreatening, and familiar–strange. Frequently, the experiencing of emotion is accompanied by some felt bodily sensation, such as an increase in heart rate, sweating, or sensations in the chest.

The conative aspect refers to motives, desires, wants, and wishes for the satisfaction of which knowledge is acquired, maintained, and used, and actions are undertaken. Most often, these motives, desires, wants, and wishes are accompanied by emotional reactions along the dimensions described above.

In simply identifying these three different aspects of the mind, we take no position on their independence from each other. In one important social psychological theory based primarily on Tomkins (1962, 1963), conation is treated as *derivative* of affects. On the other hand, the Freudian position would consider conation to be independent of either affect or cognition. In actual fact, all three aspects of the mind generally function simultaneously. From this perspective, we are never only feeling or only knowing or only wanting. One or another of these functions may be uppermost at any given time, but the other two are likely present as well. At this point, we leave aside all questions raised by the role of conscious and unconscious processes as they bear on these three aspects of the mind; these questions will be addressed below. Yet, a historical note may be useful. For a long time, psychologists found it incomprehensible that cognition could occur without awareness. Indeed, throughout the 19th century, with a few exceptions (Freud, for one), consciousness was considered to be the subject matter of psychology. However, it is important to point out that Freud vacillated about whether an *affect* could be unconscious. In his paper on the unconscious, for example, Freud hypothesized that affects were quintessentially conscious and only their *disposition* to appear under certain circumstances could be unconscious. Freud's vacillation on the subject derived from clinical experience with obsessional patients in whom unconscious guilt appeared to play an important role. The dispositional view of affect is reminiscent of a position more recently taken by philosopher John Searle (1990), who maintains that ideas, as well as affects, are dispositional in nature. The social cognitive notion of schema or script is also such a dispositional concept.

Where does cognitive psychology fit into this general view of the mind and its functioning? Bower and Clapper (1989) defined cognitive *science* as a "multi-disciplinary field with diverse goals and intellectual agendas" (p. 245). They considered cognitive psychology to be one of cognitive science's constituent disciplines, distinguishable from the other disciplines mainly by its heavy dependence on controlled experiments. Simon and Kaplan (1989) identified some of the other disciplines involved in cognitive science: artificial intelligence, philosophy, neuroscience, linguistics, and anthropology. Bower and Clapper also defined the subject matter of cognitive psychology as based on "experiments . . . [that] generally observe peoples' behavior as they are performing a specific task, such as perceiving, learning, judging or remembering something" (1989, p. 253). The methodological glory of cognitive psychology, inherited from academic antecedents going back to Wundt, has been the practice of a strict experimental approach that pays keen attention to necessary controls, precisely defined measures, and appropriate statistical analyses. Traditionally, cognitive psychology has been concerned with normal adult subjects in an alert, waking state, and has aimed to arrive at generally applicable laws of cognition. From a handful of subjects and on the basis of carefully designed experiments, one should be able to arrive at generalizations that could apply to all human beings. In this important respect, the model for cognitive psychology is similar to that of physics or chemistry, where, from a quite small sample of matter of any kind, one can arrive at lawful generalizations that apply to all matter from the smallest particle to the largest galaxy. However, as noted by Colby (Colby & Stoller, 1988):

> Most research efforts involving a computational theory of mind have been devoted to capacities we are proud of—solving problems . . . planning . . . understanding stories . . . there are other mental capacities and liabilities that we are not so proud of. Yet these departures are worth attention because they *matter* in human lives—misunderstandings, misconstruals, inhibited action, misguided desires, and a variety of displacements and deflections from the ideal design. (p. 141)

Indeed, our own research deals with such "deflections from the ideal design" insofar as we attempt to investigate the relationship between conscious and dynamic unconscious processes in psychiatric patients. It has been a time-honored practice in medicine to study pathological instances as a way to arrive at a fuller understanding of what might generally be the case. Within cognitive psychology, there is a growing interest in studying patients with brain lesions (e.g., organic amnesiacs) as a way to understand memory in general and the mental capacities of children. As we will undertake to examine in greater detail in Chapter 12, the important role of pathology and of individual differences in clarifying the nature of general principles has, in our judgment, not been given sufficient attention in cognitive psychology.

As discussed in Chapter 3 central to the conception of contemporary cognitive psychology is the information-processing paradigm based on an analogy with the computer. Bower and Clapper (1989) have stated this quite succinctly: "The presented stimulus corresponds to the program input and the subject's response corresponds to the program output; the subject executes a mental 'program' to compute the response from the stimulus. The task context is instrumental in determining the particular program the subject runs on the input" (p. 253).

In cognitive psychology experiments, the "program input" is always defined by the experimenter, never by the subject. "Programs" are presumed to apply to human beings generally, although, as noted above, there is growing interest in the study of children and of patients with brain lesions. In Chapter 3 we discussed criticisms of the "information processing" computational model and suggested alternate approaches.

THE SUBLIMINAL METHOD APPLIED BY COGNITIVE PSYCHOLOGISTS TO THE STUDY OF CONSCIOUS AND UNCONSCIOUS PROCESSES

As with any scientific subject matter, once scholarly attention is devoted to its history early forerunners are usually unearthed. This is certainly the case for subliminal perception. Readers are referred to two excellent books by N. F. Dixon (1971, 1981), in which the history of subliminal perception is traced to some of the very first researches by Pierce and Jastrow (1884) and Sidis (1898). Pierce and Jastrow reported that, when forced to guess, subjects could discriminate between weights that differed by less than a just noticeable difference (JND), the presumed basic, irreducible unit of judged sensation. Sidis reported that verbal responses experienced subjectively as guesses can be affected by concurrent stimulation below awareness. However, these early studies, and a number of others that followed, exercised little or no influence on the future development of research on subliminal stimulation. They are mainly of historical interest and, in themselves, point to the importance of a meaningful theoretical frame of reference in order for findings to achieve some lasting impact.

Attesting to the richness of research on subliminal perception, as reviewed by Dixon and others, is the fact that, since the early 1950s, a proliferation of studies of subliminal perception has extended into such areas as subception, dichotic listening, and parafoveal influences.

Within the limits of this chapter, we cannot explore the full range and variety of research in which the subliminal method has figured. However, one line of research that is particularly pertinent to our own work also has larger theoretical implications for a cognitive view of how the mind works. Specifically, this line of research is based on a distinction not acknowledged or present in most cognitive psychological research on subliminal perception. This distinction, referred to in Chapter 2, is between the cognitive and the dynamic unconscious. The dynamic unconscious involves the *interplay* of cognitive, affective, and conative factors and is not restricted to the purely cognitive. The nature of this interplay is such that certain significant psychological contents and events, because of their dangerous and threatening implications for the individual, are kept from direct access to consciousness.

What do we mean by "dangerous and threatening" and "kept from *direct* access to consciousness"? On the basis of the psychoanalytic theory undergirding this present research, explicated more fully in Chapter 2, these dangers are subjective and not necessarily objective. The individual *believes* that if he or she were to act on or even to become aware of certain wishes and desires, terrible consequences would ensue. These consequences are broadly identified in psychoanalytic theory as the loss of the object, the loss of love, castration anxiety, and loss of self-regard. To illustrate, we offer this example. When a four-year-old boy harbors the desire to possess his mother for himself, he anticipates his father's anger and retaliation as well as his father's rejection and withdrawal of love. Thus, the little boy's oedipal wish runs the risk of both castration and loss of love. For certain young boys with a particular history, it might also involve the anticipated loss of the object, that is, the father's feared departure. An example is provided in the case of Mr. A (Chapter 9). One diagnostic impression concerned the patient's beliefs about the divorce initiated by his mother, seen as resulting in the father's departure and disappearance, which occurred during the oedipal phase (Mr. A was three years old). The patient, we hypothesized, experienced this as an oedipal triumph but could not allow himself to be conscious of it because it would mean believing he had caused his father's departure and was in danger of his father's retaliation.

No brief is being offered here to support the validity of this line of reasoning, but we use this example to illustrate how the clinical theory of a subjective unconscious danger situation clarifies what psychoanalysts mean by the dynamic unconscious. We believe, however, that the results of our research supports this view of the dynamic unconscious. Readers should also bear in mind that this view of the dynamic unconscious entails an important role for cognitive factors. Certain beliefs, judgments, categorizations, and perceptions necessarily enter into the particular form and content of a given unconscious conflict in a state of repression. Indeed, as observed in Chapter 2, a *failure* to consciously classify certain stimuli as belonging together provides important evidence in favor of the role of repressive factors in unconscious conflict.

The line of research that is of interest to us began with the neuropsychological investigations of Otto Poetzl (1917/1960), a Viennese sensory physiologist. He was the originator of a method for studying dream reports as a vehicle for the recovery of subliminal stimuli. This method, for the first time, allowed the investigator to trace the *fate* of a subliminal input: Once having registered, how did it appear in some subsequent response? The importance of this methodological invention to the exploration of the dynamic unconscious is substantial. Until Fisher's revival of the Poetzl method in the early 1950s, research on subliminal processes had been done largely within an academic psychological tradition that dealt with the *immediate* effect of a subliminal input on some simultaneous cognitive act—for example, the subliminal effect on threshold determination, as in subception research, or on another supraliminal stimulus, as in dichotic listening experiments. The Poetzl method, however, incorporated responses of special relevance to psychodynamic theory, such as dreams, images, and free associations. Freud, learning of Poetzl's method and its early findings, added a footnote to the *Interpretation of Dreams* in the 1919 edition, acknowledging the importance of Poetzl's contribution: "The questions raised by Poetzl's experiment go far beyond the sphere of dream interpretation as dealt with in the present volume . . . it is worth remarking on the contrast between this new method of studying the formation of dreams experimentally and the earlier, crude technique for introducing into the dream stimuli which interrupted the subject's sleep" (1900, pp. 181–182). Parenthetically, one might observe that Freud was not uniformly opposed to experimental research, but only to experimental research that he deemed not to have any relevance to his theories.

Poetzl's complex and interesting theory as to what was going on perceptually to account for his effects has been summarized by Fisher (1960).
In this chapter, we will focus on the nature of his innovative method, its
strengths and limitations, and the way in which it was subsequently employed by others. Poetzl flashed complex visual scenes for ¹⁄₁₀₀ of a second, a
sufficiently fast exposure to abort any eye movements. He discovered that
only a part of the complex visual scene emerged in consciousness at ¹⁄₁₀₀ of a
second; the rest was presumably registered in the visual apparatus and
would be drawn on during the night and incorporated into an ongoing
dream. He presented evidence that previously unseen parts of the briefly
flashed picture appeared to emerge in dreams reported the following day. At
best, these findings can be referred to as anecdotal and suggestive but far
from conclusive, given the fact that Poetzl employed no systematic research
design involving suitable controls for response bias, chance, and the ambi-
guities involved in the way in which he identified the transformed nature of
the subliminal content in the dream. These critical limitations to Poetzl's
use of his method would, in time, be corrected in the hands of others.

In the early 1950s, Poetzl's method was taken up by Fisher in a series
of studies published in the psychoanalytic literature. As a psychoanalyst,
Fisher was particularly interested in how Poetzl's method might contribute
to understanding the nature of dreaming and its relationship to the conscious waking sources of the dream. Initially, Fisher simply repeated what
Poetzl had done, using similar complex visual scenes as subliminal stimuli.
He used the same exposure duration (¹⁄₁₀₀ of a second), obtained immediate
descriptions and drawings of the stimulus, and, on the following day, collected dream reports that were drawn as well as described. He also asked
subjects to allow images to come to mind and to draw and describe them as
a further means for recovering subliminal registrations, a response he borrowed from the earlier research of Allers and Teler (1924/1960). In his early
studies, Fisher used the same anecdotal approach as Poetzl and relied on his
own clinical assessment of what had been recovered through various transformations in the dream accounts and drawings. The individual subject
reports, as published by Fisher, were persuasive but far from conclusive.
Suitable controls were often lacking, and the various clinical interpretations could be seen as equivocal and, at times, arbitrary. Of Poetzl's earlier
work, one could say that, in the hands of Fisher, a body of anecdotal, empirical, and quasi-clinical findings was developing that called for more systematic and rigorous investigation.

These more rigorous experimental studies were conducted by Fisher as
well as by investigators at the Menninger Foundation and at the Research
Center for Mental Health at New York University. With interest growing at
several different research centers, the applications of the method broadened
but also became more rigorous and underwent substantial modifications. Two

typical studies were illustrative of this further evolution of subliminal percep-tion research from a psychodynamic standpoint (Paul & Fisher, 1959; Eagle, Wolitzky, & Klein, 1966). These two studies are of special interest because they address a cognitive issue of some importance, while remaining relevant to psychodynamic questions. The cognitive issue concerned the figure–ground organization of perception. The prevailing understanding concern-ing figure–ground organization was that the ground itself simply contributes to the formation of the figural contour and does not assume figural represen-tation in its own right. These two studies showed that, in the absence of awareness, the ground does appear to assume perceptual form. Although these studies corrected several methodological weaknesses of the Poetzl method, methodological questions remained that were, in time, addressed in further research. Indeed, the field of subliminal perception research provides an excellent example of how the dialectic between experimenters and critics has served increasingly to improve the methodological rigor of the research.

In the Paul and Fisher (1959) experiment, the Rubin's double-profile figure was used as the subliminal stimulus. Replacing the complex visual scenes used by Poetzl with a highly simplified and theoretically relevant stim-ulus constituted a significant methodological step forward. In addition, as Fisher had done in his previous studies, images were obtained from the sub-jects before the stimuli were presented as a baseline control and after the stimuli were presented. Images had the advantage of being obtainable from almost every subject, whereas dream reports were usually reported by only about two-thirds of the subjects. In contrast to dreams, images could sample recovery of subliminal elements immediately following stimulus exposure and thus could provide evidence as to how quickly subliminal effects were appar-ent. It also became possible to see whether certain transformations of inter-est to psychoanalysts required a dream state in order to occur, rather than already being present within minutes following the exposure of the stimulus.

The Paul and Fisher design called for a control stimulus in the form of a blank flash. Also, a complex scoring system devised on the basis of pilot data was applied to the images and dreams by judges who were unaware as to which stimulus the images and dream reports followed.

But significant methodological limitations remained in the Paul and Fisher experiment. These had to do with the critically important condi-tions of stimulus presentation. As was typical of experiments during this early stage of subliminal perception research, no luminance measures were provided. Mechanical (rather than electronic) shutters were used, and no calibration data were reported. Guided by pretesting results, Paul and Fisher found that an exposure of $\frac{1}{100}$ of a second, slightly out of focus and at some constant illumination, proved to be "adequately invisible." They further claimed that, at this setting, the experimenter, although knowing the nature of the stimuli, could not detect any difference between them.

However, in other data derived from a detection discrimination series in which the Rubin's double-profile figure and the control were each presented five times in random order, the correct detection percentage increased. By the fifth presentation of the figure, correct detection was at 61%; for the blank control, it was at 69%. Paul and Fisher provided evidence that the *identification* threshold—that is, seeing the Rubin's figure as a profile and the control stimulus did not occur until approximately a half-second, and, at that exposure time, only four of thirteen subjects were able to identify the Rubin's profile. Two others succeeded in recognizing it at one full second, and the remaining seven subjects failed to do so at the one-second exposure. In more contemporary methodological terms, the stimulus conditions in the Paul and Fisher experiment were at the *identification* threshold, not at the *detection* threshold.

The main method used to determine whether the images and dreams contained elements of the Rubin's profile was to have judges examine the separate sets of images and dreams and decide which sets followed the experimental stimulus, which sets followed the blank control, and which sets preceded the exposure of the stimuli. Blind judges were used, as well as the two experimenters who were considered to be biased judges, although they too were kept blind as to the stimuli associated with the images and dreams. In all instances, significantly greater than chance discrimination was made. Also of some interest is the fact that the judge who had the most experience in making these judgments, Fisher, consistently made the most accurate discriminations. These judgments were based solely on the pictorial renditions of the images.

Because of the reliance on an either/or judgment, it was not possible in this study to determine separately whether the figure-ground property of the experimental stimulus had a special effect. However, in an earlier study published in the same year (Fisher & Paul, 1959) and closely paralleling the second study, evidence was adduced to show that the "twoness" of the Rubin's profile did indeed influence the content of images. In this earlier study, a clock face, rather than a blank flash, was used as the control stimulus. In addition, a detailed scoring system based on prior pilot work was used to rate the contents of the different images. The exposure conditions were the same as in the second study, and similar results were obtained: It took approximately a half-second before subjects could begin to detect differences in the stimuli and about one second before they could identify these differences. Again, these findings would suggest that the stimuli were presented below the identification threshold not the detection threshold. In view of the fact that few judgments were obtained from subjects during the discrimination series, more recent research might make the reliability of these identification thresholds questionable. Many more such judgments are deemed necessary in order to establish the threshold. This point will be taken up later in this chapter, in the context of our own research.

Again, as in the second study, the most experienced judge, Fisher, made the most accurate judgments. This finding is of some importance, especially with respect to figural responses, because the recovery of subliminal registrations in images and dreams often involve distortions and various graphic transformations. Why this happens poses some interesting questions with respect to perceptual organization and memory formation. Poetzl was the first to point out how elements of the subliminal stimulus were transformed in the course of appearing in dreams. He likened these transformations to Freud's primary process mechanisms of condensation, displacement, and symbol formation. However, Poetzl's judgments were subject to the criticism that they could be arbitrary and ambiguous insofar as adequate controls were not incorporated into the research. However, in the case of Fisher's judgments, adequate controls had been incorporated, and his judgments must therefore be considered as evidence that these distortions and transformations do take place. How and why this happens then become significant research issues.

In the Eagle, Wolitzky, and Klein (1966) study a refined methodological effort was made to determine whether the ground in a stimulus would indeed subliminally influence recoveries of the stimulus in the form of images. The stimulus used was a silhouette of a tree stump with branches, the contours of which outlined a duck on the right side, which was part of the white background of the stimulus. Two groups were compared. For one group, the stimulus was presented at 1 second so that the stimulus was in consciousness; for the second group, the stimulus was exposed at $\frac{1}{100}$ of a second, an exposure time at which the stimulus could not be discriminated from a control stimulus. The control stimulus was a representation of a similar tree stump without the contour features that formed the outline of an embedded duck. The study was administered to 311 male and female undergraduates at local universities. Following the exposure of the experimental and control stimuli, subjects were asked to produce an image of a nature scene. These scenes were then judged for the appearance of such items as a duck, water, birds, feathers, animals, or other items that had been selected from associations to a picture of a duck obtained from a previous sample of subjects.

In a threshold determination procedure for the one-second exposure, the experimental stimulus was presented three times at the one-second exposure and the subjects were asked to carefully describe what they saw. In a second step, the experimental stimulus was exposed three times at one second with the question, "There is something in the picture in addition to the tree—what is it?" In a third step, the same question was repeated, but the stimulus was exposed for 30 seconds. In a fourth step, the stimulus was again exposed for 30 seconds and an outright clue was given: "There is a duck somewhere in the picture—find it." Subjects who had seen the $\frac{1}{100}$ of a second exposure were taken through the same procedure, with the exception that the first exposure was for $\frac{1}{100}$ of a second, presented three times. Most subjects failed to identify anything like a duck, even after 30-second exposures and the explicit clue to find a duck. At the exposure times used in the experiment (1 second and $\frac{1}{100}$ of a second), only one subject (from the 1-second group) in the threshold determination procedure identified the duck, and that subject was in the one-second group. These findings strongly suggest that, for both the supraliminal and subliminal groups, the duck outline was not in consciousness. Nevertheless, for both groups, significant numbers of subjects incorporated duck-related ideas into their images of nature scenes. Nor did it seem to matter at what exposure level in the threshold determination series the subjects were finally able to identify the embedded duck. These results imply that the important condition was an absence of awareness of the *embedded* duck, regardless of whether the stimulus as a whole was in awareness. In itself, this finding suggests that the duration for which the stimulus is presented is critical only insofar as it renders awareness unlikely; there is nothing inherent in the exposure time itself. Yet, the fact that the subliminal recovery of an embedded figure appeared following $\frac{1}{100}$-of-a-second flashes is of significance. Under these conditions, even when the *entire* stimulus is out of awareness, subliminal effects related to the embedded figure are obtained.

The original Poetzl procedure employed by Fisher was also used as the basis for a series of studies by Shevrin, Luborsky, and Stross at the Menninger Foundation (see Shevrin, 1973 for a review of this research). Shevrin and Luborsky (1958) had introduced several significant additions to the Poetzl procedure in order to more thoroughly test the nature of the method itself. As with Poetzl and Fisher, they used complex visual stimuli at approximately the same duration. However, instead of one description and drawing of the stimulus, Shevrin and Luborsky obtained two drawings and descriptions immediately after presentation of the stimulus and a third on the following day, after dream reports had been obtained. In addition to dream reports, images similar to those obtained by Fisher were elicited from subjects on the day following the exposure of the stimulus. The three drawings and descriptions of the stimulus were employed in order to test Poetzl's *law of exclusion*. According to this law, pictorial elements incorporated into the conscious perception of the flashed picture would be less likely to be incorporated into images or dreams, and the reverse would be true for those elements unreported in the initial descriptions. By obtaining a third description and drawing on the day following the image and dream reports, Shevrin and Luborsky hoped to determine whether, in fact, this law of exclusion would apply even after the indirect means of recovery had been obtained. Indeed, the three descriptions and drawings of the stimulus stabilized and did not significantly incorporate elements recovered in the images and dreams, while the images and dreams incorporated very few of the elements of the conscious perception of the stimulus. In addition to content elements, Shevrin and Luborsky devised a way to identify formal visual elements by measuring degree of angularity.

They discovered that the dreams, unlike the images, incorporated angular features of the stimulus. In addition, they had subjects rate how pleasant or unpleasant the dreams reported were. The dreams were rated as much more unpleasant if they contained more elements of the unreported aspects of the flashed stimulus. Shevrin and Luborsky (1958) reasoned that the elements recovered in the dreams, in particular, must have entered into some repressed unconscious process wherein they were rated as unpleasant.

One significant limitation to the Shevrin and Luborsky study was that no base rates were established for elements of the pictorial stimulus. Arguably, such elements as appeared would have appeared following any stimulus or no stimulus at all. This base rate problem was solved in a replication of the Poetzl procedure undertaken by Giddan (1967). In this experiment, two experimental groups were employed and each was shown a different picture. In addition, there were two control groups, each of which was shown a blank slide. In one of these two control groups, each subject was also shown the initial stimulus drawing of a randomly selected experimental subject. The blank-slide group allowed the control of base-rate recovery effects. The blank-slide-plus-matched-percept group allowed the assessment as to how much final recovery by the experimental subjects was influenced by further elaborations or associations initiated by a drawing of the original experimental stimulus. The results supported the original Poetzl findings, Fisher's results, and the Shevrin and Luborsky findings. Giddan was also able to replicate the finding concerning Poetzl's law of exclusion, for which Shevrin and Luborsky had also found support. In the Giddan study, only images were used.

A further extension of the Poetzl procedure was made by Haber and Erdelyi (1967), who used free associations following the exposure and description of the stimulus. They found that elements of the picture, unrecovered in the original description and drawing, appeared in the free associations, as compared to asking subjects to perform some neutral activity. Furthermore, there was a tendency for some of these elements that were recovered in free associations to become part of, and subsequently enter into, further drawings of the picture—an outcome that was not altogether consistent with findings supporting the law of exclusion. Associational activity appeared to facilitate the recovery of hitherto unreproduced items from the previously flashed stimulus.

The sequence of studies based on Poetzl's method—beginning with Poetzl himself and continuing on through Fisher, Shevrin and Luborsky, Giddan, and Haber and Erdelyi—documents the increasing rigor with which these researches were undertaken. Partially in response to criticisms by Eriksen (1960) and Goldiamond (1958), complex and useful controls were incorporated and the phenomenon nevertheless remained. However, these studies could still be criticized for the unsystematic way in which stimulus conditions were treated. The stimuli themselves varied considerably from experiment to experiment, as did the stimulus durations, and any reference to measures of luminance was totally omitted. Finally, no exhaustive method was used to determine how much the subject was really conscious of, following the flash of the stimulus. At most, two or three descriptions and drawings of the stimulus were obtained. It could be argued that, following the brief exposure of the complex visual scenes, subjects were at least fleetingly conscious of much more than was reproduced in the drawings and descriptions. Complex scenes are notoriously difficult to capture fully in words, and not many subjects have sufficient artistic ability to draw what they cannot put into words. Yet, fleeting awareness may function quite differently from focal awareness. This issue would resurface in subsequent, more rigorous experimentation undertaken by cognitive psychologists, to which we turn next.

Perhaps the most influential series of studies on subliminal stimulation undertaken by a cognitive psychologist were those published by Marcel in 1983 in *Cognitive Psychology*. The report of these experiments was followed by a second article, in the same journal, presenting a comprehensive and provocative theoretical account of the findings. A number of significant technical and methodological differences existed between the Marcel experiments and the Poetzl-based experiments. In keeping with many other cognitive studies of perception, subliminality was rendered by a procedure called "pattern masking." In pattern masking, subliminality is achieved by masking the subliminal stimulus with a second stimulus composed of either random parts of letters or numbers, or containing different kinds of figural properties. The critical parameter is the time interval between the onset of the subliminal stimulus and the onset of the masking stimulus. This interval is referred to as the "stimulus onset asynchrony" (SOA). At a certain critical SOA, the subject consciously sees only the masking stimulus and not the prior stimulus now rendered subliminal. The method of pattern masking is in contrast to the energy masking used in the studies thus far described. In energy masking, the masking stimulus is simply a blank field that is either brighter than the previous subliminal field or is on for a longer period of time, thus resulting in a greater amount of light energy hitting the eye. Of further relevance is the fact that, in Marcel's pattern-masking studies, the masked stimulus and the mask were presented dichoptically, that is, to different eyes. Polaroid lenses were used to occlude each eye from receiving the stimulus delivered to the other eye. Again, this is quite different from the energy-masking Poetzl studies in which the stimuli were presented binocularly, that is, directly to both eyes. This difference is of some importance because, in his 1983 paper, Marcel claimed that energy masking did not work but pattern masking did. He reported an experiment in which energy masking was used monocularly, that is, both the subliminal stimuli and the energy mask were presented to the same eye. There is little doubt, however, that energy masking does work, based on the many studies reviewed above as well as the many more reviewed in Dixon's two books and in subsequent work, some of it in our own laboratory (Snodgrass, Shevrin, & Kopka, 1993; Wong, Shevrin, & Williams, 1994). The one important difference between the Marcel energy-masking study and others is that the stimulus and mask were presented *binocularly* rather than monocularly as in Marcel's study. Nevertheless, the differences between pattern masking and energy masking are poorly understood, and further study is required. (In a personal communication, Marcel has indicated that energy masking does in fact work binocularly but apparently does not work monocularly.)

Among the many interesting findings reported by Marcel, two are especially intriguing and important. Marcel was able to demonstrate that when semantic, graphemic, and detection SOAs were compared, the order among these SOAs was the reverse of what one might intuitively expect. The SOA for the detection threshold was *longer* than for the graphemic SOA, which was, in turn, longer than the semantic SOA. In other words, a shorter time interval between stimulus onset and pattern mask resulted in more subliminal semantic priming than either graphemic priming or the actual detection of the presence of a stimulus.

Marcel refers to the second finding as the polysemous property of subliminal priming. If a word having two different meanings is used as a subliminal prime (e.g., *palm*) it will prime both meanings if it is presented subliminally and only one meaning supraliminally. This difference is produced by preceding the priming word, for example, *palm*, by the presentation supraliminally of either *wrist* or *tree*. When *palm* is masked, the word preceding it does not matter; it will prime both meanings. However, when *palm* is supraliminal, the meaning that it primes will depend on which meaning has been previously presented supraliminally.

Marcel's findings were subjected to critical scrutiny by Holender (1986), who cited several unsuccessful efforts at replicating Marcel's experiments. Primarily, however, Holender called attention to significant differences in Marcel's experiments between the SOA threshold determination procedures and the actual conditions used in the priming experiments themselves. He argued that these differences would tend to bias the conditions in the direction of producing awareness in subjects at the time the priming stimuli were presented. This criticism was further elaborated by Merikle (1992), who called attention to the fact that the chance criterion used for accepting subliminality in the Marcel studies was less than 60% (when chance was 50%). Merikle argued that, insofar as it was above the chance or objective threshold (50%), Marcel's subjects, while claiming not to see anything, nevertheless were making better than chance discriminations at what he called the subjective threshold. Merikle further claimed that were the objective threshold to be obtained, no subliminal effects would occur. Nevertheless, the subjective threshold was clearly of some importance because, as Marcel reported, qualitative differences in priming effects were obtained as compared to supraliminal primes (for example, the polysemous findings). Merikle also argued that, in order to determine the awareness threshold, many more trials would be necessary than the number used by Marcel. At the same time, Merikle underscored the importance of finding qualitative differences between unconscious and conscious processes as a critical criterion. Thus, he was willing to accept the subjective threshold as associated with some difference of qualitative importance and indeed the only threshold at which subliminal effects could be obtained.

Responses to Criticisms

The most suitable response to the Holender critique concerning the difference in criteria between threshold-setting procedures and the priming procedure is to follow threshold procedures that do not incur this limitation. In our own research, we have undertaken to deal with this potential problem in several different ways. Perhaps the most convincing way has been to set a duration that is as fast as available tachistoscopic equipment can provide. The duration we have relied on in almost all instances is 1 msec at 10 ft-lamberts. We have now accumulated extensive evidence with many subjects that, at this duration and luminance level, the stimuli we have used are at the *objective* threshold as defined by Merikle. Second, in most of our recent experiments there can be no difference between the threshold-determining conditions and the priming conditions. The subliminal effects are measured at the time the stimuli are flashed at 1 msec. Last, in one recent experiment in our laboratory, Wong, Shevrin, and Williams (1994), employed a stepwise threshold determination procedure that allows for establishing *individual* thresholds. Once an individual threshold is set, it is used in the subliminal study itself. In addition, a threshold series is administered before and after the experiment. In the Wong et al. study, the threshold that was determined initially is at the objective identification threshold and remains so in the second postexperimental check. Of further interest is the fact that, on average, these individually determined thresholds were at 2 msec, with a range between 1 and 4 msec. This information would be further confirmation that the 1-msec exposure time is indeed at or below most individually determined thresholds.

Merikle has called attention to the need for meeting at least three criteria for establishing subliminality: (1) eliminating response bias, (2) obtaining a sufficient number of threshold-determining responses, and (3) identifying qualitative differences between conscious and unconscious processes. Merikle has also made a distinction between the subjective and objective thresholds: The former is a threshold somewhat above chance (i.e., below 60% in the Marcel experiments), and the latter is at chance. Merikle advised that the response bias issue could best be dealt with by instructing subjects to give an equal number of yes or no responses to the presence or absence of the stimulus. As Marcel has pointed out, however, many subjects in subliminal experiments such as his own look on being asked to say yes when they see nothing at all as nonsensical, and they often object to the instruction. Nevertheless, there is good reason for giving subjects this instruction. Only by answering yes or no even in the absence of a stimulus is it possible to accurately determine an objective threshold or how high above the objective threshold the subject's perceptions might be. The need for many individual trials is justifiable simply on sampling grounds. Often, in subliminal experiments, too few trials (around 10 to 20) have traditionally been used to determine thresholds. Contemporary detection theory requires many more trials. In the study reported in this book, the criteria for detection can be criticized on the grounds of response bias and the number of detection trials, but the use of a 1-msec duration at 10 ft-lamberts, as previously noted, would appear to shelter us from these criticisms. In addition, in another experiment from our laboratory (Snodgrass, Shevrin, & Kopka, 1993), Merikle's criteria were followed for determining response bias and the numbers of trials at the same 1-msec duration, 10 ft-lambert luminance, and the objective threshold as defined by Merikle was achieved.[1] Thus, we can say with some conviction that our exposure conditions are not subject to either Holender's or Merikle's criticisms.

Previous Relevant Contributions from Our Own Series of Studies

The research reported in this book is, in some important respects, the outgrowth of a series of previous studies going back to 1958. Without exception, these studies have been informed by an interest in investigating the nature of the dynamic unconscious. Thus, the Shevrin and Luborsky (1958) replication and extension of the Poetzl phenomenon undertook to determine whether Poetzl's law of exclusion held up, and whether what was recovered in the dreams would be linked with unpleasant affect. Even in

---

[1] Indeed Van Selst and Merikle (1993) replicated the Snodgrass, Shevrin, and Kopka (1993) findings, further strengthening the claim that our conditions are at the objective threshold.

the first of our studies, we were not simply interested, as were most cognitive subliminal studies such as Marcel's, in content-free neutral stimuli.

A series of investigations based on a rebus-type stimulus followed the Shevrin and Luborsky (1958) Poetzl replication. These new studies attempted to deal with several of the methodological limitations of the Poetzl procedure, while building in a means for distinguishing between primary and secondary process thinking as defined psychoanalytically (Shevrin & Luborsky, 1960). The possibility of fleeting awareness was dealt with by shifting from a relatively long exposure duration (100–200 msec) to a brief duration (1 msec). These studies are summarized in Shevrin (1973).

The rebus stimulus was the pictorial representation of a word. The stimulus most often used in these studies was a picture of a pen pointed at a leg that was prominently flexed at the knee. There were several methodological advantages in using rebus stimuli. The two items composing the rebus were not associated to each other. We knew from normative association studies that knee is rarely associated to pen and vice versa. In visual scenes, on the other hand, the visual coherence of the scene (i.e., a street scene with cars or buildings) contains many closely associated elements. Contrasted with the complex visual stimuli used in the Poetzl studies, the rebus stimulus was relatively simple. At the same time, the rebus stimulus allows for three distinctly different types of subliminal effects: (1) *conceptual* level, measured by the presence of such words as *ink* and *paper* related to pen, and *leg* and *foot* related to knee; (2) *clang* level, reflected in words sharing the clang sound of pen or knee, in words like *pennant* and *any*, and (3) *rebus* level, reflected in words related to the rebus word itself (penny), such as dime or nickel. The conceptual level is very much like the level generally studied in most cognitive priming experiments. However, the clang and rebus levels have special relevance to the psychoanalytic conception of the primary process and, in particular, the use of what Freud referred to as "superficial associations" as forms of displacement. Many dynamically rich slips involve phonetically related words that are quite different and at times antithetical in meaning. When a member of an audience who has been listening to a dull speaker asks for someone to "shut the bore," the consciously intended word "door" is replaced by the phonetically similar clang-like "bore," which expresses the person's underlying feeling. Similar uses of phonetic relationships can be found in dreams and in the pressured verbal flights of manic patients. We had hypothesized that the clang-like rebus subliminal effects would appear subliminally but not supraliminally. This hypothesis was borne out by our first published rebus study (Shevrin & Luborsky, 1960).

In a series of studies combining the rebus stimulus with hypnosis, we found that rebus effects were present only in hypnotically recalled nighttime dreams and not in hypnotically obtained images. Images were better able to recover the conceptual level of the stimulus (reviewed in Shevrin, 1973). This result was further confirmed in a sleep–dream study conducted by Shevrin and Fisher (1967) in which it was found that both clang and rebus effects appeared in free associations following awakenings from rapid eye movement (REM) dreaming sleep, while conceptual level effects appeared in free associations following stage 2, nonrapid eye movement (NREM) sleep. A dream state was necessary in order to retrieve the phonetically related effects of the penny rebus. Shevrin and Fisher also found that subliminal recovery of rebus, clang, and conceptual effects was greater following sleep awakenings from their respective sleep stages than in images obtained in the waking state.

These rebus studies were also notable for their incorporation of an electrophysiological measure in the form of ERPs. We were able to show that amplitude components at certain latencies could discriminate between the penny rebus and a dummy control (Shevrin & Fritzler, 1968). Aside from some early studies by Libet, Alberts, Wright, and Feinstein (1967) with implanted electrodes and using somatosensory stimuli, ours was the first to demonstrate an ERP indicator of a subliminal visual process. We were also able to show that different parameters of the ERP were related to the conceptual and rebus level subliminal effects. The conceptual effects were highly correlated with an early voltage amplitude, and the rebus effects were correlated with the appearance of bursts of alpha approximately 1 second after stimulus exposure. Finally, by relying on Rorschach ratings of repressiveness, we were able to show that more repressive subjects showed a *smaller* ERP amplitude response to the rebus stimulus and gave fewer rebus-related associations. Findings in these experiments were all replicated at least once (Shevrin, Smith, & Fritzler, 1969, 1970).

These rebus studies dealt with what one might call a formal aspect of dynamic unconscious thought organization marked primarily by superficial associations in the form of phonetic transitions and combinations. However, these studies allowed for no examination of conflict. The study reported in this book constituted an effort to investigate the role of conflict with the use of a subliminal method. However, in this study, we have no means of identifying any of the formal or superficial shifts in thought organization as determined by the rebus experiments. At some time in the future both approaches will need to be combined.

COGNITIVE IMPLICATIONS OF OUR PRESENT STUDY

As reported in Chapter 1 and as will be explored in greater detail later, our results document qualitative differences between conscious and unconscious processes as required by Merikle. In addition, we have demonstrated that these qualitative differences bear on emotionally laden and conflictual material involving significant motivations.

We have also been able to demonstrate the important role that individual differences play in assessing the nature of subliminal effects. In contrast to the general principles cognitive psychology attempts to explore and clarify, our approach makes it necessary to consider the highly individual ways in which subliminal stimuli are experienced and processed. In Chapter 12 we will discuss the implications of our approach, not only for an understanding of individual psychology but for an understanding of how the individual brain itself is organized.

Finally, our research supports the validity of energy masking as a means for investigating subliminal perception.

The Psychophysiological Method

In Chapter 4, we discussed some of the strengths and weaknesses involved in the measurement of event-related potentials (ERPs). The main strength resides in the ability of ERPs to detect, in real time, ongoing brain processes that are related to complex psychological functions. The central weakness of ERPs derives from their inability to allow any but the most crude localization of the source of brain activity. We cited Allison, Wood, and McCarthy (1986), who characterized this weakness by way of an analogy with an arithmetic sum. The sum itself may in fact be correct, but it does not reveal the individual numbers from which it was summed. A sum of 47, for example, could be arrived at by adding 40 and 7, 30 and 17, and so on. Similarly, the same ERP could have been created by any number of component brain processes at different locations in the brain. Although ERPs cannot be used to investigate brain localization, they have proven quite useful in demonstrating correlations among psychological functions such as attention, association strength, and subliminal perception. As we will try to show in Chapter 12, the weakness in localization may yet prove to be a strength insofar as many complex psychological functions may be the result of an integration of widely distributed and parallel processes in the brain. ERPs may be markers of this integration. In other words, knowing that the sum is 47 may turn out to be quite important.

As also noted in Chapter 4, the reliance in most ERP research on voltage amplitudes at relatively fixed latencies rests heavily on two assumptions: (1) the electrophysiological significance of voltages and (2) the latency stability, or stationarity, of these voltages. We have argued that both of these assumptions are questionable. Allison, Wood, and McCarthy (1986) have raised doubts about the reliability and validity of even the voltage directions—whether positive or negative. They have shown that, depending on a variety of factors, a positive voltage might in fact be negative and vice versa. We will also try to show that the slope or rise of a voltage component is important because it is related to frequency variables.

In this chapter, we will describe in some detail the psychophysiological methods we have devised to measure the stimulus effects that are of importance to us. We do not rely on voltage amplitudes at fixed latencies; instead, our methods assume that brief energy packets with rapidly varying latencies and frequencies play vital roles in ERP signal detection. The case will be made for a time–frequency analysis method that does not assume stationarity of the signal. Readers will be introduced to the concept of an information-theoretic approach that was relied on initially in our research. The results were encouraging, but they fell short of allowing us to fully test our hypotheses. The information-theoretic approach was then incorporated into a time–frequency feature analysis based on a new method of signal analysis that will be described in some detail. This new method did permit us to test our main hypotheses, and the results were highly encouraging. Finally, the time–frequency analysis was incorporated into another method of signal analysis, the adaptive Gabor transform, which made it possible to add other ERP parameters to time and frequency. The additional parameters were time–frequency variance, energy level, and phase. Results from the adaptive Gabor transform were consistent with those from the time–frequency feature analysis, but allowed for generalizing to a more complex set of ERP dimensions. Detailed results will be presented in Chapter 8.

For readers who are not acquainted with the technical aspects of signal analysis and the necessary mathematical formulations, we will summarize the text from time to time in less technical language.

THE INFORMATION-THEORETIC APPROACH

Several different ideas are referred to with the common label "information theory." Shannon's Information Theory (Shannon & Weaver, 1963) is the best known, and it forms the basis for the developments to follow. Information is a much used and abused term. Everyone has an idea of what information is. Most people consider that information refers simply to facts, rather than to the more complete concept of information that is elaborated below. An analogy would be the common idea of statistics as baseball data, rather than the formal notion of statistics as a mathematical framework for understanding random phenomena and significant departures from randomness. *Information processing,* as often used in psychology, refers to the processing of this type of factual information. Information-processing models of the brain are based on this conception of information. These brain models are computer-like in conception and, as such, have come under much well-deserved criticism when they are carried too far (see Chapter 3). The information approach to be discussed in this chapter is almost the antithesis of the information-processing idea.

Information, as we use it and as used by Shannon, is related to uncertainty. Thus, the statement "The sun will rise tomorrow morning" would seem to have high information content to the uninitiated. However, in the Shannon sense, there is almost no information in this statement because there will be no uncertainty about it. Restating a certain fact provides no information. Paradoxically, random noise, on the other hand, has a large amount of information associated with it, insofar as it is maximally uncertain and therefore useless. A simple example from the game of "Twenty Questions" can illustrate this concept of uncertainty and its relationship to information. At the start of the game, before any questions have been asked the possibilities are limitless; thus, uncertainty and, therefore, potential information are at their greatest level—the very opposite of the sun rising in the morning, for which uncertainty is zero. Once the first answer is given, identifying the unknown reject as animal or mineral, the universe of possibilities has been reduced considerably. With the second question, "Bigger or smaller than a bread basket?" uncertainty has been reduced even further. If we imagine a game in which each question would ideally divide the range of possibilities in half, we could apply a binary rule, as when we guess whether a coin toss will result in a head or tail. Each binary decision carries up to one *bit* of information, or the amount by which uncertainty has been reduced. The greater the number of bits, the greater the information. Let us next consider a more complex example.

Suppose you were to walk along a road and collect a handful of pebbles. Suppose further that there are 128 pebbles on the road. The total information contained in this set of pebbles is equal to the total number of pebbles, or 128. Each pebble could be characterized by using a seven-bit binary representation ($2^7 = 128$). Or, for each pebble, there are seven binary choices that characterize the information contained in the pebble (i.e., big/small, round/oval, and so on). The problem in this case is that too much information is available. Usually, we wish to order things in some parsimonious way rather than simply having a large catalog or inventory. The challenge might be to sort the pebbles into, say, two classes. Suppose that 64 pebbles have diameters greater than 1 cm and 64 pebbles have diameters less than 1 cm. It is as if someone had asked, in the game of 20 questions, "How many pebbles are larger than 1 cm?" and, as luck would have it, half are larger than 1 cm, a binary answer. The information has been reduced to one bit. Pebbles may now be characterized by representing the large class by 1 and the small class by 0. Order has been found in randomness. Maybe the pebbles can also

be sorted by color—say, black, brown, white, and gray. This color classification contains 2 bits ($2^2 = 4$) or four possibilities. Now suppose that
large pebbles are found only on the north side of the road. Pebble size now
provides information about whether a pebble is on the north or south side
of the road. Observing a large pebble is sufficient to tell you that you are
on the north side of the road; You can obtain one bit of information by
this observation. Research can be launched to discover the reason for a
relationship between the pebble size and a particular side of the road.
The fact that there is much more information *not* related to the side of
the road does not matter. For example, pebble color may have no relationship to the north or south side of the road. An information-theoretic approach provides a systematic, formal system for measuring information in
any system. In our research, the stimuli have been divided into four
equally likely classes of words. We then ask the question, "Is there any information in the ERPs concerning the class from which the stimulus
word was drawn?"

The Benefits of the Information-Theoretic Approach

By using information concepts, one may combine diverse observations
about the system under study. Each of these observations is measurable by
the same yardstick—information in bits. One bit of information about
color is the equivalent of one bit of information about size. They can be
added together like numbers, even though color is measured in wavelengths
and size is measured in centimeters. Information theory allows symbolic
and numerical observations to be combined in a single framework. Thus,
one can combine sensory, behavioral, and brain activity measurements on
the basis of one metric, that is, bits.

Biological systems, such as brain processes, are often nonlinear and
nonstationary. By nonlinear, we mean that a process might accelerate over
time rather than increase by equal increments. For example, a car going
from a stop to highway speed in a few seconds is increasing its speed in a
nonlinear manner, but the same car proceeding down the highway and
gradually increasing its speed by 5 miles per hour every 5 minutes is increasing its speed linearly. The graph of acceleration would have a curve in
it; the graph of regular increase in speed would be a straight line. By nonstationary, we refer to the tendency for an event (e.g., P300) to occur at
different times (in fact, P300 really occurs in a wide window of latencies
from approximately 275 to 450 msec). An information-theoretic approach
is not affected by most forms of nonlinearity in which the transformation
is one-to-one. Most conventional approaches to measuring brain processes

depend on linearity and precise time registration, or stationarity of the signal. Information possesses several properties that mitigate the effects of this disparity between the requirements of conventional measurements and the true nature of brain processes. Among those properties, additivity is most useful.

Additivity

Even though the measurements involved in a particular study may result from highly nonlinear phenomena, the information approach will linearize the result in certain cases. We can use our earlier pebble example to illustrate this idea. Suppose that one investigator used pebble diameter to measure the size of pebbles and another investigator used pebble volume. A linear relationship may exist between some road characteristic and pebble diameter, but the relationship between that same road characteristic and pebble volume would have to be quite nonlinear because volume is estimated by the cube of the radius of a sphere, and the cubes of numbers increase nonlinearly (i.e., the cubes of the series 1, 2, 3 . . . are 1, 8, 27 . . .). Thus, the published curves of the investigators would look quite different, even though they describe the same phenomenon, that is, size. However, if information is used as the common metric, both investigators will obtain similar results. It is well-known that sensory processes transform incoming stimuli in a logarithmic or power-law fashion. The information approach would not be affected by this transformation. Furthermore, as described above, information obtained from independent phenomena can simply be added. Suppose that the county line divides the road on an east–west basis. Suppose further that black and brown pebbles are found in county A, which is east of the line, and white and gray pebbles are found in county B, which is west of the line. Pebble color then provides one bit of information about the county the pebble is in. Knowing pebble color has reduced uncertainty about what county the pebble is in. However, we already know that large pebbles are on the north side of the road and small pebbles are on the south side. Pebble color and size together now provide two bits of information. A large white pebble is found on the north side of the road in county B; a small black pebble is found on the south side of the road in county A. The bit of information concerning north or south can be added to the bit of information concerning east and west to provide two bits of information about locations. The north–south bit must exclusively signal north and south, and the east–west bit must exclusively signal east and west. If so, the information is additive. This is without regard to the linearity of the basic observations that determined the bit value (i.e., diameter vs. volume measurements). By this means, it becomes possible to convert potentially confusing nonlinear results into a manifestly linear result.

In the next section, we present a formal, mathematical description of the information just discussed in nontechnical language.

Formal Description of Information

A measure of information is required to meet certain standards, some of which have been touched on, that result in

$$H = -\log(P) \tag{7.1}$$

where P is the probability of a message state occurring. If the logarithm is taken to be base 2, then H has the units of bits. For example, if a message state has a probability of $\frac{1}{4}$, then H is two bits. If there is a set of m message states from a source x, where the ith symbol has a probability of $P(i)$, then

$$H(x) = -\sum_{i=1}^{m} P(i)\log_2[P(i)] \tag{7.2}$$

Because of the similarity of this formulation and those of statistical mechanics, this measure is often called the entropy of the source. The maximum value is obtained when $P(i) = 1/m$, in which case

$$H(x) = -\sum_{i=1}^{m} \frac{1}{m} \log_2 [\frac{1}{m}] = \log_2[m] \tag{7.3}$$

If there are two symbols of interest, say x and y, with m possibilities for x and n possibilities for y, then the entropy of the joint event is

$$H(x,y) = -\sum_{j=1}^{n} \sum_{i=1}^{m} P(i, j)\log_2[P(i, j)] \tag{7.4}$$

The conditional entropy of y, given that x is known, is

$$H(y|x) = -\sum_{j=1}^{n} \sum_{i=1}^{m} P(i, j)\log_2[P(j|i)] \, b \tag{7.5}$$

The conditional entropy of x, given that y is known, is

$$H(x|y) = -\sum_{j=1}^{n} \sum_{i=1}^{m} P(i, j)\log_2[P(i|j)] \tag{7.6}$$

Now, suppose that x is the set of symbols representing the input to the system and y is the set of symbols representing the output of the system. Then

$H(x|y)$ is called the equivocation and represents the information lost by noise in the channel.

The entropy of the input (source) is

$$H(x) = -\sum_{i=1}^{m} P(i)\log_2[P(i)] \text{ bits/symbol} \tag{7.7}$$

The entropy of the output (receiver) is

$$H(y) = -\sum_{i=1}^{m} P(j)\log_2[P(j)] \tag{7.8}$$

The information that is transmitted through the channel is

$$T = H(x) - H(x/y) \tag{7.9}$$

or

$$T = H(y) - H(y/x) \tag{7.10}$$

Equation 7.9 is probably most easily understood intuitively. The equation shows that the information that is able to pass through the noisy channel is the information available at the input minus the information lost in transmission. T is often called *transinformation*.

If one had an estimate of the H values, one could find the information that passes through the channel. $H(x)$ is easy to determine in an experiment if one takes care. If the probabilities of the input stimuli are known, then $H(x)$ may be easily computed. For example, if four classes of input stimuli are to be used and are equally likely ($P(i) = \frac{1}{4}$), then $H(x) = $ two bits.

The equivocation is more difficult to obtain, however, because it depends on the unknown output, y. The estimation of this quantity will be described next.

Estimation of Information

$H(x/y)$ may be estimated if $P(i|j)$ is known. That is, what is the probability that input i was present, given that observation of output j was obtained? Suppose that the input is a set of stimuli and the output is a brain wave voltage measurement. If an A to D converter is used, then the voltage observations will be discrete. One can more easily find $P(j|i)$. This is easily done by observing the distribution of voltage values for a given input i. This distribution is discrete but can be modeled by a continuous normal distribution for convenience in computation. The desired probability, $P(i|j)$, can be obtained by the Bayes theorem:

$$P(i|j) = \frac{P(j|i)P(i)}{\sum\limits_{k} P(j|k)P(k)} = \frac{P(j, i)}{\sum\limits_{k} P(j, k)} \qquad (7.11)$$

With the later simplification resulting from the fact that the input stimuli are equally likely, this derivation assumes that there is only one output observation for each stimulus. However, this formulation can be applied for each time sample of the output. In addition, observation j may consist of several voltage values collected from different electrodes at different times or from the same electrode at different times. In this case, a multivariate characterization is required. The probability distribution of voltages for each stimulus type is required to formulate the information model.

The approach has several problems. Bias of the estimate is a major concern. The information measure is manifestly biased. Experiments carried out using noise data sets with no inherent information produce information values. Because the measure is nonnegative, averaging of the results produces a positive bias offset. This bias has been found to decrease for larger data sets and can be shown to ultimately approach zero for very large data sets. This is not practical experimentally, however. The bias increases as one uses more observations in obtaining the information measure. A bivariate model exhibits more bias than a univariate model. Fortunately, the information obtained using the univariate model exhibits a relatively small bias effect. One has to balance the gain obtained by using more observations against the increased bias that results.

To date, the sampling distribution of the information measure has been impossible to derive or to approximate reasonably. This problem is offset in practice by simulation, category scrambling experiments, and other means, in order to assess the integrity of the results. The model assumed to date utilizes a normal distribution for characterization of the data. The normal distribution is completely characterized by its mean and variance, so any information conveyed by higher moments of the data would not be factored into the model. Some preliminary work using nonparametric statistics has been carried out with encouraging results. The normal model may also be corrected to include skew and kurtosis, an approach that yields some improvement as well. Modeling and estimating the information more effectively may improve the technique considerably.

This concludes the mathematical description of information. We next turn to a consideration of its applications, particularly those that are relevant to our data.

Applications of the Information Technique

There have been scattered brain signal studies that have utilized informa-tional concepts in some way (Callaway & Harris, 1974; Gersh, Yonomoto, & Naitoh, 1977; Vidal, 1977; Inouye, Yagasaki, Takahashi, & Shinisaki, 1981; Satio & Harishima, 1981; Kamitake, Harashima, & Miyakawa, 1984; Williams, Shevrin, & Marshall, 1987; Shevrin, 1988). The goals of these studies fall into two basic categories. They represent attempts to (a) find informational markers of external stimuli in brain waves via information measures (b) track "information flow" or directed information from one area of the brain to another. A recent study (Kushwaha, Williams, & Shevrin, 1992) attempted to combine these ideas and track information movement in the brain in response to specific categories of word stimuli.

In our studies, we have used univariate normal distributions and bi-variate normal distributions to model the distributions of voltages obtained when the four categories of word stimuli were presented to patients. The normal distributions are obtained by estimating the mean and variances of the voltages obtained for each word class from the set of ERPs evoked by the stimuli. The ERPs consist of 256 points sampled at 250 Hz. The first 32 points are obtained prior to stimulus, to establish a baseline. Thus, a statis-tical information channel model is obtained for the data set. With this model, one may examine each ERP in terms of its information content vis-à-vis the model by passing it through the model. One may find $P(i|j)$ for each voltage value of the ERP and thus compute a T based solely on that single ERP. The model is exactly the same for each ERP, so this process re-sults in a mapping of the set of ERPs into a set of information profiles that spans the same time extent as do the ERPs. Averaging this set of T's would provide an estimate of the information in the entire scheme. One may also focus on the average for a certain category of words or even groups of words within a category, in order to see where the information is contributed. The net result is that a nonlinear ruler is used to measure the set of ERPs, each in exactly the same manner, in such a way that the measurement is lin-earized according to information content.

Figure 7.1 illustrates the preliminary results obtained for three two-way category comparisons: The unconscious conflict, conscious symptom, and ordinary unpleasant categories have been compared individually to the ordinary pleasant category that serves as a control. In the analysis, the ordinary pleasant category is considered to be one set of symbols. The ordi-nary unpleasant, conscious symptom, and unconscious conflict categories are used, in turn, as the other set of symbols. The result is the information that passes through the channel concerning these pairings. As illustrated in Figure 7.1, we found information peaks occurring early (100–400 msec

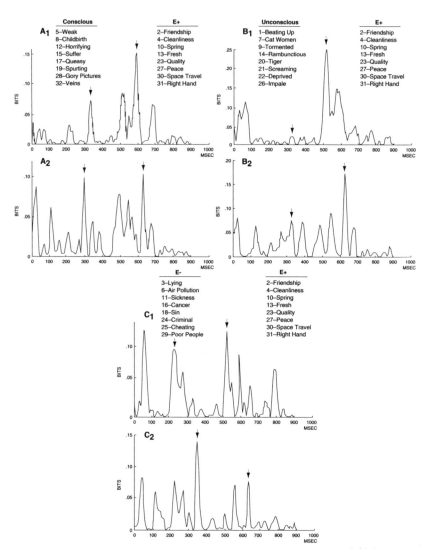

FIGURE 7.1. Transinformation two-way comparisons. The subject is a 20-year-old man suffering from a blood phobia. Each curve represents the amount of information in lists (y axis) at different times (in msec; x axis). In each pair, the upper curve is the information for the supraliminal criteria and the lower curve represents the subliminal conditions. The two-way companions are between the conscious symptom words, unconscious conflict, and ordinary unpleasant words, each is compared with the ordinary pleasant words. A_1 and A_2 are the curves for the comparison of the conscious symptom words (listed in the upper left-hand corner of A_1) and the ordinary pleasant (E+) control words (listed in the upper right-hand corner of A_1). B_1 and B_2 are the curves for the unconscious conflict words compared to the ordinary pleasant (E+) words; C_1 and C_2 are the curves for the ordinary unpleasant (E−) words compared to the ordinary pleasant (E+) words. Arrows point to the peak transformations at 100–400 msec and 404–704 msec poststimulus.

poststimulus) and late (400–700 msec poststimulus). A statistical analysis revealed that for both the conscious symptom and unconscious conflict categories, when compared to the ordinary pleasant category, information peaked early subliminally and late supraliminally. For the ordinary unpleasant words, no such difference was found.

Although these information results were encouraging, the information measure failed to distinguish between the conscious symptom and the unconscious conflict categories. We next turn our attention to another approach for identifying ERP signal properties that proved more useful. This method incorporates the information metric but goes beyond it.

TIME–FREQUENCY DISTRIBUTIONS

The focus of this chapter now changes to a different subject area that is quite new to the study of brain signals: the identification of frequencies rapidly changing over time. In the EEG literature, frequencies have been measured within broad time windows and in certain frequency bands: 1–3 Hz (delta), 3–5 Hz (theta), 7–13 Hz (alpha), and so on. A segment of EEG may be analyzed in terms of its frequency spectrum (the Fourier transform), which measures how much of the total voltage or energy is found in each of the frequency bands. When a person is relaxed or falling asleep, the EEG frequency spectrum is heavily weighted toward the alpha band; when a person is awake and alert, the spectrum shifts toward higher frequencies. This analysis, however, cannot reveal how frequencies shift *within* the time window. If, for example, the time window were 10 seconds wide and the person is relaxed and falling asleep on *average* across the time window, alpha will be the dominant frequency. However, at any particular moment within the time window, alpha may be absent. If, for example, at the sixth-second mark the person momentarily became alert, there would be, instead of alpha, momentary high frequency followed by a return to alpha as the alertness waned. The spectral analysis would not capture that frequency fluctuation. In any attempt to zero in on this fluctuation by narrowing the time window to one second, measurements would fall prey to a fundamental characteristic of the Fourier transform which dictates that durations in time and bandwidths in frequency are inversely related.

Spectral analysis of the kind just described works best (a) when the signal of interest is composed of a number of discrete frequency components so that time is not a specific issue (e.g., a constant frequency sinusoid or a regular repetitive wave), or, somewhat paradoxically, (b) when the signal exists for a very short time so that its time of occurrence is considered to be known (e.g., an impulse function). Signals that cannot be satisfactorily represented in these ways are somehow suspect and must be forced into the mold or abandoned. Thus, it is not unusual that brainwaves have been considered in terms of their rhythms or frequency components (EEG analysis) or their time domain components (ERPs).

For our purposes, we drew on a method of time–frequency analysis that can identify rapidly changing frequencies by establishing their joint time–frequency distributions (Williams & Jeong, 1989). Musical notation is one such centuries-old representation of a time–frequency distribution. Each note represents the pitch (frequency) of a sound and its duration. Complex musical pieces consist of many notes with distinct pitches and durations. The trained ear is capable of abstracting these complex relationships; efforts to devise more mathematically precise time–frequency relationships have been crude by comparison. These approaches have assumed that a tone persists for a certain length of time in order for its frequency to be determined exactly. For example, a spectrogram or sonogram is based on the assumption that the signal remains stationary for a time in order for time–frequency relationships to be determined. These methods require moving a window of fixed duration along the signal so that the frequencies of the tones lying within the window can be measured. Any variation in the frequency of a component within the window produces a confusing result. The method described by Williams and coworkers (Choi, Williams, & Zaveri, 1987; Williams & Jeong, 1989) allows for high-resolution descriptions of the time–frequency components of a signal. Using this method, one can now identify precise time–frequency components, thus unifying the previous dichotomy between time and frequency and making possible a much more accurate identification of time-varying features. This method surpasses in precision the amplitude components (e.g., P200) used in our previous research. A preliminary account of the application of this new approach to some of our data has been presented elsewhere (Shevrin et al., 1988).

The following section presents a more technical and mathematical description of the time–frequency approach.

Time–Frequency Feature Analysis

It has been quite difficult to handle many rapidly fluctuating (nonstationary) signals satisfactorily, using conceptualizations based on the assumption of stationarity. The spectrogram represents an attempt to apply the Fourier transform, or spectral analysis, for a short-time analysis window, within which it is hoped that the signal behaves reasonably, according to the requirements of stationarity. The spectrogram may be described in terms of the short-time Fourier transform with analysis window $h(t)$ and signal $f(t)$, so that

$$T_f(t, \omega) = \int_{-\infty}^{\infty} f(u)h^*(t-u)e^{-j\omega u}du \tag{7.12}$$

The spectrogram is the modulus squared of this:

$$S_f(t, \omega) = |T_f(t, \omega)|^2 \tag{7.13}$$

By moving the analysis window along the signal, one hopes to track and capture the variations of the signal spectrum as a function of time. The spectrogram has many useful properties, including a well-developed general theory; however, the spectrogram often presents serious difficulties when used to analyze rapidly varying signals. If the analysis window is made short enough to capture rapid changes in the signal, it becomes impossible to resolve the frequency components of the signal during the analysis window duration.

The Wigner distribution (WD), first described in a quantum mechanics context (Cohen, 1966), exhibits some interesting properties when interpreted in a time–frequency context. The WD is a bilinear distribution of the form

$$W_f(t, \omega) = \int_{-\infty}^{\infty} f(t - \tau/2)f^*(t + \tau/2)e^{-j\omega\tau}d\tau \tag{7.14}$$

The WD has many important properties. It provides a high-resolution representation in time and in frequency for a nonstationary signal such as a chirp. In addition, the WD has the important property of satisfying the time and frequency marginals. However, its energy distribution is not nonnegative and, because of its bilinearity, it often possesses severe cross terms or interference terms between components in different t–f regions, potentially leading to confusion and misinterpretation. If $f(t) = x(t) + y(t)$, then the WD will yield $W_x(t, \omega) + W_y(t, \omega)$ as desired, but also $W_{xy}(t, \omega) + W_{yx}(t, \omega)$, the cross terms or interference terms.

Both the spectrogram and the WD are members of Cohen's class of distributions. The WD has a unity-valued kernel, and the spectrogram kernel can be shown to be the ambiguity function of the window, $h(t)$. Cohen (1966, 1989) has provided a consistent set of definitions for a desirable set of t–f distributions that has been of great value in guiding and clarifying efforts in this area of research. Among the desirable properties are the absence of negativity of the energy values (the spectrogram has this property, the WD does not) and the property of proper time and frequency marginals (the WD has it, the spectrogram does not).

Many investigators have considered the WD to be the basic t–f distribution. Its principal faults, nonnegativity and the cross terms, have been considered to be facts of life that can only be dealt with by performing additional computations. Recent developments in our group have convinced us that there are many t–f distributions with properties nearly as desirable as the WD but with considerably reduced interference terms.

New Distributions

To be able to give a particular distribution an interpretation as a distribution of its energy in time and frequency, the distribution should possess certain properties. For example, the t–f distribution should be a real valued distribution such that the shift in time (or frequency) of a signal results in the corresponding shift of the distribution. Also, the projection of the distribution on the time (or frequency) domain should be equal to the instantaneous power (or spectral density) of the signal. Furthermore, the centroid time (or frequency) of the distribution at each frequency (or time) should be equal to the group delay (or instantaneous frequency) of the signal.

Cohen's class of t–f distribtutions is characterized by

$$C_f(t, \omega, \phi) = \frac{1}{2\pi} \iiint e^{j(\Theta t - t\omega - \Theta\mu)} \phi(\Theta,\tau) f(\mu + \frac{\tau}{2}) f^*(\mu - \frac{\tau}{2}) d\mu dt\, d\Theta \quad (7.15)$$

where $f(t)$ is the time signal, $f^*(t)$ is its complex conjugate, ϕ is the kernel of the distribution, and all integrations are assumed to be from $-\infty$ to ∞. The form of the kernel determines the character of the distribution. The kernel is a constant ($\phi(\Theta,\tau) = 1$ for all Θ,τ) for the WD. It can easily be shown that the WD and the symmetrical ambiguity function are related by two-dimensional Fourier transforms in time and frequency or

$$A(\Theta,\tau) = F_t\,[F_\omega\,[W(t, \omega)]] \quad (7.16)$$

If we define a new function of time and frequency,

$$\Phi(t, \omega) = F_\tau[F_\omega\,[\phi(\Theta,\tau)]] \quad (7.17)$$

then generalized time–frequency distributions of Cohen's class are simply the result of the double convolution in time and frequency of $\Phi(t, \omega)$ and $W_f(t, \omega)$, or

$$C_f(t, \omega, \phi) = \Phi(t, \omega)\, *_{t,\omega}\, W_f(t, \omega) \quad (7.18)$$

where $*_{t,\omega}$ is convolution in both time and frequency.

The convolution property of the Fourier transform permits the following relationship to be expressed, because convolution becomes multiplication under the Fourier transform:

$$A_F(\Theta,\tau) = \phi(\Theta,\tau) \cdot A(\Theta,\tau) \tag{7.19}$$

and

$$A(\Theta,\tau) = \int_{-\infty}^{\infty} f(t - \tau/2)f^*(t + \tau/2)e^{-j\Theta t}\, dt \tag{7.20}$$

$A(\Theta, \tau)$ is the Fourier transform in time and frequency of the WD. The function $A_F(\Theta, \tau)$ may be called the generalized ambiguity function. Understanding the relationship among the ambiguity function, the kernel function, and the generalized ambiguity function is the key to the design of t–f distributions with desirable characteristics. The kernel function may be used to change the shape of the generalized ambiguity function by virtue of its multiplicative effect in the t–f domain on the ambiguity function.

The kernel cannot be chosen at will, however, if one wishes to retain certain desirable characteristics. A number of these characteristics have been studied by Claasen and Mecklenbrauker (1980c), and the following observations come from their work. If one wishes the resulting t–f distribution to be real, then $\phi(\Theta, \tau) = \phi(-\Theta, -\tau)$, and if one wishes to have the distribution satisfy the time and frequency marginals, then $\phi(0, \tau) = 1$ for all τ and $\phi(\Theta, 0) = 1$ for all Θ. In addition, the derivative of $\phi(\Theta, \tau)$ with respect to Θ must be zero for all τ, and the derivative of $\phi(\Theta, \tau)$ with respect to τ must be zero for all Θ, so that time shift and frequency shift in the signal are represented in a like manner in the t–f distribution.

Figure 7.2 illustrates the effect of three choices of kernels: (a) the WD kernel, (b) the spectrogram kernel, and (c) a new kernel designed to shape the generalized ambiguity function so as to reduce cross terms. The kernel for this distribution is of the form

$$\phi(\Theta, \tau) = e^{-\Theta^2\tau^2/\sigma} \tag{7.21}$$

This is the kernel of the exponential distribution (ED) (Choi & Williams, 1989). Building on this kernel, we have introduced a new class of distributions that have kernels with similar characteristics. These characteristics are:

1. $\phi(\Theta, 0) = 1$ for all Θ
2. $\phi(0, \tau) = 1$ for all τ
3. $\phi(\Theta, \tau) = \phi(-\Theta q, -\tau)$
4. $\phi(\Theta, \tau) << 1$ for $|\Theta\tau| >> 0$

The virtues of the first three characteristics have been previously mentioned. The WD kernel has characteristics 1 through 3 but not 4, because the Wigner kernel is 1 for all Θ and τ. The consequence of requiring

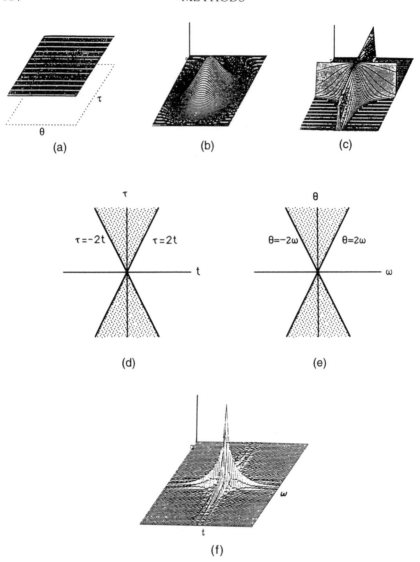

FIGURE 7.2. Kernel characteristics. (a)–(c): Ambiguity domain kernels of (a) WD, (b) spectrogram, and (c) RID. (d)–(e): Nonzero support of the RID kernel in the (d) temporal correlation domain and (e) spectral correlation domain. (f): The RID kernel in the time–frequency domain. From Jeong and Williams (1992).

characteristic 4 is to taper the kernel off to zero rapidly, away from the Θ and τ axes.

Time–frequency distributions have some additional desirable characteristics, namely, their time-support and frequency-support properties. A time–frequency distribution that exhibits the time-support property has the same time limits in the time domain as does the original signal in the time domain. That is, if $f(t) = 0$ for $t > t_{max}$ and $f(t) = 0$ for $t < t_{min}$, then $C_f(t, \omega, \phi)$ is also zero outside those time limits. If the time–frequency distribution exhibits the frequency-support property, then $F(\omega) = 0$ for $\omega < \omega_{min}$ and $F(\omega) = 0$ for $\omega > \omega_{max}$ implies that $C_f(t, \omega, \phi) = 0$ outside the same limits. These properties can be ensured by constraints on $\psi(t, \tau) = F_\Theta[\phi(\Theta, \tau)]$ and $\psi(\omega, \Theta) = F_t[\phi(-\Theta, \tau)]$. Then the constraints are

$$\psi(t, \tau) = 0 \text{ for } |t| > |t|/2 \tag{7.22}$$

and

$$\psi(\omega, \Theta) = 0 \text{ for } |\omega| > |\Theta|/2 \tag{7.23}$$

A descriptive name, *reduced interference distribution* (RID), has been given to a distribution whose kernels possess the four characteristics that lead to the much reduced interference terms coupled with the time- and frequency-support constraints. The reason for the RID approach's success can easily be seen by looking at the ambiguity domain form (Θ, τ) of the kernels shown in Figure 7.2. The ambiguity function has the form of a joint correlation in time and frequency; thus, the desired autoterms produced by a given signal component with itself fall on the Θ and τ axes near the origin. Interference terms, due to signals separated in time and frequency, generally appear away from the axes and the origin to their time and frequency separation. The WD (Figure 7.2a), with its unity kernel, emphasizes all terms in the ambiguity plane equally, so the interference terms are carried along on the transformation back to time–frequency. The spectrogram (Figure 7.2b), with a gaussian time window (which produces a 2D gaussian kernel), tends to emphasize the center of the ambiguity plane and tapers off away from the origin. Thus, the autoterms are kept, and the interference terms tend to be suppressed. The RID kernel has a radically different kernel compared to the spectrogram. The RID kernel suppresses components away from the axes, but maintains the important kernel properties required to retain time and frequency marginals. Time and frequency support is built into the RID. The spectrogram does not retain the time and frequency support properties so that the time–frequency distribution obtained using the spectrogram is smeared in both time and frequency, producing a defocused view that often obscures fine detail. The WD keeps the fine detail and nice properties, but the interference terms compete strongly with the autoterms, often making an incomprehensible mess of the time–frequency representation.

Discrete Time–Frequency Distributions

Several discrete forms are available for these time–frequency distributions. The pseudo-Wigner distribution (PWD) (Claasen & Mecklenbraucker, 1980a, 1980b, 1980c) is a discrete realization of the WD. The RWED is a discrete realization of the ED (Choi & Williams, 1989). The binomial distribution (Williams & Jeong, 1992) is a very convenient, discrete RID realization. Discrete forms of time–frequency distributions do not adhere strictly to all of the theoretical properties of the continuous forms, but they do provide a good approximation and have the virtue of being applicable on a digital computer.

Combining Time–Frequency with Information Theory

As has been obvious to us, certain time–frequency features characterize the ERPs that are evoked by the word stimuli. To quantify this observation, we used information-theoretic methods to determine which time–frequency features carried the most information about the category membership of each ERP. Five time–frequency features were then selected based on their high category information and on their efficacy in classifying the ERPs correctly in combination. A classifier was then developed using these features with the goal of correctly classifying each ERP in terms of the word category membership of its stimulus. This approach has proved successful and will be described more fully in Chapter 8.

APPLICATIONS TO OUR RESEARCH

The ED (Choi, Williams, & Zaveri, 1987) and its improvement, the RID, have been used to analyze our ERP data. We were able to discriminate between the conscious symptom and the unconscious conflict categories. The data analysis and results will be described in Chapter 8.

THE ADAPTIVE GABOR TRANSFORM

We next wondered if the time–frequency space found to be so important could be more fully characterized. Brown, Williams, and Hero (1994) and

Williams, Brown, Zaveri, and Shevrin (1994) have developed a new analysis technique based on the Gabor logon, that captures quantitatively five relevant dimensions: (a) time, (b) frequency, (c) spread, (d) phase, and (e) amplitude. As our time–frequency results suggest, the spatio-temporal relationship among combinations of brain rhythms may play a role in processing word meaning as related to conscious and unconscious brain processes. The important role of brain rhythms is underscored in recent research reported by Jagadeesh, Gray, and Forster (1992). They found, in their investigations of the cat visual cortex, that "rhythmic firing can be synchronized among cells in widespread areas of the visual cortex . . . [suggesting] . . . that the synchronization may contribute to the integration of information across broadly displaced parts of the visual field" (p. 252). Closer to our own level of analysis, Shastri and Ajjanagadde (1993) have proposed that the synchronization of the parallel and distributed brain processes involved in concept formation and categorization may be achieved through a phase-locking mechanism applied to varying brain rhythms. The short rhythmic bursts that may be involved in such phase-locking, Brown, Williams, and Hero (1994) have shown, are described well mathematically by linear combinations of Gabor logons.

The primary goal of the adaptive Gabor transform was to go beyond the previous time–frequency analysis that identified isolated points in time–frequency space and to provide a fuller description in terms of time–frequency variance, phase, and amplitude, as well as time and frequency.

Formal Mathematical Description of Adaptive Gabor Transform

The adaptive Gabor transform (AGT) (Brown, Williams, & Hero, 1994) is a signal representation that efficiently captures time–frequency dynamics of signals that are highly concentrated in time–frequency. In this representation, a signal is modeled as a linear combination of Gabor wavelets (often called Gabor logons). The mathematical description of the Gabor wavelet is

$$f(t) = \sqrt{E} \cos(2\pi(\omega - \omega_0)(t - t_0)) + \phi \exp\left(-\frac{(t - t_0)^2}{2s^\sigma}\right) \quad (7.24)$$

where the parameters are central frequency, ω_0; central time, t_0; phase, ϕ; and time spread, s.[1] E is the energy factor for the logon.

---

[1] Time spread and frequency spread are inversely related, due to the properties of the Fourier transform. The time bandwidth (time spread, frequency spread) product is a constant. That is, $\Delta t \Delta w = c$. The Gabor logon is characterized by $c = \frac{1}{2}$, the lowest possible time–bandwidth product. Thus it is the most compact signal element possible and for this reason is considered to be the quantum signal element.

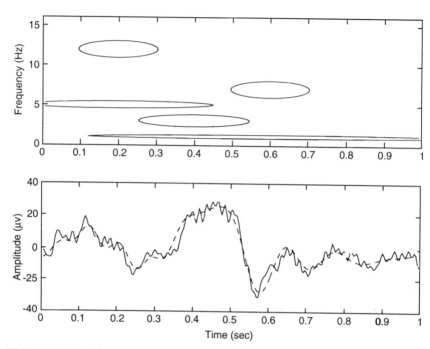

FIGURE 7.3. Adaptive Gabor transform of an ERP for one presentation of a supraliminal conscious symptom word. Lower plot shows an ERP (solid line) and the model fit (dashed line). The correlation coefficient between the model and data is .93. The upper plot shows the time and frequency location and the spread of the five logons composing the model. The contours are located at one-half the peak value of the logon. From Brown (1994).

Our studies found that five Gabor logons combined linearly could generate both the supraliminal and subliminal ERP curves and yield correlations with the original signal in the .85 to .95 range. The Gabor logon parameters were adjusted adaptively in order to fit the ERPs as well as possible. Figure 7.3 shows the fit for a typical supraliminal ERP using five logons and Figure 7.4 shows the fit for a typical subliminal ERP using five logons. This approach captures most of the detail of the ERP. The parameter values just described were derived for each ERP in the data set, using five logons to fit the data. This cluster of values was used in a pattern recognition scheme to classify the ERPs according to the class of stimulus used. Neural network classifiers were also used on these data with some improvement of results (Brown, Williams, & Shevrin, 1995).

Results from the adaptive Gabor transform will be described in detail in Chapter 8.

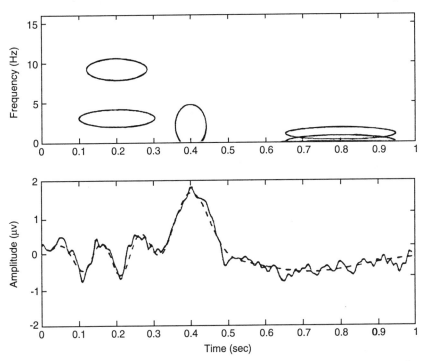

FIGURE 7.4. Adaptive gabor transform of an ERP for one presentation of a subliminal unconscious conflict word. Lower plot shows an ERP (solid line) and the model fit (dashed line). The correlation coefficient between the model and data is .969. The upper plot shows the time and frequency location and the spread of the five logons composing the model. The contours are located at one-half the peak value of the logon.

PART THREE

THE EXPERIMENT

Experimental Procedures
and Results

In Parts One and Two, we have presented the theoretical considerations informing our research and the methodological strategies that were developed to make the research feasible. We are now ready to describe the experimental procedures and results. Out of necessity, these accounts will be highly technical, drawing on standard cognitive laboratory procedures for investigating subliminal perception and a range of statistical techniques for analyzing the data. For the psychoanalytic reader who may not be acquainted with these technical means, we first provide a brief, nontechnical summary.

The conscious symptom words, the unconscious conflict words, the ordinary unpleasant words, and the ordinary pleasant words previously selected for each subject are now presented to the subject, first subliminally and then supraliminally. The ERP brain responses to these words are then submitted to a time–frequency feature analysis so that, for each subject at the two durations, a five-feature sequence of frequencies is identified. On the basis of these "brain melodies," the conscious symptom, unconscious conflict, and ordinary unpleasant words are each compared to the ordinary pleasant words to see how well these brain melodies can correctly discriminate them from the ordinary pleasant words. In this design, the ordinary pleasant words serve as a control. In a drug study, a placebo would be the control.

The first finding of interest was that the unconscious conflict words were correctly classified with respect to the control words *subliminally* only, and the conscious symptom words were correctly classified *supraliminally* only. Of importance was the finding that no difference existed for the ordinary unpleasant words between the durations, thus supporting the interpretation that the effects were related to the two types of pathological words.

The second finding of interest concerned the part played by the *highest* and *lowest* frequencies in each of the brain melodies. For the unconscious conflict words, the highest frequency occurred *early* subliminally and *late* supraliminally, but the reverse was true for the conscious symptom words (see Figure 8.1). Strikingly, for the lowest frequencies, we found the exact mirror image of the results found for the highest frequencies (see Figure 8.1). Again, we found no difference for the ordinary unpleasant words.

We also found some interesting relationships involving a measure assessing the degree to which subjects relied on repressive or obsessive defenses. A substantial positive correlation was found between the degree of repressiveness and the extent to which unconscious symptom words were more correctly classified subliminally than supraliminally. The brain melodies of repressive subjects could more correctly classify the unconscious conflict words subliminally than supraliminally, suggesting that some inhibitory process related to repression was at work supraliminally. The correlations for the conscious symptom and ordinary unpleasant words were insignificantly small, further supporting the special effect of the unconscious conflict words.

Finally, results from the adaptive Gabor transform analysis of the brain responses confirmed and extended the time–frequency feature findings. This is of some importance because the adaptive Gabor transform incorporates three more dimensions of the brain responses in addition to time and frequency, and thus provides a fuller description of the nature of the discriminating brain responses.

The findings form a converging pattern of results supporting the main hypothesis of the research, which is that dynamic unconscious processes exist and are instantiated in brain processes. The subjective clinical judgments of the psychoanalyst concerning the nature of the unconscious conflict in each subject are supported by the objective measurement of unconscious processes and their correlated brain responses.

This chapter gives a detailed account of the subjects used in the study, followed by a description of the experimental procedures and a fuller and more technical presentation of the results.

SUBJECTS

The most suitable subjects for our research would be patients who were clearly within the neurotic range and were suffering from fairly discrete ego-dystonic symptoms sufficiently discomfiting to motivate them to seek treatment. We decided that patients with phobias and pathological grief reactions would meet these criteria. Eleven such subjects have completed the experiment. Of these, eight suffered from phobias (six from social phobias, one with a blood phobia, and one with agoraphobia), and three suffered from pathological grief reactions. Of the eight subjects suffering from phobias, six met DSM-III-R (American Psychiatric Association, 1987) criteria for Social Phobia (300.23); one, a blood phobic, met criteria for Specific Phobia (300.29); and one met criteria for Panic Disorder with agoraphobia (300.21). In the ICD-9 diagnostic classification system, all these subjects would meet criteria for Neurotic Disorder, phobic state (300.2). The three subjects judged to have been suffering from pathological grief reactions were more difficult to fit into DSM-III-R diagnostic categories. Bereavement (V62.82) would be the closest diagnostic category, although in each instance the distress lasted more than two months, the DSM-III-R cutoff point for considering an alternate diagnosis. In all three cases, the main Axis I diagnosis was Dysthymic Disorder (300.4). In the ICD-9 diagnostic classification system, these subjects would meet criteria for Adjustment Reaction, prolonged depressive reaction (309.1). Seven subjects were men and four were women. All subjects were right-handed and were tested for normal eyesight (if necessary, corrected by glasses). No subject reported previous head injuries, psychiatric hospitalization, or neurological disorder. With one exception, they were all in their twenties and thirties (one woman was in her early forties). Subjects were informed beforehand that the laboratory team knew nothing about their difficulties, other than that they had a psychiatric complaint. Subjects were also told that they could stop the laboratory session at any time and ask to speak to the research director (H. Shevrin). It was explained to the subjects that they would, at times, see words that were familiar to them and that, at other times, it might be hard for them to see any words. The laboratory session usually lasted from 3 to 4 hours and was scheduled within a week of completing the clinical assessment. All subjects were referrals from various mental health agencies.

Aside from the demographics of our subjects, a number of considerations were of greater pertinence to the conduct of the clinical evaluations. How best could our research subjects, who were also patients, be introduced to the research goal of the interviewing without disturbing the clinician–patient relationship? We decided that this should be addressed up front, initially by those who referred patients to us. Referring clinicians were told to inform a potential patient that, in return for an evaluation by an experienced clinician and referral for treatment, the patient would agree to have the evaluation tape-recorded and reviewed for diagnostic and research purposes by a group of clinicians. If the patient agreed, he or she was then told to telephone the research director (H. Shevrin). The same conditions were repeated on the phone, and an appointment was arranged for an initial screening in the laboratory to determine whether a usable EEG could be obtained from the subject. Prior to the laboratory procedure, the subject was read, and signed, an informed consent agreement for the laboratory part of the research. At the start of the first clinical interview, the patient signed another informed consent agreement that included a proviso that, at some point, the findings of the research would be published with subject anonymity protected. No further use of the data would be made without the subject's consent. On several occasions, we learned that potential subjects demurred when told of the research conditions by the referrers. The usual objection was to the tape recording. No patient who decided to call the research director refused participation.

Are patients who are willing to volunteer as subjects similar to patients who are not? Were our subjects truly voluntary or paid? One could argue that our subjects were "paid" by having a senior, experienced clinician conduct the interview in return for their participation, although no actual monetary payment was made. The question of voluntary versus paid is important because it bears on the issue of subject motivation. For our purposes, there was no doubt that our subjects had to be highly motivated to participate in the searching character of the evaluation, which went well beyond simply eliciting an account of their symptoms. They also had to tolerate a lengthy (3 to 4-hour) laboratory procedure requiring them to sit with their eyes focused in a viewing box with electrodes on their scalp while, for half the time, they could see nothing (subliminal condition), and for the other half they could see many words disturbingly related to their problems (supraliminal condition). Our hope was that our subjects' desire for treatment would see them through, strengthened by whatever interest they might have in contributing to research. Our hope was borne out by our experience. Not one subject dropped out (although one subject balked at filling out some of the questionnaires). We fulfilled our end of the bargain by arranging referrals for our subjects, each of whom accepted. Their readiness to do so argues in favor of the conclusion that we had achieved good rapport with them and some understanding of their treatment needs.[1]

Laboratory Procedure

The 32 words making up the four categories selected by the clinicians were presented in a Gerbrand Model T-3A three-field Dodge-type tachistoscope with field brightness, as measured at the eyepiece and surrounding room, set at 10.0 ft-lamberts. Displays were tested for steady-state and pulse brightness to verify equivalence of the fixation and stimulus fields. The 32 words were presented in six randomized blocks for 1 msec

---

[1] Further underscoring the importance of subject motivation was our experience in the early phases of the research, when we explored the possibility of using paid, nonpsychiatric subjects as controls. We discovered that these subjects (three in number) were reluctant to be forthcoming in the interviews, and two did not complete the laboratory procedure. We decided that these data were unsuitable for control purposes.

(subliminal condition) and then at either 30 or 40 msec (supraliminal condition), depending on the duration at which the subject could clearly report seeing the words, determined by presenting two neutral words, first at 30 msec and then at 40 msec, before the experiment began. The eight words in each category were presented six times for a total of 48 presentations of each category for each of the two durations. Words were printed on 4″ × 6″ cards in Helvetica Light 18-point type. The white background had approximately four times the reflectance of the black-lettered words. The stimulus cards were numerically coded so that the assistant presenting the words did not know what they were. Subliminality was confirmed by a discrimination series of 40 stimuli presented in the form of 20 paired comparisons at the end of the experiment, flashed under the same subliminal condition as during the experiment. Subjects could not discriminate between same and different word pairs, blank pairs, or word/blank pairs at better than chance levels (50%). We have also subsequently presented two $E+$ and two $E-$ words under the same subliminal condition for a total of 120 times for each word in a forced-choice paradigm to 35 subjects. The subjects' guesses were consistently at chance levels (Snodgrass, Shevrin, & Kopka, 1993).

ERP Measures

ERPs were derived from three electrode placements with reference to linked ears: P_3, P_4, and a special placement one third of the distance from C_z to P_z ($C_z P_z$), which was found in previous research to provide data discriminating between $E-$ and $E+$ word categories (Chapman, 1979). Silver–silver chloride disk electrodes were used, impedance was below 5 kW, and an electrode at the left mastoid served as a ground. Data were collected using a 130-msec prestimulus period and continuing for approximately 1 second. Electrode signals were amplified and monitored using a 24-channel Grass Model 8 EEG. Signals contaminated with eye movements, muscle movements, eye blinks, or alpha waves were rejected either manually or, as in the case of alpha waves, automatically by the computer, and were replaced immediately. Gain and bandwidth were set at 7 mV/mm and from 1 to 70 Hz, respectively. Data were sampled at 250 Hz, using an HP 1000 computer system. All individual ERPs were preserved on disk files for subsequent processing.

METHODS OF ANALYSIS

Two methods of analysis were applied to the ERP data: (a) the time–frequency feature analysis and (b) the adaptive Gabor transform (AGT).

Each has been previously described in Chapter 7. A psychological measure of defensive organization, the Hysteroid–Obsessoid Questionnaire (HOQ; Caine & Hawkins, 1963), was also included.

Time–Frequency Feature Analysis

On the basis of our new time–frequency (t–f) analysis, the conscious symptom (C), unconscious conflict (U), and ordinary unpleasant (E−) categories were each compared in a discriminant analysis with the ordinary pleasant (E+) category that served as a control or placebo condition. The categories within a pair (e.g., U vs. E+) were divided into development and test sets, with the odd presentations (1, 3, 5) and even presentations (2, 4, 6) serving alternately as development and test sets. Thus, the 48 ERPs constituting the odd presentations for the U and E+ category pairs (24 from each category) were analyzed into their differentiating t–f features, and the first 19 of these features were rank-ordered in information units (bits) according to their ability to differentiate the two categories (Williams, Shevrin, & Marshall, 1987). Features were next combined into clusters of increasing size (2, 3, 4, . . . , 19 features) based on a patterning principle: Each feature added was selected to maximize the cluster's capacity to differentiate within category pairs, regardless of the original information ranking. According to accepted criteria for pattern recognition, with 24 members in a subset (half of the data in a set of 48), a cluster of five time–frequency features should provide maximal capacity for differentiating categories (Devijver & Kittler, 1982).

Once these feature clusters had been selected for the development set (odd or even), these same features were then applied independently to the test set for validation. Because the actual stimulus was known in each case, a 2×2 contingency table could easily be constructed for the hits and misses. Chance classification of the test data would be 50%. A percent-correct classification score for each subject for each duration and category was entered into the statistical analyses.

Adaptive Gabor Transform

This measure allowed us to include frequency spread, time spread, phase and amplitude, along with time and frequency, producing a more thorough and complex analysis of ERPs than the time–frequency feature analysis (see Chapter 7 for a full account).

Hysteroid–Obsessoid Questionnaire

In addition to an assessment of unconscious conflict, an independent measure of defensive organization was judged to be useful. We chose a well-standardized instrument for measuring a personality dimension, hysterical–obsessive, for which a reasonable case could be made that the dimension was related to stable but different patterns of defenses. The instrument chosen was the Hysteroid–Obsessoid Questionnaire (HOQ; Caine & Hawkins, 1963; Caine & Hope, 1967). We reasoned that hysteria would be associated with a repressive–avoidant pattern of defenses, and obsessionality, with an obsessive–intellectualizing pattern of defenses. A number of studies have successfully assessed these stylistic attributes, relying mainly on the Rorschach (Schafer, 1954; Luborsky, Blinder, & Schimek, 1965; Shapiro, 1965; Shevrin, Smith, & Fritzler, 1969; Smokler & Shevrin, 1979). Ludolph (1981) reported a significant, positive correlation (.78, $p < .05$) between the HOQ and the Rorschach, based on judgments of hysteroid and obsessoid styles. A high score on the HOQ indicates a hysterical personality organization, and a low score, an obsessional personality organization.

We sought to answer one main question: Would the $t–f$ features differentiate the two clinically selected pathological word categories depending on whether the words had been presented subliminally or supraliminally? In order to answer this question we planned three contrasts. The first planned contrast reflects our particular interest in whether the U and C categories would differ from each other in percent correct classification as a function of duration. The remaining two contrasts compare the U and C categories separately across durations. In statistical terms, the null hypotheses for the three contrasts would be expressed as follows:

1. $(U_{sub.} - U_{sup.}) - (C_{sub.} - C_{sup.}) = 0$
2. $(U_{sub.} - U_{sup.}) = 0$
3. $(C_{sub.} - C_{sup.}) = 0$

RESULTS

Time–Frequency Feature Analysis

The $t–f$ discriminant analysis was performed on data obtained from electrodes C_zP_z, P_3, and P_4. The $t–f$ feature analysis also made it possible to combine electrode pairs of special interest in the form of cross-energy, $t–f$ density distributions (see Appendix B for the mathematical derivation of these distributions). Insofar as our stimuli were words, we were particularly interested in the contribution of the left hemisphere as compared with that of the right hemisphere. For this reason, we added P_3 and P_4 to the C_zP_z placement found by Chapman (1979) to differentiate between the E− and E+ categories. By combining C_zP_z with P_3 and P_4 respectively, we attempted to take advantage of any commonality between a more central and a lateralized electrode.

Multivariate analyses of the percent-correct classification scores revealed that, for the C_zP_z/P_3 electrode pair, a significant category by duration interaction was present: $F(2/20) = 3.82$, $p = .039$. For the first planned contrast, the difference in percent-correct classification between subliminal and supraliminal durations for the C and U categories was significant: $t(20) = 2.82$, $p = .011$.[2] The average difference between subliminal and supraliminal durations for the U words was 5.92% in favor of the subliminal duration (54.78% vs. 49.04%) and −2.65% in the opposite direction in favor of the supraliminal condition for the C words (48.33% vs. 50.99%). This difference was statistically significant.[3] The t–f features more correctly classified the U words subliminally and the C words supraliminally.

For the second planned contrast, in which the U words were compared across durations, percent-correct classification was significantly higher subliminally than supraliminally: $t(20) = 2.79$, $p < .014$.

For the third planned contrast, in which the C words were compared across durations, the percent correct classification was not significantly different: $t(20) = -1.25$, $p > .10$.

In post-hoc testing, no significant differences appeared for contrasts involving the E− words.[4]

---

[2] The error term for this contrast is the interaction error mean square with 20 degrees of freedom. As Keppel (1982) pointed out, the interaction mean square is appropriate for use in calculating this interaction contrast unless there is reason to suspect heterogeneity of within-cell variances, which is not the case here. These same considerations apply to calculating the appropriate significance levels for the other two planned contrasts.

[3] Classification results using the development/test method of validation are highly conservative and represent a lower bound on the true performance of the method. If above-chance results are obtained, it is highly likely that the true performance of the method would be considerably better if given a much larger set of data for development and testing.

[4] Chapman (1979), using hundreds of stimulus repetitions presented supraliminally, was able, on the basis of a principal component discriminant analysis, to classify E+ and E− words significantly better than chance. With the same electrode placement, C_zP_z, and relying solely on the supraliminal presentations, we failed to replicate Chapman's findings for the E− and E+ words. However, it is important to take note of several significant differences in our procedure. We employed far fewer stimulus repetitions, the E− and E+ words were embedded in entirely different verbal contexts (other Osgood dimension words versus personally meaningful words), and a different

Because of the contribution of hemisphere to our results, percent-correct classification scores were correlated between C_zP_z/P_3 and C_zP_z/P_4. For the U words only, a significant negative correlation was found for the subliminal condition ($-.63$, $p < .05$). The correlation for the supraliminal condition was .40 (ns). When the *difference* between the subliminal and supraliminal percent-correct classification scores was correlated across hemispheres (high score in favor of the subliminal condition), the correlation for the U category words was $-.70$ ($p < .05$), and nonsignificant for the C and E− categories (.30 and .05, respectively).

How might relationships between frequency and latency in the five *t–f* feature clusters account for these percent-correct classification results? Analyses were pursued only for the C_zP_z/P_3 electrode pair. Inspection revealed that there were considerable individual differences in frequency and latency across durations within categories. It was thus decided, for the purpose of this exploratory analysis, to compare the latencies of the lowest and highest frequencies for each subject within categories and durations and to perform a multivariant analysis of variance (MANOVA) on these data with the two latencies serving as dependent variables.

In determining the relationship between the two latencies, the MANOVA program automatically seeks out the linear combination of the two dependent variables that maximize the differences among the six category-by-duration cells. In this instance, the raw discriminant function coefficients were .00687 for the highest frequency latency and $-.00561$ for the lowest frequency latency. The contributions of the highest and lowest frequency latencies were of approximately equal magnitude but in opposite directions. Not surprisingly, a significant category-by-duration interaction was found: $F(4/36) = 4.14$, $p = .007$, Hotelling's test.

Post-hoc Hotelling T^2 contrasts were computed using a power correction suggested by Stevens (1986). Three significant contrasts emerged: (a) between subliminal and supraliminal U words: $T^2 (2/9) = 15.51$, $p < .010$; (b) between subliminal and supraliminal C words: $T^2(2/9) = 7.23$, $p < .013$; and (c) between subliminal C and U words: $T^2(2/9) = 7.69$, $p < .011$. No significant differences were found for the E− category.

The direction of these differences revealed that, for the U and C words, mirror-image reversals between latency and frequency occurred as a function of duration that paralleled the direction of the percent-correct classification results. For the subliminal U words, the *highest* frequency had the *shortest* latency, but the reverse was true for the subliminal C words. For the supraliminal U words, the *lowest* frequency now had the *shortest* latency,

---

type of ERP analysis (principal component versus time–frequency features) was used. These substantial differences may account for our failure to replicate Chapman's findings.

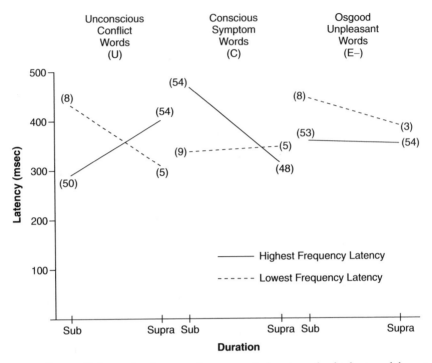

FIGURE 8.1. Relationship between latency and durations for highest and lowest frequencies by word category. Numbers in parentheses are the frequency averages.

but the reverse was true for the supraliminal C words. These interactions are displayed in Figure 8.1.

Hysteroid–Obsessoid Questionnaire Results

Where dynamic unconscious processes are involved, we would expect personality and defensive organization to play some role in the differences found between the U and C categories for percent-correct classification success and the relationships between frequency and latency. HOQ scores were available for eight of the eleven subjects; two subjects were not administered the HOQ through an oversight, and one subject refused to take the test. When the percent-correct classification difference scores between the subliminal and supraliminal durations (high score in favor of subliminal condition) were correlated with the HOQ score for the U category, the correlation was .77 ($p < .05$). For the C and E− categories, the correlations were insignificant (.16 and −.24, respectively). The hysteroid–repressive subjects more correctly classified the words related to their unconscious conflicts subliminally than supraliminally. Consistent with repression, these results could be interpreted to mean that the hysteroid–repressive subjects knew unconsciously what they had to remain unaware of consciously.

When we obtained correlations between the HOQ and the highest and lowest frequencies, we again found that, for the U words, there was a substantial tendency for the correlations to be in opposite directions in the subliminal condition. For the highest frequency, the correlation was .71($p < .05$); for the lowest frequency, the correlation was $-.55$(ns). When the difference between high and low frequencies for a given subject were correlated with the HOQ scores, the correlation for the U category in the subliminal condition was .81($p < .05$). The only other significant correlation was a correlation of $-.83$($p < .05$) between the highest frequency for the E$-$ category and the HOQ in the subliminal condition. This correlation was in the opposite direction from the one obtained for the U words (.71 vs. $-.83$). With respect to latency of the lowest frequency feature, fairly large correlations in opposite directions were found for the C words (subliminal condition: $-.95$, $p < .01$; supraliminal condition: .70, $p < .10$). It is again notable how correlations tend to go in opposite directions as a function of duration. Overall, these findings involving the HOQ suggest that personality and defensive organization do indeed play a role in the effects we have been investigating.

Adaptive Gabor Transform Results

The same discriminant analysis was performed on the data as had been performed with the time–frequency features. In this analysis, however, a four-way discriminant analysis was performed in which each category was compared against all the others, rather than the Osgood pleasant words serving as the control for the C, U, and E$-$ words. In this respect, positive results would be more generalized.

For hypothesis 1, the same significant interaction was found: $t(10) = 2.37$, $p < .020$. There was better classification subliminally than supraliminally for the U words and better classification supraliminally for the C words. For hypothesis 2, testing the differences for the U words separately, the results were in the same direction but weaker: $t(10) = 1.31$, $p < .110$. For hypothesis 3, testing the differences for the C words separately, the results were in the same direction as before but stronger: $t(10) = -2.66$, $p < .010$.

We will discuss these results and their implications in Chapter 12.

CLINICAL CASES

Three subjects will be presented in clinical detail in this part. Our intention is to show readers what the clinicians actually did, how they thought about the clinical material, and how they reached their hypotheses, especially concerning unconscious conflict.

To our psychoanalytic readers, the case material will likely not seem unusual, nor will the clinicians' way of thinking and reaching conclusions appear at odds with their own experience. We present these cases to our psychoanalytic readers so that they may judge for themselves how we went about the task of evaluating our patient-subjects. As in standard psychoanalytic practice, the interviews were not administered on the basis of any research-guided question-and-answer format, but care was taken to give the patients full rein to describe their reasons for coming, the nature of their complaint and their understanding of it, their current life circumstances, their upbringing, their reactions to the interviews and to the interviewer, and anything else that they might want to talk about. Many bases were touched, but in no particular order. By encouraging this kind of open-ended inquiry we anticipated that more of the patients' style and more ways of shaping the interviews would emerge. There would also be opportunity for surprising revelations, several examples of which occurred in the cases to be presented, that would prove to be remarkably informative (i.e., memory emerging in the third psychodynamic interview in the case of Mr. B, and the dream in the case of Mr. C).

A special word is directed to our nonpsychoanalytic readers. As we stated in Chapter 5, our aim was to treat the clinicians as experts in their own field; their experience and way of thinking about the clinical data were to be given the fullest opportunity to operate. Although the clinicians were encouraged to provide rationales for their inferences and conclusions and often challenged each other to provide these rationales, it is likely that nonclinical readers will find the clinicians' conclusions at times impressionistic and at times unconvincing and puzzling. This is often the reaction of non-experts to the way experts arrive at and present their judgments. In truth, the reason for this is not hard to find: Whenever highly complex phenomena are being judged on the basis of equally complex and not fully articulated theories, intuition plays a considerable role. Intuition is often regarded as the residue of much experience based on trial and error. For these very reasons, we chose the Delphi method of arriving at consensus judgments as the most suitable way to maximize the validity of our clinical judgments and to avoid the pitfalls of customary reliability measures, which artificially constrain the clinicians' way of thinking.

No matter how impressionistic or unconvincing the clinicians' way of thinking may seem to our nonanalytic readers, two important counterweights have been central to our design: (a) the clinicians must translate their hypotheses into word choices and (b) the sub- and supraliminal presentations of these words and their associated ERP serve as avenues of convergent validity. As mentioned earlier, this design is similar to the use of medical laboratory findings to support the validity of previous clinical diagnoses. Our own laboratory results appear to converge with clinical judgments; thus, a pattern of convergent validity emerges.

The three cases presented have been selected to illustrate three different aspects of the clinical assessments. In the case of Mr. A, a section is devoted to illustrating the interview and test contexts in which individual words selected for the conscious symptom and unconscious conflict words occurred. In the case of Mr. B, the emergence of a quite significant memory in the last psychodynamic interview illustrates the manner in which the psychodynamic method operates. In the case of Mr. C, a challenging diagnostic puzzle was addressed and required an additional psychodynamic interview. In all three cases, we hope readers will note the richness of personal material elicited from the patient-subjects, which provides the true database for psychodynamic judgments.

To facilitate the readers' ability to follow the case presentations, we list below the chronological order of interviews and discussion meetings (a full listing appears in Table 5.1). Special note must be made of the interview designated as the medical–psychiatric interview. To be certain that no significant psychiatric or strictly medical problem was overlooked, a psychiatrist conducted a more structured interview, inquiring about possible medical problems and such psychiatric illnesses as affective disorders and psychoses. The psychiatrist was also a psychoanalyst and participated as a judge, reading all of the clinical data. The order of interviews and tests was as follows:

1. Two psychodynamic interviews
2. Medical–psychiatric interview

3. Psychodiagnostic tests (conducted during the same week as the above interviews)
4. First clinical evaluation team (CET) meeting
5. Third psychodynamic interview
6. Second CET meeting
7. Fourth psychodynamic interview (as needed)
8. Third CET meeting (as needed)

The psychodiagnostic tests (WAIS, Rorschach, and TAT) were an important part of our clinical assessment, but they posed special problems in presenting the clinical data. Not all judges drew equally on the tests, although they were free to use them as much as they wished. Understandably, the psychologists (Judges 1, 3, and 4) on the clinical team had the most experience with the tests and relied on them more than did the psychiatrist member (Judge 2) of our team. Nevertheless, final judgments had to be integrated with the clinical data; the tests might point in a certain diagnostic direction or suggest possibilities that then were supported by additional data from the interviews. Occasionally, in the case presentations, test data are cited. Whenever this occurs, an explanation suitable for readers without experience in administering psychodiagnostic tests is provided. In the case of Mr. B, a more extended consideration of the tests is given, in light of their application to that patient.

From whatever perspective our readers approach this Part of the book, we would like to inform them that, in each of the three cases, a suitable referral for treatment was worked out with the patient. This point is important because the diagnostic process in a psychodynamic evaluation undertakes to deal with resistances to accepting treatment recommendations that in themselves provide valuable diagnostic information. Mr. B., for example, was resistant to the evaluation process itself, which strongly suggested diagnostically that he would be unlikely to benefit from a psychodynamically oriented psychotherapy. A behavioral treatment with Inderal[1] was prescribed in his case.

Finally, we anticipate that psychoanalytic and nonpsychoanalytic readers alike will take note of the striking contrast between the clinical and the laboratory-based methods, while at the same time appreciating that the complementarity of this contrast constitutes the strength at the heart of our method.

---

[1] Actually Inderal was first *considered* but in the actual treatment Xanax was used with *in vivo* desensitization and then the Xanax was tapered and discontinued as the treatment was successfully concluded.

The Case of Mr. A

Nature of Referral

Mr. A was referred to us from a university outpatient psychiatry department where he had sought psychotherapy because his fears of participating in social events, including everyday interactions with colleagues, were hindering his work. He readily agreed to participate in the research once the conditions were explained to him over the phone.

Subject Presentation

Mr. A was an intelligent, obsessive, 30-year-old man who looked, dressed, and behaved like an intense, helpless, worried 11-year-old boy ineptly trying to make a good impression. He spoke nervously and softly, skipping quickly from topic to topic and often laughing in a pressured, friendly manner. He had extreme difficulty being clear about what he was trying to say. Many of his thoughts were presented in a highly fragmented manner expressing confusion as to whether he really meant what he had just said and whether the affect expressed was directed from him to others or from others to him. He often spoke in vague, global, overinclusive terms. Much of what he said was hostile, arrogant, pompous, and demeaning but was offered in a little-boy manner that one could easily not take seriously.

Evaluation Procedure

Mr. A's evaluation consisted of the following sequence of procedures: first evaluation interview, psychological testing, second evaluation interview, medical–psychiatric interview, first CET meeting, third evaluation interview, and second CET meeting. Mr. A participated in the laboratory procedure about two weeks after the second CET meeting.

PSYCHOSOCIAL HISTORY

During the first few years of life, Mr. A, an only child, was cared for primarily by his father. His mother claimed that his father was better at child care than she, while she in turn was better at holding down a job. Mr. A's father was a compulsive gambler and his mother worked as a secretary. When Mr. A was around 3½ or 4 years old, after one of his father's gambling episodes resulted in the repossession of their furniture, his mother insisted on a divorce. Mr. A vividly remembered his father half-heartedly playing with him while pleading with his mother to reconsider, then abruptly leaving without saying good-bye to him. Since shortly after that event, his father never returned. Mr. A claimed to have no other memories of that time period, nor any earlier memories. When his father left, his mother was allegedly unable to care for him and work at the same time. She sent Mr. A to live with an aunt and an alcoholic uncle. This uncle and two older cousins were verbally and physically abusive to him. When his mother found out, she brought him back home and hired a sitter. Throughout his school years, for "unclear reasons," his mother felt she "had to" work second shift, which meant she was at work during his waking time at home: "food, laundry etc. were always available but no mom." When home, his mother interacted with him in a distant, perfunctory manner, preferring to retire to her bedroom where she ate alone and talked to friends on the phone. Mr. A had a few male neighbor friends, but they could not adequately fill his waking time. He always felt self-consciously "freaky"; everybody had someone to go home to, but he had no one. He felt strange around other people who seemed to have a knowledge of how to act that he lacked. He felt angry and left out by most people, though he always has had a few loyal friends. He was mad at his mother about the situation, but she "couldn't see" what he was complaining about. This made him even madder, but he was also aware that she had her own problems and was doing the best she could. Thus, his realistic rage turned into helpless rage and guilt.

At age 17, he began to get intense panic attacks, especially around separations from his mother. These attacks continued into graduate school without abatement, despite psychiatric treatment with medication, until he had had two fairly good psychotherapy experiences.

Despite these many obstacles, Mr. A earned a B.A. degree, was well on his way to achieving a Ph.D. in the social sciences, and had publications in recognized journals. He stated that his primary scientific interest was in war, peace, and international cooperation, and he felt that his actual laboratory work and development of mathematical models of social behavior were trivial. Although realistically seeking help and recognition, he "liked to take on the big boys" (i.e., the established authorities), attacking their positions and championing unpopular causes.

He usually remained at any given location for about a year and then moved on. He had always alienated most people, but he developed a few long-lasting, productive relationships at each location. Although he felt very ambivalent about all people, his predominant conscious experience of these few relationships was positive. He reported that, in several years' collaboration with one colleague, he became a controlling "ego maniac" who got into petty arguments and contested the colleague for first authorships. He once ruined a project of a close colleague by not collecting some crucial data because he was angry that a paper in which he was first author had been rejected.

He had been heterosexually involved only once, briefly, with a married woman who was psychologically disturbed herself. Intercourse was problematic for them both; each feared hurting the other while at the same time actually doing so. While discussing these experiences, he referred to his penis as sometimes feeling like an "erect . . . weapon that could destroy the universe." Once he got the sense that intercourse hurt the woman, they continued to engage in it with her assent, but he would ejaculate without any sensation.

Mr. A had sought treatment because he was worried that his terror of being with people would cause him to behave in ways that would ruin his career. He feared that his "social fears" would ruin his work and social life, that he "might become agoraphobic" as he felt he had been in the past. Although comfortable in most one-to-one situations, when a third party came on the scene he became worried that the third party would see him give off inappropriate "scare cues" revealing his insecurity, and would subject him to ridicule. Often feeling afraid to talk to people, he found himself going to great lengths "to avoid groups especially ones with peers in them." Though longing for a relationship with a woman, he was very afraid of even going dancing.

He came to the local university on a 2-year scholarship while finishing up his doctoral studies. His intention was to make important contacts with some leading scholars in his field, but he did so with the expectation that they would have nothing to do with him. Although he had enough awareness of the neurotic aspects of this fear to go to the effort of coming to the university, he nonetheless behaved most of the time as if his expectations were true. His fear of talking with the university staff kept him from making proper arrangements for his arrival, so it seemed as if he had suddenly showed up. People, including the scholars whose attention he was seeking, did make attempts to accommodate him but were soon put off by him, confirming his expectations. He then became extremely tense; he would twitch and look around, talking loudly and rapidly, or he would say nothing and be unapproachable, glaring and often producing voluminous flatus. He knew that these reactions would quickly alienate him from everyone, causing them to note to each other his idiosyncratic behavior. He was keenly sensitized to people's side comments about him. In addition to what actually would be said, which was often unclear to him, Mr. A fantasized hearing additional demeaning comments. This sense that people were closing ranks to exclude him increased his feelings of enraged alienation, exacerbating the whole cycle of perceptions and behaviors. Thus, about to graduate, seeing his hopes being dashed by his intractable, phobic behavior, feeling on the brink of realizing again his most terrifying fantasies, Mr. A contacted the clinic.

INTERVIEWER'S PERSPECTIVE ON THE EVALUATION

Mr. A had apparently the same intense transference to all the research staff members as he did to the scholars whom he wished to impress. He desperately wanted the staff to help him but was sure that we would view him as a "datapoint" and would not really be interested in understanding him. Instead, we would use him for our own ends, not caring enough to consider that we had left his needs unmet. Rather than turn away in profound despair as many would, he desperately threw himself into the task of trying to get our attention and enlist our power on his behalf. One of his redeeming strengths appeared to be that he had not given up on people; one felt a real people relatedness while with him, despite the manner in which it was shown. He found himself acutely concerned about the impressions he was making, always assessing the staff's reaction to "cues" he might be giving off. He often delivered a lecturing version of what he would imagine a therapist would say about him. He openly refused to reveal important aspects of his masturbation fantasies or to describe stories that came to mind while looking at TAT cards because he felt they were "too revealing." Despite his wishes to engage the staff, he maintained a highly competitive, critical, controlling posture, while at the same time appearing laughable, inarticulate, and frustrating to understand. Despite the above transference enactment, there were also moments of clear candid communication. Even through his confused, stilted, idiosyncratic, and verbose barrage he conveyed his neediness, helplessness, and pain in a manner that engaged the staff.

To the interviewer, it seemed that while desperately wanting to "belong," his terror of his rage at being rejected forced him into a compromise in which he related himself to a person or group by defining himself as an outsider. This outsider status kept him from being totally socially isolated, while at the same time insulated others from his perceived destructive rage, and insulated himself from their projected destructive retaliation.

PSYCHODYNAMIC FORMULATION

The preceding psychological history presents an abstract integration of the patient's material, to give the reader an overview of the prepatory to the transcripts that follow. They consist of direct patient quotes and judges' notes prepared independently before each CET meeting. At the time of their preparation, the judge's notes were not written with the thought of publication. They have been included despite their unpolished nature to allow readers access to the judges' thinking and to the group process at the time of word selection. This section has three major topics: *patient's conscious description of symptom, patient's understanding of symptom,* and *unconscious conflict underlying symptom.* In treating each case in this and the following two chapters, we will move from patient quotes to individual judges' summaries, to judges' consensus, and then to stimulus word selection. The quotes will give readers a sense of the patient, which led the judges to some of their conclusions. The judges' notes are included so that readers can see how the commonalities in judges' independent thinking prior to the CET meetings were incorporated into a consensus statement. The judges' notes are also included, to show the extent of divergence in the judges' thinking.[1]

Patient's Conscious Description of Symptom

Patient's Quotes Concerning Conscious Experience of Symptom

Excerpt 1

MR. A: Ah . . . alright . . . how far back do you want me to go . . . um . . . okay . . . I used to have a severe problem in all groups . . . I would not go to the grocery store unless it was near midnight because of the low density of people . . . I would not go on busy streets . . . umm . . . I would not go to theaters by myself . . . ummm . . . I do all of that now, but . . . I have a lot of trouble going to . . . meeting situations, groups of people, to party situations

---

[1] To decrease repetitiveness we will not restate the paragraph for the other two cases in Chapters 10 and 11 although it applies equally to each clinical case study. Instead we will refer back to this paragraph.

. . . ah . . . even to the extent where I won't want to go to my office because I might run into people and I think the key thing there is . . . peers . . . umm . . . I can walk by all sorts of strangers, which I would not do at one time, I would not take elevators at one time . . . but I now seem to rapidly become . . . a tortoise sort of when it comes to . . . ah . . . group situations with peers . . . and it's very different even if there's a third person present . . . ah . . . I can interact with people one-on-one easily, but if there's even somebody else in hearing distance, or if I so determine they are in hearing distance, I can become very nervous and find it very difficult to carry on any kind of conversation, I just want to run away . . . umm . . . so it's not the same problem it was a long time ago . . . a long time ago being about 1980 . . . ah . . . and . . . ah . . . it's not real pleasant . . . to be this way . . .

Excerpt 2 (Does not immediately follow excerpt 1.)

I: By paranoia . . . what do you mean?

MR. A: Ah . . . the original manifestation then was . . . I thought everybody could smell me and that actually begins all the way back to undergraduate school . . . ah . . . in fact, there was a severe bowel problem, that was real . . . I had trouble going for days, highly constipated, I spent hours in the bathroom, trying to go . . . and I was deathly afraid to go to places like the library . . . there was a small library . . . because I was afraid they'd smell me . . . I finally . . . my second year . . . this family I was living with basically moved on and so . . . I was . . . I was elsewhere and . . . and . . . my own little support group so to speak . . . my only contact (*chuckle*) . . . disappeared . . . it got very bad, I was crying constantly, severe depression, crying constantly . . . ah . . . I wouldn't talk to anybody, I tried to work by myself . . . but I would spend days doing nothing, just staring at the walls almost but it was difficult just to get to my office . . . hard for me to do that . . . so, I finally had to do something . . . I went to group . . . my group therapy was at counseling on campus and they said well, let's try group therapy . . . you clearly have a social . . . so I started that . . . ah . . . there was a marked improvement by . . . I was in therapy . . . group therapy approximately 5 months . . . 6 months . . . 'cause I began in the spring of the year and by then I had made friends, I had gone to one or two parties, I still don't like them but . . . usually . . . but I had gone to a few of them . . . key things, I had made friends . . . then I had to go to another school . . . one of my problems has been that my work has forced me to go to five . . . to move . . . different city five times in the past 3 years . . . things got a lot worse . . . ah . . . there . . . I had a . . . again I met one or two people . . . I had some old friends 'cause I'm from there . . . but there was a deterioration lot of the old fears were coming back . . . I should also point out that the fears didn't go away then . . . what I would do was force myself to . . . for example, walk down busy streets, regardless of the fears.

Excerpt 3

MR. A: Ahh . . . let's see . . . umm . . . yeah . . . umm . . . I would . . . umm . . . I reacted very badly to rejection . . . it's almost like abandonment . . . ahh . . . in fact it is abandonment and . . . ah . . . and so . . . I'd go through some sort of stupid thing where I asked . . . sort of asked a . . . woman out, not really but sort of and . . . ah . . . um . . . I then become convinced that everybody's talking about it and . . . I then . . . and . . . and they knew how strange I am and so then what I'll begin doing is not talking to people and glaring at them . . . in anger . . . now if you do this . . . very rapidly they'll notice that you're *(chuckle)* glaring at them in anger, you're not coming out of your office, and before you know it you'll walk by a hallway, you know, things like, you know, I just can't have you stand to look at me, it's as though it's just, you know, ice cold glares and at that point it's conceivable that what I heard really . . . was factually occurring and that reinforces my beliefs . . . umm . . . and . . . umm before you know it you're totally ostracized except for a few friends that I could . . . sometimes I went . . . why do they remain my friends, you know . . . because they had to put up with this . . . umm . . . this kind of stuff . . .

Excerpt 4

MR. A: Umm . . . wouldn't talk to anybody, I mean I . . . I was . . . I was real phobic, I mean we're talking about not going down busy streets, I . . . I wouldn't go to where my office was, I . . . I was afraid to talk to people, I would jump literally when somebody would come out of a door . . . when I was walking down a hall . . . like that . . . it was real . . . a real intense fear . . . umm . . . and . . . ah . . .

Judges' Accounts of Patient's Description of Symptom[2]

JUDGE 1: My sense is that we are not dealing in this case with a circumscribed symptom but a complicated, long-standing, and relatively severe personality disorder. I could agree that on Axis I this patient could meet the criteria for social phobia. I suspect if he was also questioned carefully he might very well currently meet the criteria for major depressive episode. I would be extremely surprised if he did not meet *in the past* the criteria for major depressive episode and I would also be surprised if he did not now make the criteria for dysthymic disorder. This I think makes it difficult to

---

[2] From time to time judges will refer to material from interviews and tests that have not been excerpted in the patient quotes.

select good conscious symptom words because he has had many symptoms over the years and the ones prominent at present, though always central in his make up, are just a part of the story. Going back and using words descriptive of some of his earlier symptoms, such as the panic attacks, and particularly those that were reduced by imipramine, seems inappropriate for our research purposes.

So, the problem is that there is no circumscribed symptom that we can give the patient's description of. When you ask this patient to describe his symptom, what he does is go back and give you an account of his history. This is actually appropriate because his problem is a long-standing and relatively severe disorder. If we are going to try to circumscribe, somewhat artificially, his symptom as the social phobic aspects of the problem that are currently present, his description would be that he fears giving presentations in his seminar, going to his seminar, going to his office where he might meet his office-mate, going to parties with peers, or in any unstructured way meeting with his peers, and dancing as one would at a party. However, this is just the tip of the iceberg and indeed, in the patient's conscious description this is just the tip of the iceberg.

I think his Axis II diagnosis is his primary diagnosis and most conservatively he definitely meets the criteria for avoidant personality disorder. I would add to this, "with narcissistic features."

JUDGE 2: He states that he believes he has had a life-long difficulty in social situations, particularly since his early teenage years. He says he never felt he "belonged," never had, in his words, the "social skills" necessary to make and maintain friendships, especially with women as he grew into young adulthood. He believes he had a panic attack at age 17 that went undiagnosed until 1983 when he was 26. He feels the panic attack and an accompanying symptom of chronic insomnia contributed to his increasing fear of being ostracized and led to his being aloof with peers, even suspicious and paranoid at times. He says he became increasingly isolated, virtually unable to make friends or date women. He also describes chronic difficulties with authority figures and a self-defeating tendency of exposing himself to ridicule or failure by biting off more than he can chew academically or by actually behaving in a suspicious, aloof, and unpleasant manner with people whose attention and company he craves the most.

He currently does not have panic symptoms, notes some improvement in social interactions, and no longer completely avoids social situations such as meetings and parties.

At some indeterminate point in his teenage years, probably when he began college, he felt assailed by the feeling that because he was constipated, he was in danger of constantly releasing gas and for a time virtually excluded himself from meetings, small rooms, etc., to ward off the humiliation and rejection he felt sure would befall him if he worked or interacted with people during the time he had his "constipation" problem.

He now feels desperate, lonely, and somewhat hopeless about his future ability to be a sexual, successful, and social adult.

JUDGE 3: This patient poses some difficulties in deciding exactly what the presenting symptom is. Because of his highly confused and confusing way of presenting himself, overly verbose, fluid, charged with anxiety, fear of self-revelation and humiliation, it becomes difficult to sort out the focus of his present difficulties. As best as one could determine at this present time, he is concerned about difficulties in his social relationships with peers, both men and women, and his great social backwardness in being able to present himself in what he considers to be an acceptable way. Although he can feel comfortable in a one-to-one situation, apparently as soon as a third person enters this scene, he becomes extremely anxious and preoccupied with what impression he is making on this third person, convinced that it is likely a negative one. He becomes concerned about how people are in general reacting to him, feeling that they consider him to be odd, "weird." Although he clearly distinguishes his preoccupation with what people are "whispering" about him from a true paranoia, at times it seems to border on that, although it isn't that he is projecting his own hostile or negative feelings onto others, but rather that he is convinced that they see through his social facade or efforts to make himself presentable to what is odd and unacceptable about him. He also finds it difficult to attend large groups, in particular parties at which there is dancing, but beyond the difficulties already noted, it is hard to pinpoint the exact boundaries of his social phobia, although it certainly seems to be a fear of certain kinds of social situations.

JUDGE 4: While the patient reports many symptoms currently and in his past, the one concerning his social phobia will be focused on here.

He alienates himself by not talking with associates, being aloof, glaring at them, provoking negative reactions in them. Sometimes they make side comments to each other, sometimes he "surmises" that they are whispering critical comments about him to each other. He is aware that he is prone to read negative reactions to him into their behaviors, so it is often unclear to him whether the critical attitudes he perceives is actual or imagined. This leaves him with an "always alone"—"walking around the block"—feeling that, as it intensifies, debilitatingly increases his socially isolating behavior and interferes with his work.

These symptoms increase in intensity whenever he has to move from one location to another. Because he has had to move a lot, he has been almost continually struggling with them for the past 9 years, since the age of 17.

Consensus on Patient's Conscious Experience of Symptom Following First CET Meeting

The judges agreed that it was difficult to determine the boundaries of Mr. A's social phobia because of the long and detailed history of a panic disorder associated with an earlier agoraphobia. Nevertheless, three of the four judges agreed that at the core of his current difficulties was, in fact, a social phobia involving a great difficulty in being with people, especially when at work in his office, or at what he referred to as dancing parties, or, in particular, whenever a "third person" would join a twosome in which he was engaged. This latter characteristic of the phobia is of special interest and so far in our experience is unique. Mr. A described his fear of humiliation and ridicule, his perception that people consider him to be weird and strange, and how, in a certain sense, he realizes he provokes that response by his avoidant behavior. Judge 1 stated that the patient's primary problem could not be considered to be an Axis I social phobia but rather an affective disorder (depression) and that the primary diagnosis would need to be that of an Axis II, avoidant personality. The patient stressed that his fears were mainly centered around "peers." There were no subsequent changes to this consensus.

Patient's Understanding of Symptom

Patient's Quotes Concerning Understanding of Symptom

Excerpt 1

MR. A: . . . [I was] about 4 . . . .there was also a period of separation from mother . . . classic . . . classic from what I . . . from what little I've read . . . classic panic disorder syndrome . . . you're . . . you're separated from your mother or other . . . very significant social . . . you know, like if you have a live-in grandmother it might be different, I didn't, I was actually shunted to . . . another state where I stayed with an aunt I hardly knew, thought she was my mother, because I remember calling her mom, then I would come back and was given to my real mother . . .

Excerpt 2

MR. A: I've spent a lot of time on this, I'm highly analytic by nature, so . . . my own analysis is that I . . . fairly . . . I meet a panic disorder . . . history pretty well . . . ah . . . one of the things that came out in some of the earlier sessions, with not her but yet one of the earlier therapists, was that I did go through a period of abandonment with my mother, it occurred when I was approximately 3½ to 4 and it was at least 6 months, my mother had no choice . . . ah . . . she . . . she was not only going through divorce, she was in severe debt because my father gambled and drank so she put me into [another state] with my aunt, who I didn't know and . . . ah . . . I was with her long enough to think she was my mother, my aunt, and when I came back . . . so as one therapist said to me, you lost your mother twice, you literally had to realign that relationship twice . . . that's what I've read . . . enough . . . not twice but the rea . . . . the problem was that kind of long-term, not just a few days or even a few weeks but a very long term . . . abandonment of the mother is very common in the history of panic disorder people . . . the other thing is that panic disorder tends to begin approximately at the age of dispersal . . . I now remember my first attacks at the age of 17, I was just getting ready to go to college . . . umm . . . and . . .

Excerpt 3

MR. A: . . . so . . . ah . . . when you . . . put on to that the fact that my mother worked nights, there were no other siblings and I'd come home to . . . an empty house and when I went to bed it was still empty . . . at the time I went to bed, from the age of 8½ to . . . whatever . . . 18 . . . whatever your prime is, you know, I left . . . ah . . . I was always alone . . . ah . . . you couple that with what I consider now maybe to be sort of like the preprogramming . . . something in the brain that makes some kind of anxiety attack easier in me . . . given . . . possibly the correlation with mitral valve pro lapse . . . ah . . . plus the abandonment history . . . umm . . . you have a man with no social skills and . . . ah . . . a man who knows nothing but fear . . . and you put those two together you have random fear attacks . . . I do remember the attacks now, quite a lot, I would have incredible problems sleeping, this was from the age of 17 to 26 when I was finally diagnosed . . . a lot of problems sleeping and I would know . . . by the . . . by . . . ah . . . about midnight I'd know it was going to be a bad night . . . yeah, rapid heart beat, sweating. . . . I just thought it was something wrong with me, weird . . . umm . . . so I would plan to have maybe 12 hours to sleep . . . I wouldn't plan to sleep 12 hours but I would want to have a period where finally I would be able to fall asleep and so I had extreme bed time, so to speak . . . umm . . . the attacks haven't recurred, I've been off the drug [imipramine] . . . the drug was . . . probably . . . ended . . . April . . . this year . . . last . . . this year . . . maybe that was about the time . . . close . . . so many things I've read . . . this was only about the time I might be expecting more . . . there is . . . six months buffer time . . . after removal of the drug, especially when you've been on it as long as I have . . . I was on just 18 months . . . [unclear] a long time . . . umm.

Judges' Accounts of Patient's Understanding of Symptom

JUDGE 1: His conscious understanding of his problem is quite complicated but would go something like this: He believes he probably has a biological predisposition to anxiety and on top of this, he suffered a series of real abandonments by his mother and the complete loss of his father at around age five. Because of his mother's peculiarities and his own fears, he lacked the opportunity for development of normal social skills. All of this led him to have the concept of himself as an outsider and to engage in behaviors that are aloof and unusual. These behaviors then become a self-fulfilling prophesy because people notice that he is behaving oddly and this drives people away, fulfilling his expectation that he is being ostracized and is a hopeless outsider.

JUDGE 2: The patient somewhat glibly and jargonistically attributes his panic attacks to early separation from his mother and father, speaks of a biogenetic predisposition to anxiety, little or no social skills training as a child, and no siblings or friends he could interact with.

He spoke at one point about his difficulty with male mentors, although he is not able to elaborate on this in any meaningful way. He seems to be aware that his educational goals are taking a beating because of his frequent moves and constant battling with peers and mentors.

JUDGE 3: One might best describe the patient's efforts at understanding as a kind of proliferation of obsessional ruminations infiltrated with fantasies of various kinds, thinly crusted over with a veneer of pseudopsychodynamic sophistication. He is very fearful of what might be discovered about him of the true causes of his difficulties because he seems to be so convinced that it is likely to turn out to be something untreatable and totally objectionable.

JUDGE 4: The patient sees his symptom as some confusing amalgam of somatically induced panic attacks, fear of abandonment, and identification with his mother. As a result of what appears to have been some effective therapy, he now questions his perceptions of the negative reactions of people and is aware that he provokes most of them.

Consensus on Patient's Understanding of Symptom Following First CET Meeting

Aside from Mr. A's considerable, highly intellectualized, and pseudodynamic understanding of what might be involved in his social phobic behavior, the judges by and large agreed that he had little true insight or appreciation as to the unconscious motivation for his behavior. One judge felt that there was a germ of insight in the patient's connecting his social phobia to his early and continuing difficulties in separation from his mother. There were no subsequent changes to this consensus.

Conscious symptom words selected

Social fears	Peers
Agoraphobic	Groups
Talk to people	Dancing
Scare cues	Tense

Some Interview and Test Contexts of Conscious Symptom Words

After we selected the relevant words, we asked ourselves: How well did the selected words actually capture the patient's conscious experience of his symptom? All interview and testing transcripts were searched for every utterance of each stimulus word. Each word was listed along with material preceding and following it. From the resulting 115-page document, we were reassured that indeed the stimulus words occurred in a context very much in keeping with what we had selected them to represent.

As an example, the following is a highly summarized presentation of the context surrounding **social fears.** Mr. A used the words *social fears* together as a unit in two places (Examples 1, 2, 3) and the word *social* in various indiosyncratic contexts (Examples 4, 5, 6, 7).

Example 1. Very early in the First evaluation interview, Mr. A gave several examples of what he termed his **social fears.**

MR. A: Umm . . . I didn't basically know anybody, I was already very agoraphobic, [I had] **social fears** of all kinds . . . ahh . . . I wouldn't go to . . . elevators . . . I'd walk up several flights of stairs . . . [to avoid people] . . . I would try to get the bus routes with the least number of people on them . . . everything like that . . . I had no friends . . . I sort of became adopted into the family [where I was living] and that helped out a lot . . . I released gas constantly and I also felt I was releasing gas constantly . . . it was associated [to the] more **socially** isolated [feeling].

Example 2. In response to the medical interviewer's question concerning the trouble he was having at work he replied:

MR. A: I don't like going to my office, I have **social fears** of going there, clear . . .

Example 3. At one point he summed up his situation,

MR. A: . . . you have a man with no **social** skills . . . ah . . . a man who knows nothing but **fear** . . .

Example 4. In describing his loneliness and feeling of being very different from everyone else as a child, he complained:

MR. A: . . . and I was going home to something on the stove . . . she was already gone. When I'd go over to a friend's house to have dinner it was an incredibly strange experience . . . I had no **social** father . . . and not only did I have a problem with having a **social** father sitting there, I didn't know what to do, then there was also the mother who had fixed dinner and they all were eating at the table. Even when my mom was off . . . we never ate at the table, I would eat . . . on a tray . . . then we got two TVs, by the time I was maybe 11 or 12 I would eat in my room and she would eat in her room.

Comment: Here *social* was used in the context of a poignant, acute awareness of how different he was from his peers. Note the idiosyncratic expression, "no . . . *social* father." Here he refers to *social* as something very important to him that he *simply* did not have in his life.

While describing his current problems, Mr. A's use of *social* referred to a capacity to relate to others and a sense of having a relationship to others that he feels he simply never had and that currently was not available to him.

Example 5

MR. A: . . . what really bothers me was that . . . there's a **social** network of gossip [unclear], which there was, I am not a member, I have no network.

Example 6. He's getting his Ph.D. in the **social** sciences, and had taught classes and done considerable published research and writing in that area.

Example 7. He was in laboratory studies related to **social** behavior and mathematical models of **social** behavior.

Comment: His use of *social* in connection with his current and future career commitment indicated the one positive aspect to his sense of "social" for him, a hope to which he had made a career commitment, that somehow the social aspect of life was masterable.

Summary of Conscious Symptom Word Selection

Although the judges struggled with the patient's complaints of many symptoms and had difficulty ordering them in terms of their importance, they did agree on the fact that one of his important symptoms had to do with a fear of being with people. There was high agreement as to the behaviors and the feelings related to this fear. These considerations guided the selection of the conscious symptom words.

Unconscious Conflict Underlying Symptom

We hope that readers will be able to perceive that there was a core agreement among the judges that the patient's conflict underlying his symptom had to do with the management of his *rage*. There is considerable disagreement as to the relative contributions from the oedipal, anal, and oral stages of development, as well as on many other issues. To help readers follow this thread of agreement, judges' comments concerning the patient's struggle with his rage are printed in bold type.

This section contains two series of independent judges' comments and consensus statements. This was necessitated by the fact that there was a shift in the judges' thinking after the third interview.

We begin with excerpts from the transcript that was used by the judges to infer unconscious conflicts.

Patient's Quotes Related to Unconscious Conflict

Excerpt 1. When asked how he felt about talking with the interviewer, the patient replied:

MR. A: . . . this is highly asymmetrical, you're learning a hell of a lot about me very quickly and you're asking [unclear] questions [unclear], I'm doing it for [unclear] reasons [unclear] done and the second reason is it's data, I really do believe something for science and all that crap, so . . . maybe . . . if you can use this in the future.

MR. A: I view this experience almost exactly the way I do the experience at [another] university hospital . . . you . . . I happen to be a data point for you and you in the process will try to help me out . . . and . . . ah . . . umm . . . and I view the fact that I'm a data point in the sense that this is [unclear] and . . . because I'm not convinced that much can be done . . . I'd just like to learn to be able to be less unhappy . . .

I: Something I'm concerned about, when you said "I'm just a data point," I'm concerned that your interviews with all of us and the therapy that may follow fits all too well with what you've been telling me about, where you are with someone for a brief period of time, then there's this big separation and you have to start all over again. I could see how you might be feeling that, once again you will go through the motions with us, we will get our data from you, but you won't get the help you are needing. I think we should talk some more about that feeling next time.

MR. A: Exactly

Excerpt 2

MR. A: Just that it's a vulnerability, it's not as though [what I say is] going to be used against me, but it's still . . . it's like, you know . . . you're not doing this to me buddy, you're sitting back there and you're just . . . you know, you're asking your questions, your being analytic and diagnostic . . . and I don't know a goddamn about you and I won't know when I leave . . . and that kind of asymmetry . . . is not made . . . it's not what we're meeting for, you know . . . that's not the way relationships are and so then I . . . naturally . . . the clinical relationship is a stress . . . I mean is sort of a stress relationship initially . . . I know the state . . . of . . . of . . . behavioral . . . science . . . you guys don't know much . . . you don't . . . and it's best if you admit it . . . you know . . . and . . . ah . . . I'm going to be moving on.

I: So even the prospects here, even though you've made contact with us, seem bleak?

MR. A: No, it feels better, I . . . I notice that I feel immediately better once I had called . . . whoever I called and asked for a referral, and then I was referred to this . . . even before I saw you guys . . . I think that's the difference, see . . . I noticed that I feel . . . I can work better if I know I'm going to go see somebody at the end of the day. I mean I'm still fairly tense . . . I felt a little more relaxed once I had made the appointments to see these . . . you guys . . . but then again, I think to myself, is this . . . what is this, some sort of giant . . . ahh . . . mothering system (*chuckle*) . . . you know, you guys are getting paid these salaries and then you know, eventually my insurance company will be paying, and they've already paid out quite a lot of money . . .

Excerpt 3

I: Well . . . what do you mean by "aloof"?

MR. A: Aloof? . . . ahh . . . ohh . . . just you assume things . . . umm . . . you're ready very quick to terminate things and . . . it's sort of like . . .

ah . . . like what I'll do is contact somebody once and if they don't contact me again I'll assume maybe they don't want to see me . . . which in the American culture is not probably the brightest thing to do . . . we're not known for punctuality, those kind of things, especially social engagements . . . ah . . . but I'll do that, I've done it . . . already . . . here . . . I just assume well, I . . . I didn't meet the . . . the quota . . . whatever it was they were looking for and . . . it's as though . . . almost as though I was so desperate . . . to connect with people that . . . I'm doing it . . . intentionally so I don't look so desperate . . . you know . . . umm . . . and it's been getting worse, I think . . . as time goes on . . .

Excerpt 4

I: And then of course, unfortunately that could be a self-fulfilling prophecy . . .

MR. A: Oh yeah, sure . . . because people see it and then they . . . well, they give up, but they try . . . even rapidly give up . . . ah . . . and . . . well, probably most people are insecure when it comes to meeting new people, and so, if they see enough negative signals they'll just shut off themselves . . . so I end up breeding a lot of . . . my own problem . . . oh well (chuckle) . . .

I: Did you have any thoughts about coming to see me today?

MR. A: . . . I never particularly want to, let's put it that way . . . ah . . . it's not just you . . . it's ah . . . it's never exactly the most thrilling in the world, also . . . really what's going through my mind lately is not this . . . it's rather, I have a fellowship and I feel like a charlatan . . . a complete charlatan, I shouldn't have gotten the money, I'm doing nothing, it's almost been two months . . . umm . . .

I: What happens that it turns out that you're not doing anything?

MR. A: Oh . . . I think it's pretty complicated . . . I think it has a function of . . . ah [unclear], location from the environment, it's a function of a lot of my work being rejected . . . ahh . . . umm . . . but I wouldn't just get no's, I get a yes and a no, I get controversial reviews . . . ah . . . I've plugged that into the whole way I look at the world . . . and . . . ah . . . I'm a hick . . . I seem to give off enough scare cues . . . there were . . . there are always a few people who will come over and try to . . . help . . . and . . . ah . . . I think I'm integrating very slowly, I don't know how to talk, I can only talk academically so to speak . . . I . . . I'm not real good at anything else . . . umm . . . but my guess is that I am . . . almost in spite of myself, slowly integrating . . . umm . . . not exactly as the most . . . gadfly kind of person in the world by a long shot but . . . but . . .

Excerpt 5. When asked to clarify his claim that he often felt "watched" he said:

MR. A: Yes . . . I think what it is is that I'm projecting what I do to other people which is that I . . . I . . . I observe everything . . . it's almost instinctive now, it's very hard not to . . . it's not as though you walk through a door and listen . . . it's just that you get incredibly sensitive to almost every cue and you also read a lot of cues that aren't there . . . umm . . . and so what I do if there is a third person in the room is very rapidly get afraid that . . . I'm not doing things correctly, that it's obvious that I'm not doing things correctly and that they already have an established relationship and I'm the outsider, so it's always as though I'm trying to break in . . . umm . . . one of my best friends as an undergraduate . . . ah . . . had a girlfriend and he went with her almost every weekend and . . . we were very close but nevertheless he disappeared on the weekends and . . . and I never had a girlfriend and . . . and so . . . I don't know if you've ever seen the old Bob Newhart show . . . umm . . . there's a character on there . . . umm . . . Howard Borden, who is the guy who lives next door, I don't know if you know it or not . . . you do . . .

Excerpt 6. When asked to describe what he meant by "needing legitimization" he said:

MR. A: Ahh . . . what it would mean in this case . . . ah . . . it . . . it's as . . . umm . . . not being trained correctly it's possible very . . . if you know how to do it . . . if you know the field it's possible to show that I'm pretty ignorant in a lot of variants . . . I haven't passed comps in [in basic areas in my field] and so if you poke right it'll . . . this . . . you can rapidly say this guy doesn't know much, I think that's possible . . . umm . . . legitimacy would be partly compensating for that, that even though a guy doesn't know something traditionally he clearly is . . . worked with somebody who is recognized as knowing the field and values him, secondly somebody who can give you . . . umm . . . some moral support literally when you're working in a field which is clearly deviant and . . . ah . . . which . . . clearly views what you're doing as very deviant even though I think in a few more years [my area] will become mainstream, it's already starting . . .

Excerpt 7. When asked about masturbation he said the following:

MR. A: Normally the fantasies are private and they're private not because they're weird [unclear], it's just that they're related to . . . in fact, see . . . I would steal a Playboy centerfold (*laughs*) . . . I used to babysit and it was really bizarre because there was this woman and she had this kid and she had no husband, she had been divorced and I got bored one night and began going through her magazines in this cupboard [unclear] not a lot but she had Playboys and I thought it was a little unusual at the time but what I began doing . . . was taking them home with me, sneak em out, you know. . . . [Then later I would fantasize that] . . . that there would be maybe three or four women living in a place and they would sort of take turns, not all at once, it wouldn't be like a gang-bang, but they would take turns, well, tonight you're going with so and so . . . and it was always easy to get [unclear], it's like okay, come on . . . sure . . . I want to do this to you . . . so [unclear] there were never any . . . I never had any fantasies of like James Bond, you chase the woman, she doesn't want you, eventually you are macho and [unclear], then I had two fantasies about being taught things . . . 'cause I didn't know anything . . . and they were sort of the same way . . . older women sort of introducing [unclear] but severe . . . I mean . . . severe meaning I [unclear].

Excerpt 8. His response to a TAT card 8 BM (depicting a young boy in the foreground with two men in the background, one standing up. The other lying down).

MR. A: *(long pause)* Ugh . . . it just took awhile because I had a lot of trouble with the boy, the boy is . . . umm . . . or young man, whatever he is . . . he's very well dressed and the background scene is one of an emergency operation, the gun makes me think that perhaps the operation involves some sort of . . . yeah, there'd been a battle, perhaps these individuals involved in some sort of armed resistance . . . ah . . . the only interpretation I can think of for the boy is . . . or whatever he is . . . a man . . . is that he represents sort of the other side . . . he's a man who . . . ahh . . . or whatever he is, he's somebody who will inherit a high social position . . . ah . . . in a sense his actions are the actions of his . . . .inheritors or the ones he will inherit from . . . are response for the scene . . . he has his back turned, he's not involved in the scene itself . . . [Tester: Okay, something about his presence in the . . .] . . . He's a representative of the system which generated the conflict . . . he gets the fruits, so to speak, while other people around him often experience the . . . unpleasant consequences . . . [Tester: Yeah, and the thoughts and feelings] . . . Well, it's sort of surrealistic, in other words . . . umm . . . the boy isn't aware necessarily of what's going on there, he's just primming [sic] up for . . . his life . . . and so in that sense there isn't a connected thought and feeling for the entire scene . . . I interpret both as doctors . . . the men . . . obviously not being cut into . . . umm . . . at least the fore one is rather old and I guess it is that he's simply carrying out his function and he's sort of more resigned, he's seen a lot of this kind of stuff, so I guess the overall impression is one of . . . apparently divorced lives . . . actually intimately affecting each other, though neither is aware of it . . . the doctor in the background is observing . . . learning surgical technique so to speak, in rather unpleasant circumstances . . . or how one goes about doing surgery in rather unpleasant circumstances without all the normal . . . umm . . . what you call its . . . ah . . . medical technology . . .

Judges' Accounts of Unconscious Conflict Underlying Symptom

JUDGE 1: For reasons similar to those that make it difficult to focus on a single conscious symptom, it is also difficult to decide on a *single* unconscious conflict. His adaptation to his problems is complex and multifaceted. When I recall that my job in this section is to describe the unconscious conflict underlying the symptom, it makes it irrelevant here to describe his conscious description of all of his problems. Let me say that I would broadly agree with the account of his problems that I gave a very brief synopsis of. [see Judge 1: Conscious Understanding of Symptom.] I want to call attention to my belief that there is a particular problem in his case of making a clear-cut separation between what is conscious and what is unconscious because he is exquisitely conscious of himself and extremely intellectualized. He gives conscious references to many aspects of his problems. Because of this, he is partially conscious of most of his conflicts, and, yet, this does not mean that there are not many associated aspects of these conflicts of which he is unconscious. **My candidate for best single unconscious conflict would concern sadistic rage or perhaps what Kohut would call narcissistic rage.** He believes all those who are supposed to help and nurture really use, abuse, hurt, and abandon those they are supposed to be caring for. This is abundantly and repetitively clear in his transference toward the staff. I might add parenthetically regarding his forgetting staff names that he forgot who his mother was and could see his impact in her collapsed face. Also, he "can never remember" the name of the older woman therapist he liked so much in Irvine. This is his sadistic retaliation for their/our mistreatment of him. This object relations paradigm is utterly clear in his description of his maternal relationship, paternal relationship, former therapists, etc., etc., etc. I would like to add here that this is also a case where the realities of a probably seriously disturbed, maybe narcissistic and schizoid mother, actual separations, actual unavailability of father, are equally important as the fantasied elaboration of these events.

Although losses are obviously central in this case, I don't think words reflecting loss would be good **unconscious** words, rather **words reflecting his sadistic and narcissistic rage over these losses and his unconscious fantasies of how these separations were really sadistic abuses that he**

deserved but wishes also to subject others to. Thus, I tried in my selection of words to leave out the tremendous number of words that are in some way related to his problems and to only include those that seemed to particularly reflect the more unconscious sadistic and narcissistic rage.

The most repetitive object relations paradigm present in this patient's test protocol involves the belief that the weak and inferior are abused, oppressed, coerced, forced, and dominated by the strong, powerful, and superior. The more conscious variations on this theme refer to himself as helpless, depressed, misunderstood and weak in relation to, on the one hand, a mother who is "oblivious" to his deepest needs, or is outright aggressively hostile toward him; or, on the other hand, in relation to a paternal object who is perhaps more positive and idealized (a "congenial mentor," or even "my hero") but still distant and unsustaining.

However, on a more unconscious level he very much identifies with the "armed resistance" that is aggressively competing for power and wishes to defeat and overthrow the effete, insensitive, "primming boy" and his whole social class. My guess **is that primary unconscious conflicts are over this aggression and its sadistic variants. He would like to be the author of this sadistic, controlling, coercive, forcing, dominating power, instead of the object of it, but such wishes need to be disguised and denied. The protocol definitely has a "pregenital" feel. Genital issues seem as yet remote, while the currently most salient issues could be construed in terms of anal power struggle or phallic competitive aggression on the one hand, or in terms of narcissistic rage and withdrawal into a narcissistic false superiority on the other.**

His defenses first and foremost depend on the obsessional use of his superior verbal skills to distance from anxiety and give himself the feeling that he is in control. Also prominent are isolation of affect from ideation, idealization, and reaction formation. A defensive narcissistic sense of superiority is also in evidence.

Consistent with this interpretation, I categorized the words I selected into three groups. The first group represents the tendency toward idealization of a paternal object and includes my hero, gadfly, and mentor. My second group of words represents his view of himself as weak and oppressed and includes the words breast, tail pointing up, mouths opening, upstretched arms, exposing myself, oblivious mother, and datapoint. The final group of words I categorized as involving the aggressive and sadistic struggle for power and this group included abuse, coerce, deprive, power, manipulation, stick tongue out, mandibles, force, boxer, predator, beady eyes, teeth, bulldog, snake tongue, huge fingernail, slash, resentment, subordinate, armed resistance and dominate. One reaction formed member of this category was "law abiding."

JUDGE 2: This patient is a man with what appears to be long-standing inhibitions and anxiety in social and sexual situations. The complicated and confusing way in which he tells his story makes it difficult to pinpoint the onset of symptoms and to obtain a reasonable history of the sequence of events that led up to his current symptomatic status. Even so, certain conclusions can be drawn with some degree of certainty and areas of ambiguity more clearly defined.

The first comment I would make is that this patient's story is remarkable for its use of jargon, intellectualization, and emphasis on either overly biological or overly psychological theories about why he has problems. As a result, his history appeared tortuous, devious, and quite untrustworthy. I believe this is a character trait in this patient by which he continually complicates, obfuscates, and otherwise renders material incomprehensible. It is his way, as I see it, of defensively warding off memories of actual events, internal and external, and instead of using denial and projection, makes it appear that his problems must surely have an external causes; i.e., mother, mentor, genetic predisposition, etc. He is enough of an academic to be able to weave current theories in a rather loose way into his symptoms and essentially present a picture not of a man with mysterious problems, but of a man with hopelessly incurable problems, i.e., he is a neurotic with the despair characteristic of patients with profound inhibitions for whom time is running out. I believe this patient's notion of maternal deprivation is somewhat contrived. Note, in contrast, later references to overcloseness to mother. She continues to mother him somewhat, intends to leave her property to him, and rather embarrassingly, from this patient's point of view, continues to insist that she should keep "an extra room" for him, as if to indicate this overcloseness—not as this patient likes to see it, the deprivation he suffered at the hands of his mother.

Further, there is evidence in the interviews of the mother supplying this patient with everything he wanted (books, etc.), again highlighting the patient's need to put distance between his mother and himself. This is not to say that this household was not dysfunctional at times, but to indicate that the so-called "deprivation" is spurious and not pathogenically related to the patient's social phobia.

A more telling developmental problem, I think, was the lack of a male figure that he could utilize as ego-ideal and further use to lessen the power of his fantasy of having gotten rid of him. The scenario that I favor would suggest that on his father's departure, he began to increasingly identify defensively with his mother (note overlap in time of goiter in mother and neck swelling in the patient, both occurring at the time of the parents' divorce, and the similarity in the complaints of abdominal distress in the patient and his mother, namely the "gas problems," and the "abdominal attacks"). At this point he had successfully gotten rid of his father and become engaged in what was to be a lifelong attempt to impose punitive and harsh rules on himself. He uses regression to anal level defenses to cope with situations that endanger his fragile sense of masculinity and threaten to bring homoerotic longings to the surface.

Phallic–oedipal issues are present, although cleverly disguised or just plain ignored at several points during the interviews. For example, it is interesting that the patient would attribute his sexual difficulties exclusively to his "lack of social skills," i.e., his being an innocent little boy, when in fact the story of his only sexual experience involved a married woman, a fact he barely mentions. The woman he tried to date recently also was someone who he knew had a boyfriend, perhaps even a live-in boyfriend. He states in this connection that he frequently finds himself the odd man out, "the third person," a clear-enough allusion to triangular dynamics.

In addition to the many crippling inhibitions he mentions, to note how when his failing defenses and subliminatory activities are unable to bolster his image of himself he resorts rather clumsily to aggressive wishes to dominate over and/or wrest power from male mentors. **He then finds himself in the furious, somewhat inept effort to carve for himself a place in academia involving unusually difficult and interminable cross-disciplinary projects as if the real reason was to merely exclude himself from any one clearly defined arena of academic rivalry or competition.**

I think, in summary, that phallic, perhaps oedipal issues and the fear of his aggressive impulses most easily explains the underlying cause of the social phobia. There are, in addition, worrisome regressions to paranoid, anal–erotic tendencies that bear further inquiry.

JUDGE 3: What to make of this patient's verbosity, the way he inundates both the tester and the interviewers with wave upon wave of words, at times very confusing and confused, at other times suddenly quite clear and even perspicacious. As I have already indicated in my comments following an examination of the tests, perhaps the best way of understanding the patient's manner of presenting himself is to consider him to be under the influence of an enormous anxiety, concern that he will be misunderstood and mistreated, both trying as much as possible to hide what he considers will put him in a very bad light and expose him to humiliation and ridicule, while wanting desperately to receive help while being convinced that none will be forthcoming. Add to this the patient's obvious obsessional style and, indeed, a breakdown of such defenses as isolation of affect in particular, and we might be able to account for the evidences of verbal peculiarity, stilted language, lapsing syntax, etc. However, I would suspect that one would need to add that there is a strong admixture in this patient of what we might call in the descriptive sense, schizoidal. He is a person, on his own account, much given to being by himself, preferring at times to isolate himself, spending long hours studying and teaching himself many things in which he takes great pride, while at the same time becoming more and more worried about his tendency to isolate himself. But it is quite obvious from much of his account that he is perhaps at his most comfortable when he is self-preoccupied, isolated, and alone, rather than when he is actively trying to be with people and relate himself to them. I think it will be necessary to try in the concluding interview to press very hard the limits of his possible schizoidal isolation and his anticipation that individuals will simply view him as a "datapoint." In this latter view of himself, presented as if this were solely in the eyes of others, one suspects that this is his own view of himself and of people in general and is, at its most withdrawn, schizoidal. Yet, there is also much more to this young man, who is struggling with might and main to somehow overcome many severe handicaps in his upbringing.

Hypothetically, at this point I would be inclined to venture the construction that there are two conflicts possibly related to his symptom: (1) Enormous guilt over what he must have experienced as an oedipal triumph and (2) an intensely troubled relationship with his mother. With respect to the first hypothesis, the patient describes, in some detail, how in effect his mother chose him over father, whom she disposed of as a weakling, and then decided not to marry another man because he might abuse her son, even though the son, on his own account, very much wanted her to marry this potential stepfather. As I read between the confusing lines of this account at that time in his life, which he presents as one in which he was lonely, isolated, and unhappy with his mother (which he undoubtedly was), there is also, I suspect, an underlying sense of triumph at having been selected as a very special child. There is an inordinate ambition in this person, who seems to be setting out to establish a field of his own, to engage in polemics with established people in the field before he has even earned his credentials, etc. This kind of underlying omnipotence is certainly part of a regressive retreat from this presumed oedipal triumph with its highly mixed bittersweet outcome. **There is no doubt that the primary fixation in his case is to be located at the anal sadistic level** with more than a strong hint of earlier oral difficulties having to do with compounded problems over separation from a mother who was pathologically bent on establishing her own life with her child no matter what. Yet, it must be kept in mind that until the parental divorce the patient experienced for the first 4 years of his life roughly a relatively intact family life. **I would also account for the patient's sexual difficulties, in particular his anhedonia, as related to an inordinate fear of his penis as a violent, aggressive, destructive weapon that can literally bring an end to the world, and, in particular, in its act of ejaculation.** Although the patient denied several times having any sadistic fantasies in any overt "bizarre" manner, the hints in the fantasy of controlling a harem of women certainly point to the central importance of a kind of sadistic control of these women who will service his needs one after another. I would further hypothesize that his current social phobia in the presence mainly of peers is to be accounted for by this inordinate ambition and his anxiety that it will "leak out" and show him to be this intensely ambitious, grandiose individual who will sweep all before him. Also consistent with this hypothesis is the peculiar version of the phobia when a third person enters the scene, which might then be a representation of a reestablishment of the oedipal triangle that interferes and reveals his special relationship with the other person, genetically speaking, mother.

With respect to the second hypothesis, there is considerable evidence, certainly on the tests in particular but elsewhere in the interviews, of the patient's repeated view of himself as subject to rejection and abandonment. Certainly the experience at 3½ when, following the parents' divorce he was sent to live with an aunt, would accord with this hypothesis. And certainly this patient has a score to settle with women on the basis of his unhappy experiences with his mother. But I am not convinced that the conflict over separation is what is mainly related to his particular social phobia. I suspect that were he ever to establish a lasting relationship with a woman, that then the conflict over separation would be the most relevant. But with respect to social phobia, I would consider the first hypothesis to be more nearly correct.

In the concluding interview, it would be important to explore the nature of this man's ambition and even grandiosity by getting into greater detail about his actual work, the papers he is trying to publish, the kinds of problems he has gotten into, and how he views himself in the field. I suspect that this would reveal something of the extent of this man's ambition and his hostile, highly competitive, and even sadistic attitude toward his competitors.

The testing presents a complex and difficult to piece out picture because of the patient's evident great anxiety during the testing and subsequent evidences of disorganization under the impact of anxiety. He was plainly very concerned about revealing too much of himself, of being put in a subordinate and helpless role and then being exposed to another person's domination and control. This seems to be the main issue that comes through from the tests. There is substantial evidence of great castration anxiety and the fear that what he will reveal will be quite small, "itty-bitty," and completely inadequate. As a result, there is much evidence of a retreat into an obsessional, oppositional stance in which he will try to withhold what the other person wants of him. This becomes the regressive defensive posture against running the risk of revealing his inadequacy and opening himself up to control and humiliation. There is so much evidence, in particular on the Rorschach, of eyes, people looking, etc., suggesting that this may play a prominent role in his symptom, taking the form of great anxiety over what people will see when they look so intently at him. It is unlikely that this person's primary conflict at this time is focused at an oedipal level but rather we see a markedly regressive picture. Again, as with other patients' test responses, we see much evidence of syntactical and verbal difficulties approaching the peculiar at times. I am tempted to explain this on the basis of the kind of stilted speech of obsessive–compulsive people in their efforts at being precise and then obsessional about word choices. I don't think this is consistent with a serious thought disorder. I would also, on the basis of the tests, rule out an exhibitionistic conflict as being related to the social phobia, but would see it instead as starting out as a great anxiety over revealing his inadequacy to public scrutiny and humiliation **that then is followed by a retreat into an intensely defiant, rebellious, oppositional stance.**

There is evidence that his obsessive–compulsive defenses are in a considerable state of decompensation. In particular, one would anticipate that his capacity to isolate affect is sorely strained and **that he is subject to the inroads of powerful, aggressive, sadistic feelings. It is also likely that he is afflicted with primitive, sadistic fantasies taking an oral aggressive turn.**

There is a good deal of evidence, mainly from the TAT but also the Rorschach, that the patient has substantial problems in his relationships to women, in particular his mother. One would anticipate much anger toward women and problems in separation.

JUDGE 4: The patient is a man of many contradictions and shows quite a span of psychological functioning. He evidences a lot of real empathic concern for his mother and her needs. He was polite, cooperative, communicative, and reasonably appropriate with me. While he behaves very strangely with his associates, he seems to have a realistic assessment of their reactions to him. Although he appears to have the capacity to engage in a rather high level of work in his field, he has extreme difficulty in getting it recognized. It is difficult for me to be sure whether his work is actually brilliant and his communication is interfered with by his conflicts, or whether his work merely consists of abstruse obsessions that "snows" some people and draws realistic criticism from others.

Not much is remembered of his life prior to $3\frac{1}{2}-4$ years when his parents were divorced. However, his life from then on was filled with many abandonments.

My sense is that although he may well have had at least a brush with the oedipal phase, the events of the divorce greatly interfered with much consolidation of that level of ego organization, which would have been shaky at best, and has left him vulnerable to functioning at quite primitive oral and anal levels.

Basically he sees himself as a depreciated "outsider," hick, smelly, incompetent, charlatan, desperately yearning to be legitimized and liked by mother, who though she chose working and other living patterns that precluded much of a relationship with him, at least provided a home for him; and more basically father, who literally abandoned him.

While he describes drinking, gambling, and abandoning behavior of his father's that would invite scathing criticism from anyone, he, even with some prompting, offered no criticism, but rather attempts to "understand" his father's behavior as genetically determined as is his. **I would see this defense against rage at father as the basis for the many projections that are rife in his current life.**

Although certainly angry at mother, he tends to blame himself for her distance from him, possibly from three motivations; out of his need not to alienate his sole support, out of his identification with father as the terribly disappointing one, and employing the same protective defense against his rage at mother as he does with father. In fact, there are some hints that the mother initially was the more disappointing person in his life and that father was the primary caregiver during those early years.

I would see the major underpinning unconscious conflict in this man to be stemming from **a regression from oedipal level functioning to very primitive oral and anal levels in which he massively denies his rage at father and projects his critical demeaning attitudes toward father onto others, then behaves in a "weird" manner as a defense against their projected criticism.**

There is not a clear differentiation between men and women as objects as well as his masculine and feminine identification for this patient.

His transference to our project and to me involves his seeing us as objects that he yearns to have be good parents to him, give him the legitimization, help, and comfort he needs, but sees himself as leaving us (identification with father), as well as sees us as taking data from him and giving him nothing in return. **I suspect that a lot of his obtuseness in the face of apparent cooperativeness with us is his way of being angry at us as well as self-protective.**

In summary, I would see his social phobia symptom as resulting from the projection used to manage his rage primarily at father though also at mother and all from whom he seeks emotional supplies and expects rejection and disappointment. I would see this symptom in a very immature character disorder with a capacity for regression to quite primitive modes of thinking and acting out. This rather bleak picture is mitigated by rather good intelligence, a conviction that there is something and someone good for him if he just keeps trying (he must have had some good years with someone: father?), he hasn't given up yet. This would form the basis for a beginning of a working alliance, which if and as his unrealistic expectations for succorance, propensity for projective identification, and acting out could be effectively worked with, might enable him to benefit from psychotherapy.

The WAIS and TAT reveal the relatively more healthy neurotic and sad aspects of his problems: His yearning for a situation where a couple would be together kissing and saying, "glad to be with you"; his yearning for an admiring relationship with father and resentment of his one down position; depiction of how he and his mother didn't communicate; his wish to be "looked for" by mother; the pastor–father "performing his functions without concern for the people"; his passively resignedly awaiting something to be forced upon him; and his moving to a higher social position as a result of a loss in some battle.

Although the relative structure of the TAT enabled him to demonstrate his more object related neurotic struggles, the relatively unstructured Rorschach revealed the huge ego gaps which leave him vulnerable to his more regressive experiences. In the face of color and ambiguity, he has difficulty allowing himself to be guided by "outside reality," and instead, rather than engage it and react to it, he keeps himself as an "outsider" to it and analyzes it from a primitive, idiosynchratic egocentric position that ultimately doesn't make sense to anyone, even him. His extreme difficulty with color bespoke his difficulty managing feelings, including use of isolation, defensive "analysis," and projection (many times used "you" when referring to his struggle with the cards). There were many indicators of sexual identity problems with a tendency toward a feminine identification. His response, "the merry-go-round with centrifugal force keeping people apart," I thought bespoke his experience of the divorce as well as his experience of his subsequent relationships with people.

The contrast between his TAT and Rorschach responses would indicate that although he is struggling with a high degree of confused perceptions, he can use the structure of human relationships somewhat to mitigate his confusion. He has already demonstrated this by the manner in which he used one of his previous therapies.

Consensus Following First CET Meeting

There was again a core agreement among the judges that the primary conflict associated with the symptom concerned the patient's difficulty in dealing with his rage. Two of the judges related this difficulty to an early regressive retreat from an oedipal triumph, when his mother sent his father packing and refused to remarry because it might be hard on her son. In this view, the patient is seen as inordinately ambitious, even omnipotent and grandiose, and these are the feelings he defends against by various efforts at reaction formation and avoidance, which contribute heavily to his difficulties in social groups, with peers, and, in particular, when a third person enters a one-on-one situation. The third person may be an unconscious representation of the patient's own strong desire to intrude on the parental pair; at the same time, the third person could represent the father as the intruder in the early mother–son relationship. A third judge, although agreeing that the patient had a "brush" with the Oedipus complex and then retreated from it, and that there were strong anal sadistic elements in the conflict over issues of power and control, left the door open to an important role for an earlier oral fixation based on an unsatisfying relationship with the mother. A fourth judge, although agreeing that the fundamental problem had to do with anal sadistic issues of control, domination, and power that the patient needed to repress and that produced a social phobia, stressed the significance of narcissistic features and saw the rage as being of early origin and directed toward an unresponsive "unmirroring" mother.

In this case, as in several previous ones dealt with at the clinic, the test picture tends to portray a more serious disorder than is revealed in the interviews. At times, the patient exhibits peculiar verbalizations, stilted language, lapses in syntax, and confused and confusing statements. At this point, we felt that these lapses did not indicate a psychotic or paranoid disorder, but rather reflected the degree of decompensation in his obsessive–compulsive defenses and, in particular, in his efforts to isolate affect.

It was hoped that the third and concluding interview could be used to throw greater light on the following issues:

1. The degree to which the patient was suffering from a regressive retreat to an anal sadistic position in which issues of power, control, domination, and fears of subordination were prominent versus an earlier developmental arrest at a more narcissistic level, which produced essentially an avoidant, narcissistic personality.
2. Concern about the possibility of an underlying psychosis in this man, taking either a paranoid or perhaps, more characterologically speaking, a schizoid form.
3. The strength and depth of the patient's ambitiousness or grandiosity: how realistic it is, how central it is to his current life, and the role it might be playing in his social phobia as related to his peers.

Judges' Accounts of Unconscious Conflict Following Third Interview

JUDGE 1: My formulation is not much changed by the third interview. With regard to the issue of underlying psychosis, I do not believe that the patient is or has been psychotic and feel that the further questioning in the third interview corroborated what my sense had been from the first couple of interviews and the testing. However, with regard to the more difficult question of a regressive retreat from an oedipal position or an earlier developmental arrest, I did not feel that there was anything decisive one way or the other in the third interview. There was material that one could construe in oedipal terms; for example, the material regarding his greater comfort with married women including the one-time relationship he had and the current office mate. However, I do not believe that this material is really reflective of primary oedipal issues. I think that this patient feels like he was robbed by both maternal and paternal figures and that he continues to seek what he felt he didn't get, but this search is continually unconsciously undermined by the sadistic and narcissistic rage he feels toward both males and females. I believe that the issues he has with the two sexes seem to overlap a great deal, although they may be slightly differentiated. I think he tends to see men a bit more competitively and as "ego posturing." However, he did see the one woman with whom he was in competition over the publication of his paper in somewhat this same light. I think he tends to see women somewhat more in terms of individuals that he can be helpful to and supportive of, however, I think he is relating to his current male foreign roommate in somewhat similar ways. One could probably make more of the differentiation between males and females than would be appropriate in this case. With regard to women, however, he seems to wish for a relationship in which he can be supportive while he is also being loved, admired, and wanted. I think this wish, however, is constantly being infiltrated by tremendous rage at his mother for abandoning him and for being oblivious to his needs. I think that he definitely shows evidence of wanting a "mentor–savior" relationship with a man *but this is constantly being* infiltrated with his rage at his father for abandoning him and showing little interest in him. He is more frequently and obviously sadistic and repudiating toward men in his academic context and I think in his relationship with us in this evaluation. I think he has now made it clear in the evaluation that he expects us to use him as a datapoint and to be able to do little for him and he feels perfectly justified in abandoning us to go away in January. Although this seems more obvious with men, I think impulses like this are there with women too but are more defended against by reaction formation in the form of his wish to be supportive and nurturing. My sense of this patient also is that he is far more deeply and chronically disturbed than I would expect in someone whose chief issues were oedipal but who had regressed to an anal sadistic position as a defense against these conflicts. I think of people having reached a primarily oedipal phase as having at least some arenas of their life that are conflict-free or relatively conflict-free. Although this fellow has achieved some things in his writing, it seems to me that he is deeply disturbed in every area of his life and has been so, chronically, since he was a child.

JUDGE 2: The third interview provides further evidence of the academic and professional strife in his life and how accurately it seems to reflect the patient's basic conflicts with authority figures. He describes desperate attempts to "legitimize" himself but in a curiously ineffective way—even as he is ostensibly trying to win approval and recognition from his peers, he is undermining himself by (1) deliberately provoking people by the use, for example, of terminology that he knows is inflammatory, (2) a secret contempt toward and envy of successful people that he seems to have no ability to conceal and is, thus, transparent in interactions with colleagues, and (3) replacing his feelings of being an outsider with grandiose notions of showing up the experts in the field when, in actuality, in his more reflective moments, he realizes is probably unrealistic and at any rate will involve much more effort and basic education than he is willing to admit to himself.

As one of us pointed out in the last CET meeting, so-called narcissistic defenses seem prominent this patient's grapple with the world of academia. Perhaps overall the patient does resort to primitive idealization and devaluation characteristic of Kernberg's narcissistic patient. However, narcissistic mortification does occur in the oedipal situation, and is not restricted, by definition, to earlier, more primitive, preoedipal dynamics. This is moot and is a good example of this problem of deciding just what psychosexual problem is central to the clinical picture in which grandiosity alternates rapidly with loss of self-esteem.

On clinical grounds, i.e., his speech, mode of interaction, and level of inhibition of phallic strivings, the patient most closely fits the model of the obsessive–compulsive with marked regressive pull to anal issues of autonomy and control with moderately severe narcissistic features, no overt psychosis but just barely making it socially. In this connection, I also have a suspicion that this patient is far more socially adept than he likes to believe. Being adept stirs murderously aggressive wishes and possibly psychopathic tendencies that he then smothers by self-recrimination, passivity, and more "goofing up."

I did not see any further evidence of psychotic, paranoid ideation in the third interview. The wish for the "mentor–savior," the idealized father who was never present for him, is a theme that he illustrates well in his description of the interactions with and expectations of peers and supervisors.

JUDGE 3: This concluding interview further underscores the extreme nature of the patient's ambitiousness and, indeed, his grandiosity. It also raises a question as to how realistic his ambitions are because it seems to be fairly evident that he is caught in a neurotic bind between wanting to achieve an enormous amount although, at the same time, remaining an "outsider." The role of the "outsider" is charged with considerable significance for him. One can hypothesize that as the outsider he is relatively safe from attack, while at the same time, as he himself put it, he can, in a vengeful way, "destroy what they have." At the same time it gives him, as he sees it, a special vantage point from which to see other peoples' limitations and for him to see something new and different. In his own words, it is "fun being an outsider." In effect, he is saying that he will triumph over all those who are legitimate and inside, and, if he does not, he will destroy what they have. His search for a "mentor–savior" is again a highly ambivalent one because he, at the same time, wishes to be protected and advanced by this mentor, while at the same time it is clear that he wants to destroy what this man has achieved. There would appear to be little doubt that the patient is caught up in this power struggle with a regressively experienced parent in which the distinction between mother and father is largely lost. He simply wishes to establish control and domination and to avoid subordinating himself and, if necessary, to destroy what he cannot have (that is, "to crap everything up for everybody else").

There are also continuing hints of his oedipal ambitions if he can but permit himself to run the risk of being bested in a competitive struggle. His attraction to married women whom he considers to be "safer" than single women would be an example of what I have in mind. It is as if he is saying that he is seeking a mother who is safely married and, therefore, not someone he would compete with another man for. Yet, at the same time, we know from his experience with Suzy that that was exactly what he undertook to do, although with Suzy it seemed as if the husband was pretty much in reality out of the picture. Perhaps, as he indicates, it is the woman who is in distress whom he attempts to save. I suspect, however, that the distress the woman is in is something that he has himself gone a long way to create.

The interview does not further substantiate any concern about an underlying psychosis in this man either of paranoid or schizoid nature.

JUDGE 4: While overly ambitious, the patient does have realistic talent. He is actually more intelligent and structuring of his speech than the transcript reveals. He punctuates and structures through nonverbal voice modulation and physical gestures. These also made the interviewer feel more related to him than would occur from reading the transcript.

Although he is severely obsessional, at times to the point of distorting both his perceptions and communications, and he uses projection and externalization, he has some awareness of what he is doing. He is very terrified of his sexual and aggressive wishes.

I saw him as more firmly planted in the oedipal phase, with his current adaptation a massive regression to oral but, primarily, anal phase defenses. He is very ambivalent toward both sexes, though the ambivalence is more severe and its severe aspects more repressed toward women. He approaches men for recognition and validation, although at the same time feeling locked into competition with them. He projects his own competitive needs to posture, etc., onto them and then tries to counteract it. He projects his fear of his "dangerous" sexual wishes onto women and becomes frightened of the women.

In some ways, he comes across as an "exceptional character," compensating and feeling owed for the wrongs done to him as a result of the divorce, at the hands of his abandoning father, and as a result of the early and life long abandonment by mother.

Consensus Following Second CET Meeting

There was a core of agreement that the unconscious conflict related to the patient's social phobia concerns his great problem in managing rage toward figures, male or female, whom he sees as standing in the way of his grandiose ambitions and efforts to control others. He cannot permit himself to become conscious of these rageful, sadistic, and controlling feelings because they would create enormous anxiety and conscious guilt, as well as immobilization in the pursuit of his goals. Instead, the symptomatic compromise involves an effort to keep a social and literal physical distance between himself and his "peers," who are the primary target of his destructive wishes. This conflict is quite evident in the sexual sphere, as revealed by his relationship with Suzy—his last heterosexual experience. Suzy complained of his having hurt her when he finally felt he could become "aggressive" in the sexual act. From that point on, although he could maintain an erection and consummate intercourse, he could no longer feel the excitement and pleasure of orgasm. It was as if he dissociated himself from the feeling; he described the consummatory sexual act almost as if it were an automatic, reflex action of his pelvis, so that he would not feel the guilt and responsibility for hurting the other person. His special difficulty in attending what he refers to as "dancing parties" is consistent with this understanding because, at such parties, he would have the opportunity to be in close physical proximity with women whom he fears his sexual impulses would damage. His sexual feelings are greatly colored by sadistic and hostile wishes.

When we compared what we considered to be this patient's symptom-related conflict with those of other social phobic patients, it seemed that, in general, the nature of the conflict in these different instances was varied. Thus, for one subject, we agreed that the main conflict related to the symptom involved exhibitionistic and voyeuristic impulses; for another subject, we felt that it had to do with a phallic competitive struggle with an authority figure. In these instances, the phobic objects or situations appeared to be displacements from earlier infantile ones. In the case of Mr. A, the fears and anxieties experienced in the social phobia appeared to be results of projection of his angry, hostile, rageful impulses on others, whom he then had to avoid. Also, an element of anticipation that others would see through him to his unacceptable wishes toward them created a feeling in him that he was a charlatan who was unworthy of their company.

Beyond this core of agreement concerning the unconscious conflict related to the symptom, there were disagreements as to the locus of this conflict in the patient's psychosexual economy and character organization. We have come across this problem before. Three of the four judges felt that the main locus of the conflict was at an anal sadistic level, although one of the three felt it was highly contaminated by oral sadistic and earlier grandiose and omnipotent feelings. A fourth judge continued to feel that the problems were not primarily those resulting from a regressive defense and indeed a wholesale regression to an earlier level of fixation, but that they were primarily the outcome of an earlier arrested development at a narcissistic stage. Nevertheless, all four judges agreed as to the particular focus of the conflict and what contributed to producing the symptom.

All of the judges agreed that the last interview laid to rest any concerns that the patient was struggling with a psychosis, had been psychotic at some previous time, or was schizoidal in character.

Unconscious conflict words selected

Ego maniac	Penetrate
Erect weapon	Power
First author	Take control
Hurt Suzy	Violence

The selected unconscious conflict words fall into three categories: (a) fear of primitive aggressive fantasies, (b) fear of competitive strivings, and (c) fear of aggressivized sexual wishes.

Fear of Primitive Aggressive Fantasies

Every aspect of Mr. A's life appears to be oriented toward warding off his hostility, perceived by him as terrifyingly destructive. In a limited aspect of his work, he had been able to make a realistically productive niche for himself and find abiding relationships with men and women. Even concerning his life's work, he stated that his primary scientific interest was in war and peace, and he felt that his laboratory research and mathematical model development of social behavior were trivial. These assessments reveal both his desire to somehow fit into the social scheme of things and his need to deal with his inner violent fantasies in a highly isolated manner far from the realm of human interaction. The words that represented these concerns were **power** and **violence.**

Fear of Competitive Strivings

Mr. A had collaborated on several articles with a male senior colleague who was close in age, and he had engaged several women in terms of academic issues. However, with the senior male colleague, he struggled with intense, ambivalent, controlling, competitive strivings, as revealed in his having found himself feeling "ego maniacal" and getting into many "ego fights" over who should be "first author"—to the point where many other colleagues advised the friend not to have anything to do with him. The words representing these concerns were **ego maniac, first author,** and **take control.**

Fear of Aggressivized Sexual Wishes

Mr. A's heterosexual relationships were burdened by bigger-than-life, sadistic, hostile fantasies. He revealed in one fantasy that sometimes his erect penis felt like a "weapon that could destroy the world." Again, as with so many social activities that bring most people mutual spontaneous pleasure, for Mr. A, they were completely subsumed by his struggle with his hostility. The words representing these concerns were **hurt Suzy, penetrate,** and **erect weapon.**

Interview Contexts of Unconscious Conflict Words

A highly summarized version of the context involving the words **hurt Suzy, erect weapon,** and **penetrate,** representing Mr. A's fear of his aggressivized sexual wishes is presented in the following text.

Fear of Aggressivized Sexual Wishes

Examples 1 and 2. The two words **hurt** and **Suzy** do not appear contiguously; however, when talking with the medical interviewer about his problems with women, Mr. A said, "hurt her" on two occasions, clearly referring to Suzy. Here is one of those passages:

Mr. A: I **hurt her** in bed . . . I never enjoyed . . . well, I didn't unenjoy it but I didn't have orgasms and I ejaculated. I'm pretty certain . . . I discovered that ejaculating and having orgasm have nothing in common . . .

I: You mean you were not aware that you had ejaculated?

MR. A: Not really . . . no, no big feeling . . . to it at all . . . I was initially dysfunctional like probably most males were the first time, and so I was very scared to know what to do and so she was more aggressive . . . one night when I finally became aggressive I felt as though it would be okay, so . . . you know . . . evidently I . . . I just . . . tried to enter too fast and I **hurt her** and so . . . after that I noticed that I was always . . . every time I . . . we would finish I'd always think, I'm sorry . . . and . . . umm . . . after that I never felt, I mean the penis never felt like, it's going to be okay tonight guy.

Other references to **hurting** included situations in which someone unintentionally got **hurt** in a variety of situations and it usually wasn't clear who hurt whom: patients and therapists, parents and children, and he and **Suzy;** even "professional training can hurt you as well as help you, it can blind you."

There were seven references to **Suzy.** Four had to do with his having **hurt** her, one had to do with her having hurt him, and two had to do with her being in some pain or state of consternation.

The two words, **erect** and **weapon,** although not occurring contiguously, did occur within the same speech. He had been nervously talking about his relationship with Suzy and intimating that she had accused him of something horrible.

Example 3

I: Like what did she say you did?

MR. A: . . . I didn't know what I was doing . . . to my mind an **erection** was not necessarily something which . . . *(pause)* . . . okay . . . sometimes when you're watching movies or whatever, you have the feeling it's like this great **weapon** that can be used to destroy the universe, but to me . . . it was . . . horrible, it's like . . . I need something and [unclear] so . . . I didn't do much at first, that bothered her . . . but when I finally one night began to actively start something she became very passive . . . and when I tried to **penetrate,** she . . . she went Ow . . . Ow, you're hurting me and I . . . stopped, she said she just wanted to . . . be very passive, because she had been doing **everything** before that . . . umm . . . that **hurt** a lot . . .

He used the word **penetrate** only once. To recapitulate: he was with Suzy, for the first time in his life at age 26 attempting intercourse, feeling his penis to be some "erect . . . weapon that could destroy the world." As he penetrates her, she yells, "Ow, ow, you're hurting me." This does not cause him to try to work out with her some way to penetrate without hurting or deter him from repeating the act; rather, he continues "to hurt her" while isolating any physical sensation, only to feel like a "sex maniac" when she later asks to discontinue intercourse. In the debriefing following the laboratory word presentation, he volunteered that the words **penetrate** and **erect weapon** "must have really gotten the old heart beating." He also felt we were really on track with **hurt Suzy** as well.

In summary, in the context surrounding his use of the unconscious conflict words, we see a world in which the ones with whom he wants to exchange pleasure, succorance, guidance, and soothing, hurt him and are hurt by him. His experience with Suzy crystallized that sense of the world. To hurt Suzy by penetration with his erect weapon represented, for Mr. A, the epitome of acting out his aggressivized sexual fantasies.

Although perhaps more able to intellectualize about his conflicts in the above areas than most patients would be, he was clearly not aware of the actual feelings and fantasies involved, which were defended against by isolation.

DEBRIEFING MEETING FOLLOWING LABORATORY SESSION

The patient's comments concerning the words during the debriefing further support the relevance of the stimulus words.

Without being asked anything, he said that the phrase **first author** had struck him and he immediately wondered whether the words had been tailored for his particular case. The interviewer told him he was right, and Mr. A then added that he was glad that the interviewer had told him that the laboratory people did not know anything about his circumstances. He then mentioned very quickly the **hurt lady,** then added **Suzy** and **social fears** and commented that there were two words that he couldn't quite figure out: **pocket road?** He just couldn't read the second word. The interviewer informed him that it was "radios." Other words that stuck out for him were **agoraphobia** and **social cues,** and there were other words that he knew really were "dummies" or fillers: **right hand, spring,** and **fresh.** He said, with a weak smile, that the word **penetrate** must certainly have "gotten the old heart beating." He could well see why that word was there. He then also mentioned, with the same weak smile, the words **erect weapon.** He thought that we were trying to combine or, as he said, merge an analytic with a laboratory approach, and the interviewer agreed with him on that.

He then volunteered that he had no feelings of anger, annoyance, or anything like "How dare you!" It all "made sense" to him. He also thought that we were on the "wrong track" with some of the words, although he could see why. Unfortunately, he could not remember any of these wrong-track words. He said we were really "on track" with **first author, hurt Suzy, and penetrate.**

LABORATORY RESULTS

For hypothesis 1 the total percentage of classification success in the expected direction for the conscious symptom words (supraliminal greater than subliminal) and the unconscious conflict words (subliminal greater than supraliminal) was 11.46% (group average = 8.5%).

The Case of Mr. B

NATURE OF REFERRAL

This subject was referred by a psychiatrist at a clinic on the campus where he was attending school. The psychiatrist was informed about our research and was on the lookout for patients with social phobias because that was the subject group with which we were working. She also was aware that, in exchange for a subject's participation in our research, we would provide a thorough psychological evaluation at no charge, and a specific referral for treatment.

SUBJECT PRESENTATION

The subject was a 21-year-old, single, white male in his junior year at a large, state-supported university. He was a big, muscular, boyish fellow of 210 pounds, who accurately referred to himself as "always the jock." He was attending the university on an athletic scholarship and stated that he would not have been accepted had it not been for his athletic ability because his high school grades had not been good enough for acceptance into the university. However, his intelligence was in the above average range (WAIS-R Verbal IQ 109, Performance IQ 114, and Full Scale IQ 112), so he certainly had the intellectual ability to do university work. He usually came to a session dressed in athletic shorts and a T-shirt, or other casual "jock" garb. He was given to occasionally acting on adolescent, college-boy impulses—for example, he and a friend decided, on the spur of a moment, to have all their hair shaved off, an action that had the quality of a friendly dare issued by one male to another.

He tended to speak in brief, unelaborated statements and to feel at a loss when the interviewer encouraged him to engage in more sensitively articulated explorations of his personal, subjective reactions. Indeed, he was the only subject not considered an appropriate candidate for psychodynamic therapy and was eventually referred for behavioral plus pharmacological treatment. Perhaps associated with this undeveloped capacity for psychological-mindedness, he frequently complained of feeling out of place in classes in which the subject matter was intellectual or aesthetic. Although individuals of his type might look down on their more intellectually inclined fellow students, he felt more apologetic, as though he were the one to be looked down on.

Later in this chapter, we give a thorough description and discussion of this subject's symptomatic reason for seeking treatment, but this introduction of the subject would be incomplete without at least a thumbnail sketch of his symptom. The subject's reason for coming for help was his repeated experience of distressing anxiety whenever he was in a social situation in which he feared he might become nervous, sweat inappropriately, and then be humiliated by having others see him sweating. Prime examples of this type of situation were: being seated in a forward row of a class where he could be observed by students behind him, and being called on to speak in front of a class.

EVALUATION PROCEDURE

Our usual sequence of steps was used in this evaluation (see Table 5.1). No special problems were encountered and no extra interviews were needed.

PSYCHOSOCIAL HISTORY

Mr. B, at age 21, was the youngest of six siblings in a Catholic family described by him as close-knit, conservative, and stable. He grew up in a midwestern town, where the family had always lived. His father, now 63, had been a tradesman but had taken early retirement for health reasons (diabetic neuropathy and a bout with colon cancer), although his health currently was described as being relatively good. His mother, approximately the same age as his father, was described as "a hardworking mom." Mr. B's siblings were described as follows: a brother, 40, who was "a production manager at a big firm"; a sister, 35, who was "a sales representative"; a brother, 33, who was an athletic director at "a great big high school"; a brother, 32, who worked at a large corporation and was a personal aide to the well-known founder and head of the company; and a brother, 27, who was "in construction." The 33-year-old brother, the high school athletic director, had gone to the same university as Mr. B, competed in the same sport, and was described as a "mentor."

The siblings having been so spread out in age and Mr. B having been 7 years younger than the next eldest contributed to the way he experienced his family, as illustrated in the following excerpt:

I: Tell me what it was like growing up in your family.

MR. B: Well, it started out . . . I was the youngest . . . all of my brothers and sisters were at home and it was really busy, you know, all my brothers were always doing their sports and . . . ah . . . my mom lived at home, my mom was a housewife, my dad always came home, he worked every day, and . . . ah . . . there was always lots going on and . . . then gradually everybody started slipping off to college and . . . ah . . . by the end of elementary school there was just me and [one] brother.

I: Who is how old?

MR. B: He's 7 years older than me, he's 27 right now . . . and . . . ah . . . then just about when I finished elementary school and went to junior high he left for college and there was just me, and I was always . . . I was almost like an only . . . only child all of a sudden . . . and . . . ah . . . just me and my folks at home . . . and . . . things kinda changed a little bit, you know, I was growing up . . .

Mr. B described his father as having been "hardnosed," "authoritative," and someone to be feared when the father was younger, but his father was seen as having been weakened and made more mellow after his bouts first with diabetes (when Mr. B was about 7 years old) and later with colon cancer (when Mr. B was about 14 years old). The father was, he said, a friendly and caring "guy" who was also strict and tough. The older siblings told Mr. B stories about how much rougher their dad had been on them, including beating them as punishment, but he thought they had really exaggerated these stories to impress on him how easy he had it. His mother was described as "very busy taking care of us as kids, she was always making the meals and stuff, she's very devoted to keeping the house together and the kids fed. She's still like that. . . . She's kinda selfless, always working hard for everybody else." Mother was not "what I'd call affectionate, always physical touching and everything. No, she's not like that, but she's always tuned in to how people are feeling, you know, she catches their moods."

It sounded as though the family norm tended toward being stoical and did not include a great deal of emotional self-disclosure. The parents "were never really affectionate around each other, but, then again, they never really argue in front of us kids. My dad wears the pants. My mom takes care of the family. My dad makes the decisions."

Mr. B stated that he "was used to having my brothers to talk to . . . my dad was kind of strict." Mr. B felt that his friends were given more freedom by their parents than he was given by his, and that his dad and mom "pretty much thought the same way" on this issue of strictness.

Mr. B seemed to appreciate the family's norm of male mentorship, whereby the older males in the family showed the younger ones the right path. For example, Mr. B described how his dad and brothers refused to let him compete in athletics when he was little. The message was, "You're too young for all that competition." "They'd seen a lot of little kids who've done that get burned out and end up not wanting to do it when they get into high school. . . . I kind of agreed with them. I could see their point."

Athletic competition was very important among the males in the family and indeed was quite central in Mr. B's life. He made his friends through athletic activities and experienced his greatest triumphs in athletic competitions. For example, he had been the only sophomore on one of his high school athletic teams, and he described himself as "all happy about that."

Junior high school was referred to by Mr. B as "that tumultuous period" in his life. As mental health professionals, we know this is a time of pubertal changes, but Mr. B had quite a few additional difficulties to deal with: His father had colon cancer and was believed to be near death. "They almost didn't bother operating." However, as will be discussed later, Mr. B seemed to need to deny any knowledge of his father's cancer until the day before his father's operation. Mr. B recalled other changes he underwent around this same time: "I think my personality changed a lot too." He recalled changing from "class clown," always upsetting the teachers, to adjusting more to the group and getting along in school. Interestingly, though, Mr. B refused several attempts by his interviewers to link some of these personal changes with his reaction to his father's illness. During this same junior high period, he also had some serious problems attendant on his physical growth. "My bones were growing irregularly." First the bones in his heels kept him "hobbling around," and then his spine was "kinda growing crooked." These physical problems plagued him for as long as two years until he "grew out of it."

Mr. B was uncomfortable about answering questions about his sexual experience; his replies were rather clipped and, for the most part, he denied any problems. He acknowledged masturbating prior to his first experience of intercourse when he was a senior in high school. He reported that, prior to having intercourse, he used to worry, "Am I ever going to have sex?" He also worried about whether he would be able to do it right (not an uncommon performance anxiety, but at least worth noting in the context of his presenting problem, which is itself a variety of performance anxiety). He reported that the first few times he had intercourse he was "kind of shaky," but once he had some experience everything was fine. He reported that his sexual relationship with his current girlfriend was satisfactory.

As previously stated, he was accepted at the local university on an athletic scholarship and his grades were not good enough for him to be admitted to the regular academic programs. His grade deficiency led him to feel inferior to many of his college peers. He had worked hard to develop his athletic skill and had hoped to be a starter the year he presented himself for treatment, but at the last minute he was beaten out by an older and more skillful athlete. He was quite disappointed by this. Because of the performance anxiety symptom that eventually brought him to treatment, he had avoided taking some courses he needed for his major (e.g., a public speaking class). Thus, he felt his personal powers were badly weakened by his psychological problem. After considerable personal anguish over whether to call for professional help, he finally decided to see a psychiatrist on campus, who referred him to our research project.

INTERVIEWER'S PERSPECTIVE ON THE EVALUATION

The patient was extremely uneasy throughout the evaluation. It became evident that he was quite ashamed of needing help. He made it clear that he would not want his parents to know about these visits because they would think of him as weak, although he also confessed that, despite how he thinks they would react, they probably would be concerned and sympathetic; the difficulty was more how he felt about himself as someone with an emotional problem. At one point he exclaimed, "I don't like myself . . . listening to myself spill my guts like this!" Because of his reluctance to "spill his guts," the interviewer had to resort to more question-and-answer exchange than is usually employed. This exchange in the second psychodynamic interview captures the nature of the problem the interviewer faced:

I: You're still feeling a little uneasy about coming here to talk to me?

MR. B: Yup . . . (*chuckle*) . . . filling up this dead time, you know . . . don't know what to say.

I: . . . Are there things that are on your mind that you would like to bring up? [In the previous medical–psychiatric interview, he had told the interviewer that he had forgotten to tell the present interviewer about his junior high acne.]

MR. B: No.

I: So, when there is this dead time, how do you feel?

MR. B: I'm wondering if I'm supposed to be saying more (*chuckle*) . . . if you want me to elaborate more on what I'm saying.

I: Well, if you want to, fine.

MR. B: No, I don't (*chuckle*).

I: You don't want to . . .

MR. B: I'm done, done talking.

It also became evident that the patient did not possess much psychological-mindedness and preferred mainly to see his problems as nonemotional in nature, although genuinely puzzling to him. Another excerpt illustrates this point:

MR. B: . . . He [his coach] treated me great when he thought I was going to be starting (*chuckle*) . . . I was his buddy and . . . I don't know, I think he . . . ah . . . my stomach's growling like crazy . . . Oh, I think he realized that I really wanted to get in the lineup, but . . . ah . . . there was nothing he can do, 'cause you just have the tryouts and you don't win . . . that's tough, but there's no favoritism . . . by the coaches . . .

I: Any reactions to your stomach starting to growl there?

MR. B: No . . . it was getting pretty loud (*chuckle*) . . . every time I was talking.

I: Any idea why it would growl so loudly?

MR. B: I don't know, I just ate (*chuckle*) before I came over here, I don't know.

I: That's one possibility . . . do you think that talking about this might get to you, might make you a little . . .

MR. B: I didn't think of that . . .

I: How does that strike you now that I have mentioned it?

MR. B: . . . Ah . . . I mean . . . just . . . be a little nervous, coming over here and everything, I don't know, maybe . . . but I think it's just . . . ah . . . I had a kind of . . . greasy lunch (*chuckle*).

An interesting and instructive difference began to emerge between the patient's reactions to the psychodynamic interviewer and the different medical–psychiatric interviewer. The former was an older male. In the first CET meeting, the patient appeared to be more at ease with the medical–psychiatric interviewer than with the psychodynamic interviewer. In the concluding psychodynamic interview, the patient, when asked, confirmed this impression. He accounted for the difference by referring to the medical–psychiatric interviewer as more "relaxed" and "laid back," while he felt that the psychodynamic interviewer was more "authoritative," by which he seemed to mean that the interviewer impressed him as more of an authority figure in whose presence he felt uncomfortable. He had also conveyed that he could experience his phobic uneasiness and might even begin to sweat, the most embarrassing aspect of his social phobia, if he felt himself on the spot with an authority. However, he denied feeling that way in the interviews. The transference link to his disciplinarian father, which became evident as the evaluation proceeded, constituted a good example of how the patient's interaction in the course of the evaluation could provide significant diagnostic material.

Pychodynamic Formulation

In most respects, the way in which the clinical team arrived at the psychodynamic formulation was similar to how it was achieved in the case of Mr. A. Noteworthy in Mr. B's case is the way in which the third and concluding psychodynamic evaluation interview elicited what the clinical team believed to be vital new information with respect to the unconscious conflict.

Three features of this case presentation will not be found in the other two cases: (a) a fuller explanation of the patient's account of his symptoms and *his* understanding of them (b) a fuller presentation of the words selected and the importance assigned to each of the words by the clinical team, and (c) a section on the psychological tests.[1]

Patient's Conscious Description of Symptom

Patient's Quotes Concerning Conscious
Experience of Symptom

MR. B: Well, it seems like I have ah . . . a prob . . . I get embarrassed too easily and . . . ah . . . I don't have any reason to get embarrassed, it's like I'm trying to make an impression on somebody, I'm worried that they'll have a negative impression, before I even meet them, just having them around me, just to look at me or something, gets me really . . . really nervous.

I: What happens . . . you say you get nervous, what happens?

MR. B: I get nervous that I'm going to get embarrassed so I get embarrassed, I start to sweat, and it'll just be so intense that . . . ah . . . I mean I'll start sweating and my heart will start racing and . . . ah . . . I got to leave, I got to get where . . . ah . . . I'm out of sight . . .

I: Yeah . . . can you give me an example, a recent example of that.

MR. B: Just being in class . . . ah . . . being in the middle of a class, not at the back where I like to sit, in the middle of a class, having people behind me . . . it might not happen for . . . maybe a half hour into the class,

---

[1] Refer to page 153 in Chapter 9 for an explanation of the subsections that follow.

and all of a sudden I'll just . . . ah . . . start wondering if people are looking at me, it's not like I'm paranoid, they're not looking at me, I know that (*chuckle*) . . . but maybe they'll catch me and I'll . . . start getting embarrassed or something.

I: You are worried about the people behind you?

MR. B: Yeah, who can see me. . . .

I: I see. . . .

MR. B: And I'll start getting really hot and I'll . . . my heart will start racing.

I: Hot . . . meaning?

MR. B: Hot, physically hot . . . touch. . . .

I: Really . . . .

MR. B: And . . . ah . . . start breaking out in a sweat and it's . . . I go in there worried that I'm going to start sweating, not being embarrassed, 'cause I have no reason to be embarrassed (*chuckle*), but it's like . . . ah . . . the result is worse than what I fear . . . is being afraid, or . . . embarrassed.

I: The result being . . . the sweating, or what.

MR. B: Yeah . . . so it's no longer just . . . being embarrassed if people look at me, I'm embarrassed if people see me sweating.

I: Uh huh . . .

MR. B: And that's from embarrassment, it's just a big cycle, it's . . . a vicious cycle (*chuckle*).

I: Yeah, when you break out in a sweat, where do you mainly sweat, where do you notice . . . ?

MR. B: Forehead and . . . ah . . . arms . . . mostly on my forehead and everything, so it just starts dripping . . .

I: Starts dripping . . . what gets to you about that, what makes you especially . . . ?

MR. B: That's embarrassing as heck 'cause . . . I mean . . . it's so noticeable, can't hide that.

I: Oh, I see . . .

MR. B: Can't hide that, and it's very apparent . . . but that usually doesn't happen 'cause . . . I stay out of those situations like that.

I: What do you do in class?

MR. B: Sit in the back.

I: You make sure to sit in the back?

MR. B: I make sure to sit in the back . . .

I: And if you sit in the back and you don't think anybody is noticing you then, are you okay?

MR. B: Fine . . . relaxed as can be.

I: Uh huh . . . what happens if you have to do some . . . ?

MR. B: If I have to sit in the front of a class, or . . . people around me . . . I can't concentrate, just . . . every . . . every bit of my energy is focused on . . . not . . . just trying to stay calm.

I: Are there any other circumstances or situations where you feel this way?

MR. B: No . . . just . . . it's mainly projecting my image, when other people see me.

I: So, for example, if you were sitting in the back of the class and feeling comfortable, but let's say, you were called upon to say something. . . .

MR. B: *(sort of a snicker)* That would be a big . . . big event, I'd be . . . pretty nervous.

I: Uh huh, same way?

MR. B: Oh yeah . . . I couldn't take that . . . I'd be. . . .

I: Does it happen that way, that when . . . when there are occasions when you need to say something in class . . . ?

MR. B: Yeah, I break out in a sweat . . . I'd have to get out of there . . .

I: Uh huh . . . has that . . . ah . . . how has this affected you, how has it affected your school work?

MR. B: Doesn't help *(chuckle)* . . . and I pick my classes . . . thinking of ah . . . how I can stay out of the situations that make me feel uncomfortable . . . I'm not gonna . . . I could do a lot better if I were . . . if I didn't have this problem . . . and I . . . like communications class, I could . . . I wouldn't take that, you know, if you paid me *(chuckle)*.

I: Yeah, where you have to stand up and talk . . .

MR. B: Yeah . . . and give presentations in class, that's . . . that's the worst . . .

I: How about other social situations, like . . . like mixers, parties . . .

MR. B: At parties I do good . . . have a great time in 'em . . . I'm not shy or inhibited at all . . . a lot of people think I'm kind of a crazy person that . . . just . . . wouldn't have a shy bone in their body *(chuckle)* . . . but I do, and I just do a good job of hiding it.

I: Uh huh . . . so it seems . . . would it be correct to say that it's entirely limited to classroom situations?

MR. B: No. . . .

I: Oh, where else?

MR. B: . . . Possibly even . . . ah . . . if I wasn't coming to see you, maybe this might . . . something like this.

I: Uh huh . . . like . . . like . . . meaning what?

MR. B: Face to face, talking to somebody like this, you know . . . I mean I've gotta be here with you . . . if I was . . . if I was just walking by, you know, talking to somebody in the hallway, you know, I could talk and everything, but . . . kinda being the . . . when you know you have to be somewhere.

I: You mean if you have an appointment to see an instructor, a faculty member about a paper or something. . . .

MR. B: Possibly, if I had to sit down, but not always . . . it depends on how threatened I feel or . . . if I . . . ah . . . if I start to think that I'm giving a bad impression . . . then it . . . then that starts . . .

I: Yeah . . . well when I said that it isn't limited to the classroom you said . . . you agreed that it wasn't, but I'm not yet clear from what you tell me where else it pops up.

MR. B: Ahh . . . it's happened in church . . . going up for Communion, I always hated doing that 'cause you're walking up the aisle and people are on both sides of you and I'm in line, I can't get out . . . and I'm kinda . . . I have to be up there for a while . . . sometimes . . . I start sweating up there.

Judges' Accounts of Patient's Description of Symptom

JUDGE 1: The subject experiences significant anticipatory anxiety regarding being observed publicly and sweating profusely in situations where there is no socially acceptable reason for sweating. Examples include being in the middle of a classroom and being observed by those behind him, being in line for communion at church, and being in front of a group speaking. A significant associated aspect of this experience is that he feels he must stay where he is, and, thus, there is no socially acceptable way to escape. When he can be active physically, either moving around athletically or "milling around" in a party, he does not experience his fear of embarrassing himself by sweating. Just thinking of a situation where he may be observed and not be able to escape makes him very nervous.

JUDGE 2: Patient is afraid of people looking at him from behind and "catching him" being embarrassingly inadequate, revealed by inappropriate sweating. The prospect of people seeing him in this helpless state and his not being able to extricate himself from it makes him all the more anxious bringing on a "sweating attack" during which he "gets hot," his "heart starts pounding," and he "starts drippin." This experience can occur in groups or in a one to one situation; the key factor is that he cannot escape and hide when he feels an attack coming on. It first occurred while giving a speech in class as a high school sophomore. It has severely limited his social life, his choices of college and career, and left him feeling very alone, having told only his girlfriend. He has not told his folks out of fear that it would overburden them.

JUDGE 3: The patient describes his problem as acute embarrassment when he feels he has to make an impression on people. He notices a pounding heart and becomes fearful that he will sweat profusely and that people will notice how embarrassed he is. He further characterizes these episodes as occurring in classroom situations and other social situations where he feels "trapped," for example, church or rooms with no readily available exits. He says he becomes hot and sweaty at these times, finding relief only when he feels he has the freedom to get away, as for example, when he is sitting in the back of the classroom or at a party where he can easily excuse himself.

JUDGE 4: The patient describes himself as having a problem with people looking at him, in particular in a classroom situation, if he is sitting in the midst of the class or in the front of the class. He fears greatly being embarrassed, in particular if, as he anticipates, he were to break out in a sweat because of his anxiety and that people would see him sweating. He is aware that it is all focused on his sweating now, but he doesn't know what started it. The symptom itself had its onset in high school when he had to give a talk in a communications class. The anxiety has been getting worse, in particular within the last year. He experiences the signs of anxiety, including the pounding heart, sweating, great nervousness, etc. Although he mainly talked about his phobia in a classroom situation, he indicated that in certain face-to-face situations, in particular with an authority, he would also be fearful of breaking out into a sweat and embarrassing himself in that way.

Consensus on Patient's Conscious Description of Symptom Following First CET Meeting

No major discrepancies among the clinicians was present in assessing the patient's experience of his symptom. The clinicians agreed that the phobic symptoms were mainly experienced in classroom situations and that the patient had displaced much of the anxiety involved in the underlying reason for the phobia onto the anticipation of sweating. He could obviate this anxiety to some degree if he sat in the back of the room where he could make an easy escape if he were to begin to sweat. It was noted that he identified the onset of the symptom in a communications class as a sophomore in high school when he was called on to give a presentation. The patient also indicated that he anticipated the same problem if he had to be in a "face-to-face" situation with an "authority." On the other hand, in other social situations in which he is free to come and go as he pleases, he experiences no such phobia. Although he is fearful of being seen to sweat in the classroom situation, it is no problem at all for him to be observed sweating when he is in an athletic competition.

Summary Concerning Patient's Description of Symptom

As is usually the case, there was virtually no difference between the formulations of CET judges regarding this patient's conscious experience of his symptom. This subject is an excellent example of what DSM-III-R designates as a "social phobia." The diagnostic criteria include "a persistent fear of one or more situations . . . in which the person is exposed to possible scrutiny by others and fears that he or she may do something or act in a way that will be humiliating or embarrassing. . . . The phobic situation(s) is avoided, or is endured with intense anxiety . . . . The avoidant behavior interferes with occupational functioning or with usual social activities or relationships with others, or there is marked distress about having the fear. . . . The person recognizes that his or her fear is excessive and unreasonable" (American Psychiatric Association, 1987).

The subject's conscious experience included the following. He worried that he would get nervous about people who might be looking at him—people sitting behind him in a class or standing on either side of him as he waited in line for Communion in church. He anticipated that this anxiety would lead to his sweating noticeably from his forehead and arms, that sweat would start "dripping" down, and that this would project a "negative image" to those watching. Feeling anxiety of this sort would be accompanied by his heart racing and he would become "really hot." This possibility was embarrassing and he felt a powerful urge to escape the situation. "I got to leave, I got to get where I'm out of sight." The thought of sweating is "embarrassing as heck 'cause it's so noticeable, can't hide that." This fear led him to sit only in the back of the classroom where he would feel unobserved and more comfortable. If he were called on to say something in class, his anxiety would rise and he would have to get away. He had avoided taking Communications because speeches in front of a class were involved, although the course was required for his major. However, he was comfortable at parties, where he projected an image of not being shy but rather "kind of a crazy person," that is, a cut-up or a clown. At parties, he felt comfortable because he could always duck out if he got anxious.

His concern that others might have a "negative image" of him was quite significant. He did not want his parents to know that he was coming to the clinic for help, and he had never told them about the problem although it had lasted for about five years. He wanted his parents to think of him as a "happy kid, well-adjusted and . . . ah . . . just . . . they can be proud of me." *Immediately* after the latter remark he went on to describe how his concern with his image was also elicited by the interview that he was presently engaged in. "This whole problem comes down to me and my image . . . that I'm projecting . . . . And I'm just taking everything down and letting you see that I've got hang-ups I need some help with. . . . You know me like other people don't and I just met you (*chuckle*)." His symptom was associated with a fear that others would see him in a weak and vulnerable state, "just a big sweaty heap. They wouldn't want to have anything to do with me. . . . I'm totally useless to do anything else." Later, underlining this sense of discomfort with exposing the vulnerable side of himself and again showing that it applied to the current interview as well, he said, "I don't like listening to myself spill my guts like this."

Patient's Understanding of Symptom

Patient's Quotes Concerning Understanding of Symptom

I: Tell me, do you have some ideas about what's . . . what's bringing . . . causing this . . . unhappiness for you, have any ideas at all?

MR. B: . . . I don't know, I think it's just kinda built up over time.

I: Oh, how long has it been going on?

MR. B: Well, I was always kinda shy to speak out, no, no I wasn't (*chuckle*) . . . I was always kind of shy to give, like speeches in front of class . . . or . . . meet new people, but I never really had that problem, I never had that problem until like . . . ah . . . high school.

I: It started in high school?

MR. B: Yeah.

I: Do you remember about when it started?

MR. B: It was in a communications class.

I: Yeah?

MR. B: One . . . of my first speeches I gave I just . . . broke out in the . . . most tremendous sweat *(chuckle)* . . . it was dripping off me . . . it was quite memorable . . . it was the first time I ever had . . . like a sweating attack.

I: What were you talking about, do you remember?

MR. B: It was just a speech.

I: About what?

MR. B: . . . I really don't know.

I: You don't remember?

MR. B: No.

I: This was when, when you were a sophomore, junior?

MR. B: Yeah, sophomore . . .

I: Sophomore . . . that's the first time, as you remember, that you experienced anything like what's . . . ?

MR. B: Yeah . . .

I: Began happening more and more . . .

MR. B: Yeah, and it's kinda built up, it wasn't so bad . . . in fact, through high school I could always . . . ah . . . sit in the front of the class, and I wouldn't mind being seen . . . maybe I'd get a little nervous, but . . . now it's . . . it's . . . it's so much that fear of sweating.

I: That's the main thing.

MR. B: That's it.

I: That's the result that you feel is worse than what you fear actually.

MR. B: Yeah, that *is* what my fear is now.

I: Now your fear is that you are going to sweat and that will be noticeable.

MR. B: Uh huh . . .

I: Yeah, so it started in your sophomore year and you can pinpoint it to this communications class and the first time you gave a presentation in that class.

MR. B: And now I . . . ever since then I started to avoid certain things . . . I think maybe it's . . . maybe avoiding all these chances to interact . . . maybe . . . make it now so . . . it's such a big event when I do interact that it kinda heightens everything . . . heightens.

I: You mean in a classroom?

MR. B: Well, I'm talking about these situations where people are . . . looking at me.

I: Yeah, so it doesn't have to be in a classroom, that's where it happens mainly but it could be anywhere where you feel people are looking at you . . .

MR. B: Right . . . looking at me when I . . . when I'm not . . . passing by, you know, when I'm there and I have to be there, it's more I'm sitting down.

I: But yet, people looking at you in a social situation, like at a party, that doesn't bother you . . .

MR. B: Not as much . . . not really.

I: Why do you think . . . ?

MR. B: I'm moving around.

I: It has something to do with moving around?

MR. B: Well, if I . . . if I felt anything coming on I could just duck out of the room, or I could move . . .

Judges' Accounts of Patient's Understanding of Symptom

Next, we present each individual judge's account of the patient's conscious understanding of his symptom, as written prior to the first CET meeting.

JUDGE 1: Subject doesn't have much of an explanation of the symptom except that he always felt a bit shy about being in groups and about the acceptability of his appearance, for example, his acne as a teenager was a problem for him. However, he marks the true beginning of his problem when as a sophomore in high school he had a single dramatic experience of, in fact, becoming very nervous and sweating profusely when giving a talk in front of a communications class. He seems to feel that this experience sensitized him to this possibility of embarrassing himself through sweating in public and he has become more sensitive about it through elaborating it in fantasy and reinforcing this by avoiding situations where he fears it might occur. He also associated his symptom with a longstanding feeling of being somehow different.

JUDGE 2: Patient believes his symptoms have to do with being judged by people and his fear that he will come across as incompetent, bumbling and weak if people see him in distress. He believes his anticipatory fear of, for example, sweating profusely, actually does produce sweating.

JUDGE 3: He has very little understanding of the symptom in any psychological sense. His understanding has been mainly concentrated on his belief that he cannot tolerate people seeing him sweat. As he put it at one time, they would think of him as a "heap of sweat."

JUDGE 4: No account of this patient's conscious understanding of his symptom presented by Judge 4.

Consensus on Patient's Understanding of Symptom Following First CET Meeting

The judges agreed that the patient had little psychological grasp of the significance of his symptom. The symptom was mainly displaced onto his anxiety over sweating. Note was made of the secondary consequences of the symptom, which the patient was able to identify as his anxiety over appearing weak, but they were not seen to represent any profound psychological understanding of the meaning of his symptom.

Summary Concerning Patient's Understanding of His Symptom

This patient's personal explanation of his symptom had the following elements. He recalls always having been kind of shy about giving speeches in front of a class or when meeting new people. This trait was perhaps present from childhood on. However, he marked the beginning of his symptom proper (i.e., fear that he would publicly embarrass himself by sweating) as an experience in a Communications class when a sophomore in high school. "One of my first speeches I gave I just broke out in the most tremendous sweat *(chuckle)*. It was dripping off me. It was quite memorable. It was the first time I ever had like a sweating attack." His explanation went on: "It's kind of built up. It wasn't so bad. In fact, through high school I could always sit in front of the class and I wouldn't mind being seen. Maybe I'd get a little nervous, but now it's so much that fear of sweating. . . . Ever since then I started to avoid certain things. I think maybe it's . . . maybe avoiding all these chances to interact maybe make it now so . . . it's such a big event when I do interact that it kind of heightens everything. . . . I'm talking about these situations where people are looking at me."

In probing his understanding further, the interviewer asked about other necessary conditions for the potentiation of the symptom. The subject made it clear that the situation had to involve his feeling that he could not easily escape, "I'm there and I have to be there." Thus, parties, even though social situations, were tolerable. "If I felt anything coming on I could just duck out of the room, or I could move." Also, being observed by an audience when involved in a sporting competition was tolerable. "I like to be watched [in sports competition], it's just that I don't like to be sweating . . . when I'm not supposed to be sweating [e.g., in class]." Although not consciously integrating this observation into his own explanation, he noted something further about circumstances that modified his symptom: He was able to sit in the front row of a class once when his girlfriend was there with him. "[I] kind of felt more at ease when she was around." However, he then added some other observations that raised questions about the significance of the girlfriend's presence: "But it was kind of a dark room. It was a big lecture, so it's still kind of anonymous."

We might summarize the subject's understanding of his symptom as a kind of commonsense behavioral-conditioning prototheory. He suggests the possibility of a predisposition to react anxiously to social performance situations since childhood (i.e., his shyness). As a high school sophomore, he had an intense experience of feeling overwhelmed with anxiety during a speech before a class. A kind of one-trial learning takes place, and he is hypersensitized to situations in which this experience might recur. Gradually, his anticipatory anxiety spreads to a somewhat wider variety of situations; for example, he must sit in the back of the classroom even though he is not giving a speech. He experiences a reduction in anxiety when he avoids stressful situations and this leads to increased avoidance and "heightened" anxiety when he considers not avoiding. If he feels flight and escape are readily available, he can tolerate a social situation, but if he feels he might have to passively endure increasing anxiety, something approaching panic probably ensues. The presence of his girlfriend might calm him. If conditions are such that people cannot observe him (e.g., in an anonymous dark lecture hall), he feels relatively comfortable. If sweating is socially expectable, as in an athletic competition, he even enjoys being watched.

Conscious Symptom Words

The first column in Table 10.1 is a list of the eight selected conscious symptom words. However, the next four columns need explanation. After the eight conscious symptom words had been selected but before the judges had any knowledge of the laboratory ERP responses to these word stimuli, the four CET judges were asked to rank *these eight words* on a scale where a ranking of 1 meant "best representative of the conscious symptom" and a ranking of 8 meant "poorest or most distant representative of the conscious symptom." The results are given in Table 10.1, where the third column lists the average rank across the four judges, and the fourth column gives the standard deviation (*SD*) across these four rankings. The *SD* is included to give a rough idea of how much agreement or disagreement there was among the four rankings. For example, "sweating" was a word that had the highest average rank and the smallest variance. A moment's consideration shows

TABLE 10.1. Judges' Rankings of Conscious Symptom Words from Strongest to Weakest

Conscious words	Number of judges nominating	Average rank across four judges	Standard deviation[a]	Source[b]
Sweating	4	1.25	0.43	I
Heart pounding	3	2.25	0.97	I
Speech	4	3.75	1.30	I
Really shaking	1	4.75	1.09	I
Nervous	3	5.50	1.50	I
Embarrassment	4	5.75	0.83	I
Class	2	6.00	2.45	I
Communion	2	6.75	1.64	I

[a] Standard deviation of four judges' word ratings.
[b] I, Interview.

that three of the four judges rated **sweating** 1 and one judge rated it 2 (the only way a mean of 1.25 could have been achieved). This degree of unanimity certainly is understandable, given that **sweating** was the most feared aspect of this patient's symptomatic experience.

Table 10.1 also gives a simple count of the number of judges who, on reading the interview and psychological testing transcripts, *nominated* that word or phrase as a candidate to be rated by all the judges as to its "belongingness." Because the transcripts were read independently, this number gives an idea of whether all four judges independently selected this word out of the thousands of words in the transcript, as was the case with **sweating, speech,** and **embarrassment,** or whether as few as one judge nominated the word but later all four judges recognized it as a good representative of the conscious symptom and rated it highly. (This was the case with **really shaking.**) The final column shows the *source* of the word (i.e., whether it came from an interview or a test). All the conscious symptom words in this case were selected from the interviews. Although conscious symptom words almost always come from the interviews because this is where the symptom is discussed, unconscious conflict words are sometimes selected from the psychological tests.

From the previous descriptions of the subject's symptom, it is clear in most instances why a word or phrase was selected and then rated as a good representative of the conscious symptom. **Sweating** was, for the subject, the very essence of his problem, and an occurrence of this, observed by others, was what he had come to fear most. **Heart pounding, nervous, really shaking,** and **embarrassment** were all responses that he associated with the anxiety state that resulted from fear of sweating. **Speech, communion,** and **class** were all situations in which he had experienced his anxiety symptom.

Unconscious Conflict Underlying Symptom

The formulation of the putative unconscious conflict underlying (i.e., assumed to be at least in part *causing*) the symptom is clearly far more speculative, controversial, and inferential than the mere description of the symptom or of the subject's understanding of the symptom. Indeed, it was precisely the psychoanalytic contention that symptoms *had* underlying unconscious conflicts that was strongly rejected by Eysenck (1960) at the beginning of the behavior therapy revolution (Bond, 1974). One of the consequences of the highly inferential nature of the formulations of the unconscious conflict is that it is much more difficult to select brief excerpts from a patient's own words that exemplify the evidence the judges use in arriving at their formulations. In reality, the judges read the transcripts several times and consider their earlier clinical hunches in the context of having read several interview transcripts and a psychological testing transcript repeatedly. In other words, the *whole* transcript record, as well as the judges' evolving hunches, are the basis on which they make their final formulations of the unconscious conflict. Nonetheless, in the following section, we wanted to present at least a fragment of the patient's own words from the three interviews and testing that took place prior to the first CET meeting.

Patient's Quotes Related to Unconscious Conflict

I: How about your father, tell me about him.

MR. B: Ah . . . well, he's kinda changed, he's gone through some stages, he used to be really . . . ah . . . really a hard-nosed kind of guy, you know, kinda author . . . authoritarian . . . ah . . . authoritative . . . with all those kids . . . and he was really friendly and everything *(chuckle)*, but he we always kinda feared . . . feared him a little bit . . .

I: In what way?

MR. B: I mean, don't mess . . . I mean . . . when I was a little kid, you know, you get into mischief and I wouldn't want my mom to tell my dad what I did because he'd get mad at me.

I: About what now?

MR. B: Well, little mischief I did, if I threw apples at the neighbor's house or something, whatever . . .

I: What were you afraid he would do?

MR. B: Well, when I was a real little kid, maybe . . . maybe he'd spank me . . . ah . . . after that it was just . . . he could just yell at me and scare me *(chuckle)*. . . .

I: Was he a scary kind of guy for you growing up?

MR. B: Well, kinda . . .

I: Strict.

MR. B: Yeah . . . but . . . ah . . . then . . . he got diabetes and he kinda had to I don't know, he had to change his diet, he wasn't so . . . ah . . . physical anymore, he didn't have a kind of physical nature to him.

I: Because of the diabetes?

MR. B: Yeah, he had to lose a lot of weight.

I: When did he . . . when was that discovered?

MR. B: I was about 7 years old.

I: When you were 7 years old?

MR. B: When I was 7 years old, yeah . . . and . . . ah . . . then he kinda became (chuckle) . . . more . . . ah . . . understanding, I don't know, he just . . . all the . . . all my brothers and sister say how . . . they always make up these big tales about how strict he used to be when they were young and how easy I have it now.

I: What kind of tales do they tell?

MR. B: Well, yeah, he just used to beat me and . . . senselessly . . .

I: He would beat you?

MR. B: No, beat them . . . that was just untrue, how he would be so strict with them . . . and how I never got hit . . . but . . . ah . . . he kinda became more understanding and then he got cancer and then he was really sick . . .

I: Oh, when did he get the cancer?

MR. B: When I was about . . . in junior high . . . that was kind of a depressing period (chuckle), because he was that close to dying . . .

I: Really, what kind of cancer?

MR. B: Colon cancer . . .

I: So this was just a few years ago?

MR. B: Well, junior high, yeah . . .

I: 19' . . . ?

MR. B: Late '70s.

I: Late '70s . . . can you tell me about that, about his cancer?

MR. B: Well, I really didn't know he had cancer until after they had the successful operation, I knew he was really, really sick, they never told me he had cancer . . .

I: Nobody told your family about it?

MR. B: Nobody told ME. . . .

I: Oh, they didn't tell you? . . . So, from your point of view he was just in the hospital?

MR. B: From my point of view I knew he was close to dying, but I guess they didn't want me to . . . just get this picture of cancer, like he was . . . um . . . terminal . . . (*chuckle*) . . .

I: How sick had he gotten?

MR. B: They almost didn't bother operating (*chuckle*) . . .

I: Umm . . . so it was pretty serious then . . .

MR. B: Yeah . . .

I: Now, was he looking emaciated or run-down?

MR. B: Yeah, he was down to about 120 pounds . . . he weighs about 180.

I: Umm . . . and so finally, what happened in the hospital?

MR. B: They . . . they removed it all and he slowly got better . . . but that was just kind of a depressing time (*chuckle*).

I: What . . . how . . . ?

MR. B: Junior high, you know . . .

I: How did you respond?

MR. B: . . . I don't know, it was kind of like a dark cloud was hanging over . . . over me . . . so everything was kind of depressing . . .

I: Do you remember what you were most upset by . . . at those times?

MR. B: . . . Well, everybody was gone from my family, I just kinda felt alone a little bit, my dad was, you know, really sick . . .

I: Oh, you were the only one at home, you mean . . . at the time . . .

MR. B: Yeah . . .

I: When did you find out that he had cancer?

MR. B: Ah . . . well, I guess maybe . . . I knew . . . the day of his operation that he had cancer (*chuckle*) . . . like that day my brother went and told me . . .

I: If you look back now to that time, would you say that your anxiety was connected in any way with . . . ?

MR. B: No, not at all . . .

I: With that . . . ?

MR. B: Not at all . . . oh, that's probably the time when I started . . . junior high was kind of a different phase . . . in my life, you know . . . things really changed then . . . I think my personality changed a lot too . . .

To conclude these brief excerpts related to the unconscious conflict, we present three brief Thematic Apperception Test (TAT) stories Mr. B made up in response to being shown a picture of a scene and being asked to "make up a story" including "what's happening in the picture right now, what led up to it, what the outcome will be, and what the characters are thinking and feeling." Because these TAT stories are sometimes referred to by the judges in their formulations, it may be helpful for readers to be familiar with a couple of concrete examples. However, the story cannot fully be appreciated without access to the stimulus picture.

Excerpt 1. Story to TAT Card 7BM. ("A grey-haired man is looking at a younger man who is sullenly staring into space" [Murray, 1971, p. 19].)

MR. B: . . . Well, this is a father comforting his son . . . his son just got the note that he didn't get accepted to law school . . . he was kinda worried about it, that he wouldn't be accepted but now . . . he has to face up to the fact that he's not going to go to law school and he's had to get . . . get some other kind of job . . . and his dad's a lawyer . . . the kid's really broken up about it but his father knows he'll do good . . . whatever it . . . once he . . . once he gets started on whatever else he's going to do . . . this guy's going to be depressed for a while, when he starts going out looking for other kind of . . . another line of work . . . but ah . . . eventually he'll find his niche and . . . he'll have forgotten all about this disappointment . . .

Excerpt 2. Story to TAT Card 8BM. ("An adolescent boy looks straight out of the picture. The barrel of a rifle is visible at one side, and in the background is the dim scene of a surgical operation, like a reverie-image" [Murray, 1971, p. 19].)

MR. B: . . . Well, this is a little Jewish boy and . . . ah . . . in Germany . . . umm . . . right at the beginning of the rise of Hitler . . . his father was . . . ah . . . very ill and he needed to get medical attention but . . . none of the German doctors would take him because he's Jewish . . . like I said, this boy is thinking about this, okay, . . . so, he almost . . . his father has to go underground to get . . . operated on because . . . ah . . . these doctors who are operating on him have to do it in private 'cause they could get in big trouble if any of the authorities found out . . . ah . . . this boy is really worried right now because he's worried that . . . they'll find out but he's also nervous about how his dad will turn out . . . he's also worried because he just saw the repression that's placed on his people right now . . . That's it . . .

Excerpt 3. Story to TAT Card 12M. ("A young man is lying on a couch with his eyes closed. Leaning over him is the gaunt form of an elderly man, his hand stretched out above the face of the reclining figure" [Murray, 1971, p. 20].)

MR. B: . . . Well, this boy, who is laying down, he's . . . he left home . . . a little early . . . and . . . ah . . . he went off by himself looking for work and . . . ah . . . this is back in the '20s, during the Depression, late '20s, but . . . ah . . . he finds work on this man's farm, this man just has a little farm, and this guy asks him if he could help, if he needed a hand, and the guy said, "Well, I can't pay you much, but I could use some extra work . . . a worker . . . and I'll pay you a little and you can stay . . . stay in the attic." . . . so this . . . the old man, he had to leave town for a few days and . . . this boy has been trying to take the place of both of them while he's gone and he's been working himself silly and this man just got back into town and . . . he . . . got home and he saw how much work had been done and everything and he couldn't believe it and he went upstairs to see the boy, up in the . . . the boy's room and he sees the boy is all collapsed . . . on the . . . in his bed, just so tired from all that work . . . and he's going to try to wake him and thank him for . . . you know, all he's done for him . . .

Judges' Accounts of Unconscious Conflict Underlying Symptom

JUDGE 1: Let me begin by saying that developing a coherent psychodynamic formulation seemed a lot more difficult for the interviews than for the testing. Somehow, the testing seemed to be more easily organized into a set of coherent themes. The patient's symptom seems to be especially a concern lest he reveal some sort of weakness to others and fail to maintain the "image" he wishes to project. Apparently this latter image is someone who is strong, popular, and carefree. He seemed to show significant increase of anxiety during the interviews because he felt he was "spilling his guts." Apparently, he feels that his weakness will be revealed most readily when he is physically passive and must stand or sit in one position while others observe him and there is no socially acceptable means of escape. He seems to use vigorous masculine activity to ward off a sense of weakness for example, he was the only sophomore on his high school varsity team, he took a job as a bouncer in a bar, and he is physically active and uninhibited at parties. Apparently, when he is able to engage in such physical activity he does not even feel shy, much less have the fear that he will break out in a sweat embarrassing himself.

It seemed to me that there was the possibility of some significant anxiety regarding fantasies concerning his father. There were indications of

increases of anxiety while discussing his father during both of the psychodynamic interviews. He has the idea that his dad would be disappointed in
him if he found out about his problem. There was also the suggestion that
he experienced some considerable anxiety regarding his father's health. He
seems to have been quite struck by his father's loss of physical strength and
presence, resulting apparently both from his earlier discovered diabetes and
his later bout with colon cancer. The theme of masculine competition is
represented in the material regarding his recent loss to a competitor in his
chosen sport. One way to organize this material would be to stress phallic
competitiveness as the key conflict with defensive regressions to an anal
level where he takes a more passive and unconsciously homoerotic position.
There are a number of indications that he has always felt more closeness to
males, for example, his brothers. It was interesting that his fantasy sex symbol was Heather Locklear. If I am not mistaken, she is a relatively tough female type who, as well as being very sexy, is involved in body building. She
seems to combine feminine and masculine qualities.

Although themes of competition and the idea that his symptom is
considerably blocking his active pursuit of his own aspirations are present, I
don't see much evidence of triadic oedipal material. Although I don't have
a strong sense of the specific nature of his conflictual unconscious fantasy,
I would place the conflict at the phallic competitive level with regression to
the anal level. In selecting words reflecting the unconscious conflict, I tried
to be guided by my sense of words that captured phallic competitiveness or
suggested homoerotic submission.

JUDGE 2: What emerges from the three interviews is the picture of a
young man whose social phobia began 5 years ago, probably around the time
of his father's colon cancer (although patient explicitly denies any psychological connection). Other precipitants were his self-consciousness due to a
temporarily disfiguring blow to his face and acne that he felt kept him from
engaging in closer interaction with peers.

Putting together the information we have from his childhood years,
one is struck by the ambivalent relationship with father. Undue strictness
and possible physical abuse/punishment from father seems likely although
defended against. In early latency, it would appear that the patient's murderous thoughts toward his father came to the fore, and he needed to believe that he was defective or weak and, therefore, nonthreatening.

However, there appear to be other features of this anxiety that require
further explanation. Is the patient's fear of being watched, especially from
behind, an indication of the extent of the negative oedipal, projective
mechanisms at work? Is his fear of being trapped and being unable to free
himself a clue to claustrophobia, i.e., separation-individuation conflict deriving from an over-close "only-child" relationship with mother? Is the fact

that his performance anxiety at its height occurs in more or less academic settings an indication of (1) hyperactivity in childhood, (2) genuine scholastic difficulties arising from a learning disorder, etc.?

JUDGE 3: There would appear to be at least two main explanatory factors, each of which may play some role in the underlying unconscious conflict: (1) a strong and inhibited exhibitionistic desire to show off his body and appearance in general, and (2) a strong wish to outshine everyone else and to be "number one."

As he said at one point, he does not have any problem with sweating when engaging in athletics and, indeed, enjoys being "looked at" under those circumstances. At parties he is a live-wire and described himself as "wild" and "crazy" under those circumstances. This in turn is reminiscent of his description of himself back in elementary school when he was something of a cut-up and a behavior problem in school. But things appeared to change in junior high school as a result apparently of two main reasons: (1) a severe case of acne, and (2) father's illness, bout with cancer.

The patient acknowledges the acne as a source of great embarrassment and pain for him; he does not cite father's illness at that time as playing a part in his symptom, but he is willing to identify that as a kind of turning point for him. With respect to the second possible factor having to do with his strong wish to be number one, there is much evidence to support this in his frustrating position as number two on his athletic team. He has wanted very badly to be number one, but there is this one person ahead of him, who simply is better than he and who has defeated him in the tryouts. He was hoping that his rival would select another position, but when his rival decided not to do so, the patient was stuck with being number two, which is enormously frustrating to him. He is anticipating that when his rival graduates he will at last become number one and be able to represent the school in interscholastic competition. The patient also views his symptom as making it impossible for him to realize his ambitions for himself to get a better education so that he can go into business and be a manager and a "leader." There is a 7-year-older brother whom he looks on as a mentor, who is in the same sport but has achieved success as the director of athletics in a high school. The patient describes his father as a strict person and a disciplinarian. Nevertheless, information concerning the patient's relationship to his father is rather sparse and one must infer a good deal from the kind of material just cited about his enormous ambition. At one point, he did say that he was able to grow out of "father's reach," which was something of a slip, because he meant to say that he got old enough to leave home to go to college. Also, he anticipates father would be most disappointed to learn about his phobia because it is important for him to appear strong and capable in his father's eyes.

On the whole, I would lean toward the combined importance of the exhibitionistic striving that would amount to showing off his phallus and not to feel ashamed of it, and the importance of his phallic and oedipal competitiveness with the top man, whom he wishes to outdistance. The tests may prove quite valuable here in helping us to weigh which of these alternatives is more important in understanding the unconscious conflict related to his symptom.

One possible speculative reconstruction that would pull together a number of things is to place the beginning of the patient's difficulties during junior high when father became seriously ill. At that time, he was acting up in class, getting poor behavior reports, defying the teacher's authority, etc. One could also suppose that there was a strong phallic oedipal element in this defiance that was reflecting the underlying unconscious wish to show up the authority and be number one. Father then becomes terribly ill, and the patient feels guilty and stricken by this turn of events. He becomes much more inhibited and shy, also at a time when he becomes pubescent and develops a severe case of acne. His growing sexuality, thus, becomes embroiled in this guilty conflict over father's illness. Also, of some interest in this respect is that the father loses a considerable amount of weight at this time. This may be related to the patient's current struggle with his rival whom he had wished would lose weight so that he, the patient, could be number one. The focus on the sweating as the displacement from the cause of the true anxiety may not only reflect the reversal of his exhibitionistic wishes, but also his uretheral ambitions. The "sweat dripping" is, thus, a disguise reversal of the unconscious wish to show what a mighty urinary stream he has and to show off his phallus and his physique.

Note also that at the time his father developed cancer, not long after that the patient developed some physical problems of his own with his back and with his feet, which might, in fact, have been a reaction to father's serious illness.

JUDGE 4: It would appear that the patient has never had a chance to work through a traumatic assault on his sense of well-being and masculine identification development caused by the nearly fatal and severely incapacitating colonic cancer discovered in his father when the patient was in junior high. The patient had strong needs to be tough and strong stemming in part from the fact that he was the youngest among a sibship ranging over some 19 years in which the next oldest brother was seven years older than he. When he wanted to enter athletic competition his family all said it would be too much for him. When his father was ill, nigh unto death, he was not told what the illness was. The patient then developed some physical problems that made him appear awkward, as well as acne which made him look ugly. Although he realistically asserts that even if his athletic experience had been more satisfying he would probably still be struggling with his problem, nonetheless despite "paying his dues" by hard, dedicated work as an athlete he remains one person short of first string on the team. It would appear that his intense need to be a high achiever athletically is a desperate attempt to ward off an identification as a weak, helpless, ugly woman. I feel that not achieving his athletic goals, currently, revives this threat. His intense concern about disappointing his parents, especially father, arises from projecting his own disappointment in himself (his stomach gurgled when talking about his failures wrestling and with women) for all that has entailed being the little kid in his family as well as his devastating disappointment in his father who was so struck down by diabetes and cancer. I wonder if there is something current like eye problems that has increased his worries about having diabetes and/or cancer.

He is also struggling with homosexual fantasies that he feels are demeaning and humiliating. His athletic activity is a good sublimatory outlet, however, he may feel more comfortable "being the big man on top." I wouldn't be surprised if he struggled with thinly veiled, if not explicit, homoerotic masturbation fantasies. I felt that this was acted out in the transference during the interviews by his taking a passive withholding stance, asserting himself very little and very guardedly responding to highly structured questions.

It is clear that he is terrified of these fantasies, but it is not clear how much his symptom is a regressive reaction to the trauma in junior high and how much it represents very early ego disturbance. The seriousness of the poor Rorschach percepts was somewhat mitigated by the interview history of body damage to father and himself, as well as a much more object related sense of himself, parents, and girlfriend.

Consensus on the Unconscious Conflict Following First CET Meeting

On the whole, there was substantial agreement with respect to the unconscious conflict. Two main points emerged: (a) the critical role played by the father's colon cancer when the patient was a young adolescent in junior high and (b) the central importance of the regression to a homoerotic position as a defense against phallic competitiveness and anxieties over castration. A third point, conflict over exhibitionistic tendencies, was stressed by Judge 3 and was agreed to by the other judges once it had been brought to their attention. A clear relationship exists between Mr. B's exhibitionistic tendencies (and the conflict over them) and the conflict with his father, which must have been greatly exacerbated at the time of his father's serious bout with cancer. There is little doubt about the intensity of the patient's competitive ambition—his striving to be number one ("top man") and his extreme frustration, in particular with respect to his athletic career, at finding himself "number two." He has not been able to handle this conflict over phallic exhibitionism and competitiveness successfully and advance into a more oedipal level; indeed, he has resorted to a regressive course in which he is in danger of assuming a much more "feminine" or passive position vis-à-vis a dominant male. Indeed, one can speculate that the phobic symptom is a compromise formation in which all of these elements play a prominent role. The phallic exhibitionism is reversed in terms of his anxiety over sweating, and the desire to shine forth and to be top man is replaced by an anxiety over being found weak and passive.

For the third interview, the judges felt that the following areas should be more fully explored:

1. The earlier relationship with both parents, in particular the father and his role as a disciplinarian vis-à-vis the patient.
2. The time of the father's serious illness.
3. The possibility that the patient suffered from a hyperactive syndrome as a child, which gave rise to the behavior problems he mentioned and, also, to his need to defend against this.
4. How his siblings reported being beaten by the father, and whether he had witnessed any of this or was himself the butt of his father's rage.
5. His foot and spine difficulties at the time his father was suffering from colon cancer.
6. His relationship to his girlfriend, because we anticipate there should be more difficulty in that relationship than the patient has thus far reported.
7. Why the patient has not opted to live in a dormitory but remains at home, which might point to either separation anxiety as a contributor to his problems or a choice to leave himself embroiled with father.

With respect to treatment recommendations, the judges felt that the patient might benefit from focal psychotherapy but his lack of psychological mindedness—and, indeed, his need for quick action—might make the psychotherapy difficult. The patient himself seemed to lean toward a desensitization approach, although this is something he has come across in books and in various classes, or might have been informed about by the psychiatrist he saw initially at Health Services. Inderol might be another alternative insofar as it would diminish his main complaint—the sweating.

The judges felt that the best approach to this patient would be to present him with these three alternatives—psychotherapy, desensitization, and Inderol—explore them with him, and be guided by his reactions to the alternatives offered or their combination. With respect to his psychological mindedness and responsiveness to the psychotherapy, it might also be advisable to attempt a mild interpretation with respect to the difference in the material he was able to describe to the medical–psychiatric interviewer as opposed to what he was telling the psychodynamic interviewer. It is striking to us that he revealed to the medical–psychiatric interviewer a good deal about the tough time in junior high when his father became ill, but could not, in the psychodynamic interview that followed, say anything at all about those important circumstances, even though he did make reference to that time in junior high as difficult. One hypothesis is that the transference with the psychodynamic interviewer is more of a paternal one and the one with the medical–psychiatric interviewer is more of a maternal one. By gently confronting the patient with this difference, an interviewer might see whether he can respond to it and develop some kind of appreciation of his different feelings toward the interviewers.

Patient's Quotes Related to Unconscious Conflict, from Third Evaluation Interview

I: I see . . . now just so I get the sequence correct . . . now you learned about your father's illness when . . . do you remember when?

MR. B: Gees . . . well, it was in 7th grade 'cause I was right . . .

I: Right at the beginning . . .

MR. B: Uh huh . . .

I: Of junior high . . . and you were the last in the family to find out, right, that he . . . did you find out after he had his operation?

MR. B: Well, I think it was the . . . day before.

I: The day before . . . do you recall how it was explained to you?

MR. B: . . . I knew that he might die in the operation (*chuckle*), but I didn't know he had cancer . . . I thought the . . . the operation was kinda tricky and . . . I really don't . . . I didn't really . . . have that great a grasp on what the surgery was all about and . . . ah . . . but my brother, me and him were driving around, just went for a drive in the country, my brother, the next oldest to me, the next closest to me . . .

I: How much older is he than you?

MR. B: Seven.

I: He's the one who is 7 years older, yes . . . he was the one who told you about it?

MR. B: Yeah . . . he just said . . . ah . . . you know, dad has cancer . . . I said "whew" . . . so . . . but . . . that really didn't . . . it kinda changed things, but . . . how I felt, but I . . . it was still life or death . . .

I: Yeah, so then you knew for the first time that it was possible . . .

MR. B: Yeah, and just a few days later . . . you know, after his surgery, they thought they got it all and . . . that was right, I'm 21 now, that was back when I was 13 . . .

I: 13 . . . about 8 years ago, and he hasn't had any problems since then?

MR. B: No.

I: I remember you telling me early on that he suffered from diabetes, right?

MR. B: Yeah.

I: How did it show itself, how did you know?

MR. B: . . . Ah . . . Oh, he used to be kind of big and everything, always eating . . . and then his eyes started going bad and everything . . . he had diabetes and he had to change his diet all around and the family . . . we had to start eating kinda different because we used to eat really elaborate meals, and . . . we started eating plainer foods . . . I really didn't notice it was that bad, I didn't even think diabetes was that bad, all I thought was that you couldn't eat snacks all the time . . .

I: Yeah . . . did you . . . when you learned from your brother, about your father having cancer . . . ?

MR. B: Well, there was one time . . . let me just . . . I just remembered this . . . and it was pretty weird back then . . . I don't know if this would have anything to do with my problem, but . . . ah . . . a few years after I found out my dad had diabetes, I . . . I overheard a conversation on the phone . . . and it was so stupid that I . . . interpreted this way . . . but I was in the kitchen making myself a . . . a milkshake or something, and I heard him talking on the phone and he was talking to some friend of his at work about he only had seven years to work and I thought he said seven years to live (chuckle) . . . like he only had seven years to live and I felt . . . well, it was such a shock, I didn't tell anybody . . .

I: Yeah, that was a shock . . .

MR. B: (chuckle) . . . and I thought about that every day for about a year . . .

I: Now . . . when did this happen . . . ?

MR. B: Gosh, I can't remember . . . umm . . . fourth grade . . .

I: When you were in fourth grade . . .

MR. B: Yeah, it was bad back then, but . . . I can't see any connection between that and . . . this . . . I just kinda realized, one day I thought to myself, Hey, he was talking about work, not . . . not his life, he was talking about his retirement . . .

I: But once you had that feeling, as a little kid, that your father was saying he had seven years to live, did you turn . . . did you talk it over, did you say anything to anybody, your mother . . . ?

MR. B: Oh . . . no . . . ah, . . . I used to . . . just . . . I used to get kinda depressed, just thinking about that . . . for about a week or so after that I was just really bummed out; . . . didn't feel like going out and playing or anything . . .

I: Yeah, but you didn't tell anybody?

MR. B: No.

I: But it really affected you? . . . In fact . . .

MR. B: Yeah . . . I mean . . . the fact that . . . I was a little depressed for a while there . . .

I: Yeah, but you didn't figure it out for some time . . .

MR. B: Yeah . . . *(sigh)* . . .

I: How would you say, as you were growing up back in those years, when you were in fourth grade or even younger or . . . how do you look back and feel your relationship with your father was like . . . what was it like?

MR. B: . . . Well, I . . . not really . . . we weren't really that close . . . 'cause he's, you know, he's kinda old . . . when . . . both him and my mom, they were old when they had me, both about . . . probably about 45 . . . but I . . . I had all these brothers around to hang around with . . . Oh, I just kinda wondered . . . they had raised up all these kids, and those kids knew the ropes 'cause they had seven other . . . all their little brothers come up, so . . . they could probably just . . . teach me the ropes, you know, like sports and everything . . .

Judges' Accounts of Unconscious Conflict Following
Third Interview

JUDGES 1 AND 4: Made no changes to their original formulations of the unconscious conflict.

JUDGE 2: The last interview supports the formulation that the patient has struggled with ambivalent feelings toward his father and in displacement of authority figures in general. It seems clear that father's diabetes, discovered when the patient was seven years old, played a decisive role in the development of the patient's problems. Already burdened by the image of a cruel and punitive father, either real or perceived, fostered by his siblings, he arrives at the point when he mishears the telephone conversation by his father in an especially revealing way that confirms the great intensity of his death wishes toward his father. After that follow two somewhat disabling physical ailments that reinforce for the patient the castrating power his father wields over him. (It would be interesting to find out if the patient's treatment for these conditions was itself painful in any way and denoted the father's wrath.)

As if this was not enough, the patient's father then falls ill and comes close to dying and the patient's description of the events of this period are revealing in the way he avoids thinking about or trying to understand what happened. The material in the last interview, as well as in the earlier interview with me, abounds in contradictory negations and partially articulated truths about even the sequence of events that occurred. For example, it seems as if he did not know of the seriousness of his father's condition until his brother finally told him, and, yet, on careful reading of this paragraph, it seems clear that the patient knew quite well that his father was dying or close to death and that the diagnosis of cancer was what he learned through his brother. I interpret this somewhat confusing description by the patient to mean that he has needed to remain confused about his father's illness and his own feelings. By appearing to hear the bad news from his brother, he magically makes his brother the guilty party while at the same time he disavows any knowledge in reality that confirms his frightening wishes to do away with his father. This part of the material is all the more striking because nowhere else (in this or other interviews) does he really have trouble in telling a coherent, sequential, and logical story.

Overall, this interview confirms, for me, that competitive and phallic level conflicts are the primary determinants of his social phobia. There are also hints that his boisterous (? manic) behavior in school was a defense against depressive affect brought on by the resurgence of hostile and guilty feelings about his father's illness.

JUDGE 3: Much more emerges about anxiety over father's well-being (e.g., incident in fourth grade overhearing father on phone and misinterpreting what he said). His misinterpretation may have been prompted by an unconscious wish; consciously he may have been concerned about father's diabetes and his age (parents were older people). Although much denial directed at father's impact on him, he did come up with the fourth grade memory and its impact on him, which was considerable. At same time, he was acting up in school, while being quiet at home—his rebellion toward authority displaced. Also note, when asked about differences between interviewers he referred to the psychodynamic interviewer as "authoritative" and becomes relatively noncommunicative. This may be due to repressed desire to "sound off," "speak out," "show off," but this can kill father.

Consensus Following Second CET Meeting

The judges felt that the material elicited in the third interview largely supported the formulation arrived at during the first CET meeting. In particular, some important new material emerged concerning the earlier relationship with the father that supported the original formulation. The patient reported that when he was in the fourth grade (approximately 9–10 years old), he overheard his father speaking to a friend on the phone and he misheard the father saying to the friend, "I have seven years to live," when, as he later figured out, his father had really said that he has "seven years to retirement." Nevertheless, that mishearing resulted in an extreme reaction on the patient's part—he described himself as having gotten very depressed for at least a week and as not able to get that out of his mind for the better part of a year, although he could turn to no one in the family to convey his worries. It seemed that, at that time, the father already was afflicted with diabetes and the patient knew this. Even though in an earlier interview he had denied that the diabetes meant anything to him, referring to it as simply meaning that his father couldn't snack as much as other people, it was clear from this misinterpretation that it must have been on his mind. This period of his life was when the patient was a cut-up at school, which would fit with our general understanding of the nature of his conflict with his father and its bearing on his social phobia, which, in particular, manifests itself in classroom situations. Mother continues to be described as the homebody who looked after the family, the house, and the cooking. Discipline was entirely in the hands of the father.

When he was asked further about reports he got from his older siblings that they had been "beaten up" by the father, he could add little further detail. He stated that he had never witnessed his father beating any of his siblings, and that he himself was never hit or beaten by his father. He dismissed the accusations as "stories" that were exaggerated by his siblings.

Even though the patient did come up with the earlier memory from the fourth grade, he continued to deny that his father's difficulties could have any bearing on his own. He described his problems with his feet and spine, which occurred during junior high, as something having to do with his needing to "grow up" more physically rather than as reflecting any state of worry or anxiety, or any hint of a psychosomatic disorder.

In this third interview, the girlfriend remained for him a source of support, someone he is quite seriously involved with and hopes someday soon to marry, and she reciprocates his sentiments. There appears to be little overt indication, certainly consciously, of any conflict with the girlfriend or sexual difficulties of any special note. The only negative thing he would say is that, at times, she is a little bit slow in getting ready to go places.

When he was asked why he still remained at home when he had the option of living in a dormitory or apartment of his own, he said that, in fact, he had done so for two years but had not been satisfied with the arrangements he could work out. He enjoys many things about living at home: He can come and go as much as he pleases, watch TV whenever he wants, and have his food prepared, and he knows he gets along with his parents. Apparently, they do not, according to his account, challenge him very much about where he is going and how late he will stay out, as long as he comes back during the 24-hour period. He said that he could come back at late as 7:00 in the morning without any questions being asked, just as long as he returns.

When treatment recommendations were discussed with the patient, he was particularly fascinated with the prospect of Inderol as a medication because it gave promise of ridding him of his main worry—the sweating—although he had many questions about whether it would affect him otherwise, in particular his ability to maintain his physical condition and his sports prowess. However, he gave evidence of a surprising appreciation of the value of psychotherapy for him, which he defined as helping him get to the "root" of his trouble. When we discussed the possibility of desensitization, he again tended to dismiss it.

In our discussion of his treatment prospects, we agreed that it might be useful as a start, both for his own benefit and for research purposes, to combine Inderol with a mild form of desensitization, both administered by the psychologist therapist with help from a psychiatrist. Psychotherapy would be kept in reserve for some later point as indicated.

A further point, about the nature of his conflict over his father, has to do with the fact that an actual trauma was involved—the father's brush with death, which the patient denied really knowing about until he was informed by his brother. It seems unlikely that he did not have some awareness that his father was in serious difficulty before he was told by the brother exactly what the father was going in for—an operation for his colon cancer. This awareness is especially likely because we now know that, at an earlier point, he was quite worried about his father and misheard what his father said over the phone. We would therefore infer that he was already, at that age, quite preoccupied with his father's physical health and what it signified to him. The presence of a possible trauma would only serve to exacerbate the intensity of the underlying conflict.

Unconscious Conflict Words Selected

As described more fully in Chapter 5, which is devoted to the word selection process, the judges nominated a total of 198 words or short phrases for
this subject (181 plus 38 Osgood words made up the 219 rated first [see
Chapter 5], and 17 words or phrases were added from the third evaluative
psychodynamic interview). Each of these words was rated repeatedly for its
degree of "belongingness" to the category of words reflecting the conscious
symptom and unconscious conflict. Table 10.2 shows the eight words or
phrases finally selected as best representing the unconscious conflict. As in
Table 10.1, the judges' average ranking of the words for "belongingness" are
given, along with the standard deviations and the number of judges who
nominated the word.

Table 10.2 shows that all of the unconscious conflict words in this case
were selected from the interviews. A comparison with Table 10.1 shows that
the conscious symptom words were easier for the judges to agree on because
seven out of eight of these words were nominated by more than one judge,
and five out of those seven were nominated by three or four judges. In contrast, five out of eight of the unconscious symptom words were nominated
initially by only one judge. However, as the deliberative process proceeded,
judges began to rate these words higher and higher as unconscious conflict
words, so that by the final word ratings, they had risen to the top of the list.
(In deciding how many judges nominated a particular word, approximately
equivalent words are counted as duplicates—for example, embarrassed and
embarrassment, class and communications class, speech and giving
speeches, colon cancer and cancer.)

Because the selection of unconscious conflict words is a matter of clinical inference, it is not always clear why the judges rated a word as a good

TABLE 10.2. Judges' Rankings of Unconscious Conflict Words from
Strongest to Weakest

Unconscious words	Number of judges nominating	Average rank across four judges	Standard deviation[a]	Source[b]
7 years to live	3	1.00	0.00	I
Colon cancer	4	2.50	0.50	I
Diabetes	2	3.50	1.50	I
Lost out	1	5.00	1.00	I
Top guys	1	5.25	2.17	I
Hardnosed	1	5.75	1.30	I
Disrespectful	1	6.00	1.00	I
Wild	1	7.00	1.73	I

[a] Standard deviation of four judges' word rankings.
[b] I, Interview.

representative. For **seven years to live, colon cancer,** and **diabetes,** much of the judges' inferential process is apparent from the discussions and quotations from the subject's own words. These words reflect the judges' belief that the subject's father's illnesses and the subject's hostile–competitive and guilty–frightened unconscious fantasies involving these illnesses were central in understanding his symptom. **Lost out** and **top guys** reflect phallic–competitive themes involving either defeat or victory. Additionally, **top guys** might imply a **bottom guy** and, thereby, unconsciously implicate the homosexual theme all judges discerned. **Hardnosed** can be seen as a "nodal" word that expresses a variety of themes simultaneously via a condensation-like process. **Hardnosed** was a term used by the subject to describe his father's personality prior to his illnesses. The word represents the harsher, more punitive image of his father. At the same time, "hard" has phallic connotations and "nose" could unconsciously symbolize the phallus. **Disrespectful** and **wild** were selected because they seemed to reflect a kind of displaced rebellion against the father. Although the subject was a good boy at home, he had another side to his personality that came out at school as a youngster: He was wild and disrespectful, always clowning and rebelling against his teacher-authorities. His parents would be quite surprised to find his grades concerning comportment at school to be a problem when he brought home his report cards.

Summary and Conclusions Regarding Formulations of the Unconscious Conflict

Although the outline and format for each of our clinical presentation chapters is the same, each chapter also highlights at least one issue that was not dealt with in the other chapters. Here, some observations are made about the different interpretive perspectives of a psychodynamic judge who is at first only provided psychological testing transcripts and results, as compared with a judge who reads interview transcripts first and only then goes on to evaluate the testing.

Of the four judges on the CET, two are asked to read the tests first and base a psychodynamic formulation on the results; the other two read the interviews and write formulations before they look at the tests. Following are some of the results that were based on this initial separation of assignments.

An issue of significance to the research as a whole is interestingly illustrated in the initial formulations based on the testing. Psychodynamic inferences about an individual's unconscious conflicts can be based on varying amounts of data ranging from: the individual's responses to psychological tests alone—the typical situation when a psychologist is consulted for testing only; to testing plus a few interviews; testing plus interviews plus a clinical team meeting; testing, interviews, a meeting, plus a follow-up interview to clarify outstanding questions, and so on. Ultimately, a lengthy and reasonably complete psychoanalysis consisting of hundreds of sessions should provide data on which the most complete formulation of unconscious conflicts could be based. What are the potentialities and shortcomings of dynamic formulations based on *lesser* amounts of data? A partial answer to this more general question comes from comparing the formulations of the judges who read only test responses with the formulation of the psychologist judge who read the test responses only after having already read transcripts of the first two psychodynamic interviews and the medical–psychiatric interview.

Unconscious Conflict Formulations Based Only on Psychological Testing

Between the two judges who read the tests first, there was a substantial amount of agreement on the salient conflictual elements (however, these formulations were not reproduced above). Both judges identified unconscious homoerotic wishes as primarily conflictual. Related to this, both judges noted a rather negative internalized image of women. Both judges further agreed that prominent aspects of the subject's defensive attempt at adaptation included a tendency toward impulsivity of action and some kind of difficulty integrating primary process impulses into reality-adapted secondary process; indeed, *based on tests only*, both judges raised questions about the possibility of some sort of decompensation. In one area, the ambiguity of each judge's wording made it difficult to identify whether their views overlapped or disagreed. This ambiguity concerned the subject's internalized image of males. One judge wrote that "[m]en are somehow some strange deprecated caricatures of misspent phallic assertiveness. He longs to be taken over by a phallicly powerful force but finds in its place a clownish powerless farce." The other judge wrote that "[r]elationships between males seem more idealized" but added that a male might exploit a "female only to become closer to 'the boss' or perhaps defeat the boss."

These test-only formulations seem rather patchy and schematic. For example, although they agree on the salience of homoerotic wishes, they do not say whether these are seen as regressions from phallic or oedipal level conflicts or construed otherwise.

Unconscious Conflict Formulation Based on Interviews and Testing

Against the views just described, it is interesting to compare the psychodynamic formulation of Judge 3, who came to the tests only after studying the interviews. The most outstanding aspect of Judge 3's formulation is that, although he too saw the indications of homoerotic impulses in the tests, he clearly placed these in a more comprehensive formulation based on his reading of the interviews. The impulses are seen as "a retreat into a more homoerotic submissive position vis-à-vis a frightening, overwhelming, male figure. . . . He fears an attack from the rear because of his powerful phallic ambitions." This judge adds that the subject's defense against phallic ambitions is to hide these by disguising rebellion as clownish antics and by presenting himself as a male who is weakened and exhausted and, thus, no threat to the superior male. If the subject were to act on his ambitions, he fears castrative retaliation or terrible remorse if he should defeat the other. Judge 3 saw little "in the way of oedipal issues in the testing, leaving the emphasis mainly on the phallic and anal."

Judge 3 also noted that the tests presented a "more somber picture than the interviews." Indeed, it has usually been the case with our subjects that the tests are interpreted to present a more pathological picture than the interviews. In this connection, recall the suggestion of Judges 1 and 2 of possible decompensation for this subject based on tests only.

CET Formulations of the Unconscious Conflict Based on Initial Interviews and Tests Prior to First CET Meeting

Here, we compare areas of agreement and disagreement among the judges, regarding the unconscious conflict. First, let us place what follows in perspective. When the first formulations were written, all of the judges based their formulations on the same interview transcripts (those of the first two psychodynamic interviews and the medical–psychiatric interview) and the psychological testing. The judges' first formulations were written independently; that is, prior to the initial CET meeting, there was *no* discussion among the four judges concerning the case. Moreover, the instructions to the judges were very general (i.e., "Give your understanding of the unconscious conflict underlying the symptom—if you cannot explain the psychodynamics of the symptom, discuss the patient's prominent conflicts and ego-status since these factors might be related to the symptom." Because the judges were asked to produce a free-form discussion of the patient that was guided only by general instructions, great leeway was allowed that could well lead to idiosyncratic formulations (i.e., result in maximal interjudge *dis*agreement). If one has had experience with the difficulties involved in obtaining interjudge agreement in far less inferential and more highly structured tasks (Seitz, 1966; Bond, Hansell, & Shevrin, 1987), it becomes clear how much room for disagreement there was in this case. Thus, it is interesting to see which aspects of the "elephant" the "blind men" emphasize and which areas of agreement emerge. Remember that the amount of agreement varies, depending on how complicated the subject's psychopathology is. Social phobia, like other diagnoses, is a "fuzzy set" involving prototypical cases at the center and gray-area cases toward its borders. The case described here is a less complicated case, which probably facilitated greater agreement.

The key elements of this subject's symptom included his intense fear that his personal weakness and vulnerability would be publicly revealed by his breaking out in a profuse and noticeable sweat. While sweating, he would have to remain passive and immobile. He could not escape through flight or disguise the reason for sweating with vigorous physical activity. He imagined that the audience observing him would pity, ridicule, and utterly reject the "big sweaty heap" that they saw.

When initially formulating the unconscious conflict that might underlie the symptom, *every one* of the four judges placed *sole* emphasis on the subject's relationship with and fantasies about *his father*. Because it is usual for us to attempt to understand the unconscious conflict in terms of its relation to difficulties at one or more psychosexual stages (i.e., oral, anal, phallic, or oedipal), it is noteworthy that all judges emphasized a more dyadic (father–son) and thus phallic-stage understanding of the conflict, as contrasted with a more triangular (father–mother–son) and thus oedipal-stage understanding.

The salient facts of the paternal relationship were described by the subject, and most or all of these facts were emphasized by each judge. Up to at least the age of seven, the subject recalled his father as a very "strict," "authoritative," "hardnosed" individual whom "we always kind of feared a little bit." His father was someone he did not "mess" with because "when I was a real little kid maybe he'd spank me. . . . After that he could just yell at me and scare me *(chuckle)*." However, when the subject was seven, his father was diagnosed as having diabetes and was perceived by his son as going through a change. "But then he got diabetes and he kind of had to change his diet. He wasn't so physical anymore. He didn't have a kind of physical nature to him. . . . He had to lose a lot of weight. . . . He kind of became *(chuckle)* more understanding." At this point in the interview, the subject appeared to have made a slip. Intending to tell how his brothers and sister would say how much harsher dad was in disciplining *them* with beatings, as compared with the subject, who was the youngest child, he said, "He just used to beat me [sic], and senselessly." The subject immediately went on to finish the story of his father's health and his own construals of it. When he was about 12 (in seventh grade), his father "got [colon] cancer and then he was really sick. . . . That was kind of a depressing period *(chuckle)*, because he was that close to dying." Because the subject was the youngest, he was not told what his father had or how serious it was until a brother told him on the day of his father's operation. His father lost one-third of his body weight during this illness, going from 180 to 120 pounds. Fortunately, his father's operation was successful and he slowly got better, but the subject described the experience as "like a dark cloud was hanging over me, so everything was kind of depressing."

How did the judges initially conceptualize the unconscious conflict supposedly underlying and, at least in part, causing the symptom? Three of the four judges placed emphasis on the subject's conflicts over his hostile and competitive wishes toward his father. Presumably, he had such wishes, and when his father was first weakened by diabetes and later nearly died from cancer, the son may have felt guilt as well as fear of retaliation. One unconscious resolution to such conflict might be to experience oneself as weak, and thus no threat to the father, and as defective, and thus punished for one's proscribed wishes. After his father's brush with cancer, the son had his own physical problems with the deviant growth of the bones of his feet—he felt "hobbled"—and later he suffered temporarily from curvature of the spine. He also developed a bad case of facial acne that was exacerbated in high school by becoming infected and caused him to stay in the house, out of sight, for one whole summer. Just before the acne became infected, he developed his symptom (i.e., as a sophomore in high school). An additional way of unconsciously resolving such conflict would be to entertain, even if only unconsciously, fantasies of homosexual submission to his father wherein he is a love object for his father's pleasurable use instead of a hostile and competitive threat. All four judges discerned themes that suggested unconscious homosexual wishes in relation to the father.

One of the three judges who construed the conflict in phallic–competitive terms also emphasized phallic–exhibitionistic themes. The subject was seen as wanting to outshine everyone else and be number one, but also to show off his body, including his powerful phallus. This judge suggested the possibility that the subject's unconscious "selection" of sweat dripping as the central component of his phobia might be a compromise formation (Brenner, 1982). Sweat dripping might be "a disguise reversal of the unconscious wish to show what a mighty urinary stream he has." In other words, the dripping sweat might unconsciously express a wish to exhibit a mighty urinary stream while at the same time functioning as a renunciation of and a punishment for this wish, because the sweat leads to imagined ridicule and humiliation. As such, sweat could be a compromise in that it expresses impulse, defense, and superego motives in a single action: the competitive and exhibitionistic wishes (impulse), the need to disguise and thus ward off these wishes from consciousness (defense), and the need to be punished for having proscribed wishes (superego or conscience). Another judge also explicitly formulated the sweating as a compromise formation, although somewhat differently. This judge placed the sweating in the context of homosexual fantasies. It was speculated that sweating might be the unconscious psychic equivalent of masturbatory ejaculation during an exciting and yet frightening fantasy of winning the love and approval of a desired man. In this conception, the subject's body is an unconscious equivalent of his phallus, and the sweating attack is a frightening and uncontrollable ejaculation. Here, sweating again is a compromise of a proscribed impulse (homosexual longings), which is disguised (defense), and which is associated with punishment because he fears getting caught (superego).

A third judge, although emphasizing the same father–son issues, organized them in a somewhat different fashion. The subject was thought to have "never had a chance to work through a traumatic assault on his sense of well-being and masculine identification . . . caused by the nearly fatal and severely incapacitating colonic cancer. . . ."

None of the judges gave much emphasis to the subject's relationship and fantasies concerning his mother or with females more generally. The only comments on these matters included a suggestion that "his intense need to be a high achiever athletically is a desperate attempt to ward off [what he construes as] an identification as a weak, helpless, ugly woman." Finally, one judge raised a question about the possibility of a pregenital contribution to the subject's problem: "Is his fear of being trapped and being unable to free himself a clue to claustrophobic, i.e., separation–individuation conflict deriving from an overclose . . . relationship with mother?"

The preceding paragraphs describe the salient areas of agreement and the differences in emphasis expressed by the four CET judges when they *independently* formulated the unconscious conflict each believed to underlie the symptom, that is, prior to the first CET meeting. It seems fair to say that, in this case, there was relatively little disagreement. The judges were unanimous in tracing the subject's symptom back to his relationship with his father and his reaction to his father's illnesses. All judges stressed the dyadic, phallic-stage origins of his difficulties, and all discerned conflicts over homosexual fantasies. There was a difference in emphasis in that one judge stressed issues of masculine identification and the other three stressed the drive–defense configuration of phallic–competitive and exhibitionistic drives along with homoerotic regressive defenses.

CET Formulations of the Unconscious Conflict Following Third Psychodynamic Interview

Two of the four judges, feeling that the consensus after the first CET (see pp. 213–214) was not significantly changed by the third psychodynamic interview, did not write new formulations. The two remaining judges wrote additional formulations but they agreed that the third psychodynamic interview primarily reinforced the conclusions reached during the first CET. One judge stressed the subject's "ambivalent feelings toward his father and, in displacement, toward authority figures in general." This ambivalence was thought to involve the subject's "image of a cruel and punitive father," evidence suggesting "death wishes toward his father," and subsequent "guilty feelings about his father's illness" as well as a need for self-punishment. The final judge emphasized virtually identical elements: the subject's "repressed desire" to challenge his father as well as his resulting fear that "this can kill father or incite his wrath." This judge also noted the "transference" repetition of the subject's conflict in that the subject used the same word to describe the older, male psychodynamic interviewer as he used to describe his father: "authoritative." The subject was noted to be more withdrawn and noncommunicative with the psychodynamic interviewer, who was construed as "authoritative," as compared with the medical–psychiatric interviewer, who was construed as more "laid back." Finally, the judge who had raised the possibility of pregenital "separation–individuation" issues involving the mother stated that "any suggestion about an unusual closeness to mother or fear of separation from her is not borne out by this interview."

As frequently happens, one of the subject's recollections elicited during the third psychodynamic interview struck *all* judges as especially revealing of the nature of the subject's unconscious conflict. Both of the judges who wrote additional formulations laid great emphasis on this one-paragraph recollection in a 29-page transcript. Three of the four judges nominated exactly the same four-word phrase from this paragraph, and this short phrase, "7 years to live," was finally selected as one of the eight word stimuli best representing the subject's unconscious conflict. The interviewer had been inquiring about the subject's reaction to his father's colon cancer and whether that wasn't a "turning point" in the subject's life. As if to emphasize the discrepancy between the way the clinicians were understanding the subject's problem and the subject's own understanding, the subject immediately replied, "I really don't think that's important." When asked why not, the subject explained that his father's critical condition lasted too short a time, "maybe a month and then he got better and it really didn't seem to leave that big an impression on me." However, at a later point, the subject was again describing the father's diabetes.

MR. B: . . . Ah . . . Oh, he used to be kind of big and everything, always eating . . . and then his eyes started going bad and everything . . . he had diabetes and he had to change his diet all around and the family . . . we had to start eating kinda different because we used to eat really elaborate meals, and . . . we started eating plainer foods . . . I really didn't notice it was that bad, I didn't even think diabetes was that bad, all I thought was that you couldn't eat snacks all the time . . .

I: Yeah . . . did you . . . when you learned from your brother about your father having cancer . . . ?

At this point, the subject interrupts the flow of the give-and-take to report a memory that suddenly came back to him.

MR. B: Well, there was one time . . . let me just . . . I just remembered this . . . and it was pretty weird back then . . . I don't know if this would have anything to do with my problem, but . . . ah . . . a few years after I found out my dad had diabetes, I . . . I overheard a conversation on the phone . . . and it was so stupid that I . . . interpreted this way . . . but I was in the kitchen making myself a . . . a milkshake or something, and I heard him talking on the phone and he was talking to some friend of his at work about he only had seven years to work and I thought he said seven years to live (*chuckle*) . . . like he only had seven years to live and I felt . . . well, it was such a shock, I didn't tell anybody . . .

In contrast to what the clinicians would see as *minimization* of the impact of his father's illnesses on him, expressed in the denial that the father's colon cancer left "much of an impression on him," and the statement that he "really didn't even think diabetes was that bad," the subject goes on to recall this "weird" memory in which "it was so stupid that I interpreted this way" and reports that his mind played a trick on him and inexplicably *exaggerated* the seriousness of father's health problems. As if to emphasize the role of what the clinicians would see as evidence of defensive processes, the subject states, "I don't know if this would have anything to do with my problem." The clinicians unanimously and independently inferred that this mishearing was so inadvertently revealing of the subject's unconscious conflict that they selected it as an experimental stimulus. Indeed, when the eight unconscious stimuli were ranked, this phrase was ranked 1 by all four judges, that is, as most representative of the subject's unconscious conflict.

DEBRIEFING MEETING FOLLOWING LABORATORY SESSION

Mr. B professed that he did not know what was going on during the first half of the laboratory session, the time during which the stimuli were being presented subliminally. When he began seeing the words during the supraliminal part, he was surprised that some of the words were related to him; he thought the words would be "random." When asked what words stood out for him, he replied, "I was kind of thinking, well, you wanted to see my reaction to seeing these words, like . . . sweating . . . embarrassment . . . colon cancer, seven years to live . . . Communion." It is notable that three of the words came from the conscious symptom category and two from the unconscious conflict category.

When asked for further thoughts about his reaction to these words, he said that the first words he saw that he thought were especially for him was the seven years to live stimulus. When he was asked if he had any thought as to why that phrase was selected, he replied that "it had an impact on me so . . . you probably wanted to see . . . what the reaction I'd have to that would be." When he was asked if he had any reaction, he chuckled and replied that he probably had. He then realized that the "words were focused directly at me . . . and I probably got a little surprise out of it . . . the scale probably jumped (chuckle) on your little meter . . . whatever."

The memory that turned up in the third interview, which all the judges felt was so significant, seemed also to be significant to the patient, although he could not clarify exactly why.

LABORATORY RESULTS

For hypothesis 1 the total percentage of classification success in the expected direction for the conscious symptom words (supraliminal greater than subliminal) and the unconscious conflict words (subliminal greater than supraliminal) was 3.03% (group average = 8.57%).

The Case of Mr. C

NATURE OF REFERRAL

The patient, a young man of 20, was referred to us by a university psychiatrist to whom he had come complaining of difficulty in eating in public places, such as the dormitory cafeteria. The patient had spent the previous months investigating possible physical causes for his difficulty, and none was discovered. He readily agreed to participate in the research, after the conditions were explained to him over the phone.

SUBJECT PRESENTATION

Mr. C was a slightly built but athletic young man with a graceful, fawn-like bearing suggestive of mildly androgynous qualities. Throughout the evaluation, he was quite anxious and, at times, overtly frightened, yet he was quite forthcoming and remarkably reflective, and was eager to deal with his problem.

EVALUATION PROCEDURE

Mr. C's evaluation was longer than those of the other two patients, owing to the complexity of his difficulties, his difficulty in communicating to the evaluator, and the diagnostic concerns of the judges.

Mr. C's evaluation consisted of the following sequence of procedures: first psychodynamic evaluation interview, psychological testing, second psychodynamic evaluation interview, medical–psychiatric interview, first CET meeting, third psychodynamic evaluation interview, second CET meeting, fourth evaluation interview, third CET meeting.

Psychosocial History

The patient is the third of four children born to a lower-middle-class family in a small city. The patient has two older brothers, two years and one year older than himself, and a sister two years younger than himself. The father is a building tradesman and the mother is a health professional. The father is described by the patient as an alcoholic who was a strict disciplinarian given to beating his children. However, the patient describes himself as having escaped these beatings because he was his father's favorite. (Nevertheless, in a revealing slip, the patient said, the father "beat *me*" when he intended to say "beat *them*," meaning his siblings.) The family moved to a farm when the patient was five, and it eventually fell to the patient to do most of the work because his older brother was lazy. The father would pay the patient all of the money that was supposed to have been divided between himself and his older brother. More recently, the patient and the father have worked together in a weekend business that earns the patient extra money for his schooling.

The patient has always felt closer to his mother than to his father, and, indeed, has treated her as a confidant. As a high school student, when he had questions concerning relationships with girls, he turned to his mother for advice and counsel. The father would often return late from his drinking bouts after work, so the time he could spend with his father was limited. The patient also reported that his parents frequently argued over money.

The patient described the three brothers as constantly bickering and fighting with each other in an effort to establish a pecking order among the three of them. When he was smaller, the oldest brother would "lord it" over the other two brothers and make them his "slaves." All three brothers would force their younger sister into being their joint "slave." Although a mediocre student in elementary and high school, the oldest brother did earn a degree in a profession, and he practices in a nearby city. The next older brother is attending college and working toward a degree. The patient always did better in school than his siblings; in particular, he was an academic and athletic star in high school. Indeed, from the patient's account, high school was a quite gratifying experience for him. His social life blossomed as did his academic and athletic career. When he graduated from high school, he enrolled in a technical institute some distance from home, planning to follow a profession related to his father's own interests and background. After two years at this relatively remote school, the patient decided to transfer to a larger university to complete his degree in the technical field he had chosen. At the university, he started to encounter difficulties. His academic ranking began to slip, and he began to do poorly in many of his courses and on his examinations. His social life became quite limited, and he no longer enjoyed relationships with young women as he had during his high school years and, to a lesser extent, at the technical institute he attended prior to coming to the university.

The family is Catholic and the patient considers himself to be a devout Catholic. He attends church as often as he can and tries to follow the church proscriptions of premarital sex and masturbation. Although he has engaged in sex with a number of young women, he does so with guilt and often suffers from premature ejaculation. He sees women who would sleep with him as morally loose and assumes they are probably sleeping with other men. He would not marry a woman with whom he had had sex. With some considerable anxiety, he described masturbating in high school, but he has not masturbated since. He denied having any homosexual experiences.

As a junior with a barely passing average he gave thought to changing to some other field, a move that he believed his family would support. At the same time, he was quite unclear about the field for which he should prepare himself. The phobic symptom developed in March of his junior year, following a disastrous performance on his final examinations and a brief vacation at a resort. He first noted the symptom while sitting with several male friends in the dormitory cafeteria. One of his friends had bought some fish and when he cut the fish open a foul odor emerged. The patient was revolted by the odor. When he attempted to swallow his own food, he began gagging. Over the next several months, his symptom grew worse. He couldn't tolerate being in any public eating place without experiencing considerable anxiety marked by shortness of breath, racing heart, nausea, a severe headache, and generalized tension, all of which would disappear immediately after leaving the public eating place. At first, the patient thought there was something physically wrong and visited several doctors. Nothing physical was discovered to account for his symptom. Finally, he went to see the psychiatrist at the student health service, who referred the patient to us.

INTERVIEWER'S PERSPECTIVE ON THE EVALUATION

Of particular note were several characteristics of this young man's behavior with the interviewer. Quite evidently, he was frightened. His voice would often falter and become a whisper. He seldom allowed himself to expand on his responses even when invited to do so. For the most part, he assumed a passive stance toward the interviewer, willing to respond to questions but with the fewest words possible. One did not sense that this was done defiantly or angrily; rather, he was made anxious and frightened by the position in which he perceived himself. Exactly what that position might have been was clarified by two further events during the course of the evaluation.

Both events occurred with respect to a quite meaningful dream he started to relate in the first psychodynamic interview. It was an anxiety dream in which a frightening male figure emerged from behind a chimney with a pistol while the patient was asleep. The patient screamed, awakening his brother who was sleeping nearby. The patient then imparted to the interviewer that he had a "feeling" in his throat that extended from his temple to the neck and he indicated the extent of the sensation with his hand. He added that it was a sensation similar to the one he experienced when he attempted to swallow while eating in a public place, except that the sensation was pleasant rather than unpleasant. In the second interview, he reported that he had become so upset after the first interview that he had approached a female residential assistant and, for two hours, recalled more and more of the anxiety dream, accompanied by much crying and relief. He had recalled that the figure behind the chimney was his best friend, John, who had actually come from behind the chimney with a sword while the patient was asleep, stuffed something in the patient's mouth to silence him, and then thrust the sword up through the bed and through the patient's throat. The patient had taken a girlfriend away from John not long before, but once she became interested in him the patient lost all feeling for her.

Several things are notable about these two events (the experience in the interview with its link to the phobia and the seeming abreactive retelling of the dream to the residential assistant). First, in contrast to the patient's laconic and inhibited style with the male interviewer, it was evident that he could more easily open up when confiding in a woman. This view was further supported by his description during the interviews of how his mother was often the confidante to whom he imparted the details of his relationships with girlfriends. These confidences placed his mother in a quasi-incestuous role. Second, one could infer from the reexperiencing of part of the dream in the office, with its explicit link to the phobic experience, that this was a transference in which the interviewer was experienced as the threatening male figure behind the chimney. If so, then the prevailing transference seemed to have taken the form of a passive homoerotic relationship employed defensively to fend off a retaliatory attack for his attempt at a displaced oedipal victory. More speculatively, one could surmise that he feared that the oedipal rival would thrust his penis into the patient's mouth, an action both desired and feared, for which the food he could not swallow was a substitute formation. At the same time, the oral locus of the symptom constituted an upward displacement from the more anxiety-arousing attack on his genitals, represented by the sword being thrust through the bed that he was lying on in the dream. As will be seen in what follows, there was additional evidence to support this understanding of the transference and the light that it threw on the unconscious conflict related to the symptom.

PSYCHODYNAMIC FORMULATION[1]

Patient's Conscious Description of Symptom

Patient's Quotes Concerning Conscious
Experience of Symptom

Excerpt 1

MR. C: Well, it . . . umm . . . at first . . . umm . . . I had trouble eating
. . . foods like meat and fish . . . inside the cafeteria . . . I lived in the . . . in
a dorm . . . last year . . . and . . . ah . . . gradually I couldn't . . . or . . . gradually the only foods I could eat were like cereal . . . and . . . umm . . . toast
. . . and then . . . around exam time I couldn't even eat at all . . .

Excerpt 2

MR. C: Umm . . . well, let's see . . . I think it started after I got back
. . . I went to south for the . . . for spring break . . . and . . . I think it started
after that and . . . well, the first . . . the first . . . umm . . . occurrence I can
remember . . . was . . . as . . . a friend of mine was eating fish . . . in the cafeteria and . . . umm . . . he took a bite of it and another person said, as a joke
you know, I can't believe you're eating the fish because . . . you never know
. . . where it came from . . . and . . . umm . . . well, and then he cut it open
and this awful smell came out and . . . umm . . . I thought I was going to
throw up *(chuckle)*, you know, after seeing my friend eat, you know, eat
that food *(chuckle)* . . . And . . . I guess that's the first time I can . . . remember . . . losing my appetite there . . . Umm . . . well, I lost my appetite
. . . and, I guess I felt like gag . . . I felt like gagging, sort of . . . like I wanted
to throw up but I . . . I knew I couldn't because there were so many people
around . . .

Excerpt 3

I: How do you feel when you take a bite?

MR. C: . . . Sort of claustrophobic . . . umm . . . and I guess I feel like
. . . umm . . . people are watching me too . . . Ah . . . like they're staring . . .
like . . . umm . . . everyone of them is staring at me, while I eat . . . and then
I tense up . . . and . . . I start swallowing a lot . . . but I'm not swallowing

---

[1] Refer to page 153 in Chapter 9 for the introduction to Psychodynamic Formulation and our use of judges' notes and patients' excerpts.

anything while I'm swallowing . . . Ummm . . . I have shorter breaths . . . umm . . . and I feel like going outside . . . and I get a headache . . . right here (*indicates temple*) . . .

Excerpt 4

I: And then what happens, once you're outside the cafeteria . . . what happens?

MR. C: . . . My appetite comes back . . . and . . . I lose my headache . . . and I feel fine . . .

Judges' Accounts of Patient's Description of Symptom

JUDGE 1: The patient's primary symptom is difficulty (and sometimes inability) swallowing food when he tries to eat. He was able to describe the initial circumstance in which he noticed this difficulty, that being in the dormitory cafeteria with two male friends, where one was eating some fish, the other friend was kidding the first about eating the fish, and when the first fellow cut open the fish pattie, the patient said "an awful smell" came out of the fish which made him feel like gagging or throwing up and he could no longer eat and had to leave. The patient is vague and unclear about the development of the symptom after that, though he says on some occasions when he attempts to eat he cannot swallow, he gets a headache in his temples, he feels like throwing up, his breathing is short, and he gets a "claustrophobic" feeling, meaning a wish to escape the situation and, particularly, go outside.

It should be noted that this primary symptom is a physiological or psychosomatic symptom; he sometimes couples it with anxiety over people watching him while he is attempting to swallow his food. However, he is quite equivocal about the connection between the symptom and the social context, sometimes seeming to say that he only has difficulty eating when people are watching and can eat alone but at other times saying that the difficulty with swallowing food occurs even when he is alone.

JUDGE 2: The patient describes experiencing a choking, gagging sensation upon eating, especially nonliquid food such as meat, for the past 6 months. To a variable extent, the problem has been compounded by a fear of eating or swallowing in public, leading, at times, to complete avoidance of cafeterias and restaurants and eating alone. Currently, however, he states it is less of a problem and that he can eat most kinds of food. It is hard to more exactly describe the patient's current symptom picture because he gave somewhat contradictory accounts of it.

He describes anxiety symptoms of increased heart rate and shallow breathing when attempting to swallow in public. He also feels watched and scrutinized in some way by people around him.

JUDGE 3: The patient mainly described his difficulty in swallowing foods, especially foods requiring a lot of chewing (steak and cheeses). He is able to identify the occasion on which the symptom began: He was sitting in the dormitory cafeteria with several of his friends, one of whom who had just opened a fish in preparation for eating it and then an awful smell was emitted by the fish which revolted the patient. He had to leave, unable to sit in cafeterias, feeling a tension in his throat, a kind of swelling up, a claustrophobic feeling that would prompt him to leave as he developed a headache, shortness of breath, racing heart, and possibly nausea as well. He also described general shyness, especially with his peers, some social phobic difficulties in classroom situations and at churches during such occasions as weddings.

JUDGE 4: Patient reports having trouble swallowing food especially food that he has chewed in public places. He feels "claustrophobic" in that he feels people are watching him eat, staring at him. His breathing changes, he tenses up, and gets a headache. His discomfort is alleviated as soon as he can get outside. He has lost 15 pounds owing to the restrictions imposed by his symptom.

Consensus on Patient's Conscious Experience of Symptom Following First CET Meeting

The patient described himself as having difficulty in swallowing foods in public, especially chewable foods such as steak and hard cheeses. The symptom began when he was sitting with two male friends in the dormitory cafeteria and one male friend "cut open" some fish in preparation for eating it and a foul odor was emitted by the fish. The patient felt revolted and from that point on his difficulty in swallowing became worse. He could not eat in the cafeteria at all after a while, although he could eat in his room. He described a variety of anxiety indicators such as shortness of breath, racing heart, nausea, and headache, all of which were relieved if he left the cafeteria. Nevertheless, some question remained as to the current status of the symptom, which had begun about 6 months before, as well as its character as a social phobia. There was some indication, to be followed up in the third psychodynamic interview, that he may not be suffering from the symptom at this time; there is also some evidence that the difficulty in swallowing at times also was present when he was eating alone, which would undermine the strictly social character of the phobia.

Patient's Understanding of Symptom

Patient's Quotes Concerning Understanding of Symptom

Excerpt 1

MR. C: . . . Well, in the last 6 months I've been having trouble eating food . . . well, at first I thought it was physical . . . but I went to many doctors and . . . ah . . . everyone . . . every doctor has said the same thing, that there is nothing wrong . . . physically . . . umm . . . and the last doctor that I went to thought that my problem with swallowing might be . . . through stress . . . and he recommended me to come here . . . .

Excerpt 2

MR. C: . . . it was exam time, I just . . . ah . . . ignored it, until the exams were over and . . . ummm . . . then I went . . . I went to a doctor in my home town, the family doctor, and he thought that it could be a . . . umm . . . a . . . hy-eenal [sic] hernia . . . which is a weak muscle in the diaphragm and . . . ah . . . the tests for that were negative and . . . umm . . . he thought that it was either mono or something else in the throat so he sent me to some other doctors . . . and they tested for . . . umm . . . well, no doctors could see anything physically wrong . . . umm . . . at all . . . *(chuckle)* . . . I had all sorts of tests and everything was negative.

Judges' Accounts of Patient's Understanding of Symptom

JUDGE 1: At first he thought he must be having a medical problem and he went to physicians for medical work-ups. He believed the glands in his throat were swollen and so a doctor gave him penicillin for this swelling and Maalox to help him with his food. He believes that the penicillin reduced the swelling in his glands but this did not cure the problem. Eventually it was suggested to him that it might be due to stress so he went to a mental health professional. He was impressed after our first interview with a possible connection between a recurrent anxiety dream he was having and both the tension in his throat when he has difficulty swallowing and the fear of people watching. Nonetheless, it did not seem that he had any further understanding other than merely an attention to these parallels between the symptom and aspects of the dream.

JUDGE 2: The patient has no real explanations of his symptoms except to relate his tenseness, crying, and disturbing dreams together in a loose fashion.

JUDGE 3: The swallowing difficulty the patient does not understand at all, although during the course of the first interview he recalled one dream in particular that he related to the swallowing difficulty because he began to experience a similar muscular tension from "his temple to his throat," which reminded him of the tension in his throat leading to the swallowing difficulty. However, in his recall of the dream when he experienced this muscle tension, he described it as actually feeling better than the tension during swallowing at mealtime and implying that the throat tension that he suffers from seemed to be alleviated when he was recalling the dream. The patient saw a relationship by way of his experience but did not seem to have any understanding as to why the two might be related. On the whole, one could say that the patient has little or no understanding of the underlying psychological causes of his symptom. Initially, and for some time, he thought the difficulty was physical and had it checked out on a number of occasions, only to discover that there seemed to be no physical basis for his symptom, but he was advised that likely the 'cause was "stress."

JUDGE 4: "NIL."

Consensus Following First CET Meeting

The judges agreed that the patient had little insight into the psychological causes for his swallowing difficulty, although he appeared to have some intuitive sense that it was related to dreams he has had off and on for the past several months. He volunteered one dream in particular, having to do with a young man watching him from a chimney and then pulling out a pistol and pointing it at him. It was especially important that during the time he related the dream to the interviewer he experienced a particular sensation in his musculature from the temple to the "center of the throat" that he felt was reminiscent of the kind of tension he felt in his throat when he could not swallow. At the same time, however, this particular kind of tension felt "better." Aside from this relationship by way of a somatic experience, it could not be said that the patient had any understanding of the reasons for his symptom.

Conscious symptom words selected

Shorter breaths	Cafeteria
Heart faster	Headache
Rotten fish	Nauseous
Swallowing	Tense up

The words selected for the conscious symptom category describe both the phobic setting (cafeteria), the elements of the phobic experience (swallowing and rotten fish), and the phobic anxiety state (shorter breaths, heart faster, headache, nauseous, and tense up).

Unconscious Conflict Underlying Symptom

Discerning the salient aspects of the unconscious fantasies underlying the symptom was particularly difficult with this patient, owing to the complexity of his pathology and the defensive manner in which he presented himself. To overcome these difficulties, an extra evaluation interview and CET meeting were required. During the four evaluation interviews and the subsequent three CET meetings, there was a shift in the judges' opinions: early, they saw him as potentially vulnerable to psychotic regression; later, they felt he was highly conflicted and regressed from oedipal-level conflicts. The judges agreed on the existence of a wide discrepancy between tests and interviews; the patient's potential for decompensation; his sadistic fantasies, social inhibitions, homoerotic conflicts, and oedipal fantasies. To facilitate readers' following the threads of agreement, the judges' comments concerning the above content are printed in bold type in the transcripts.

As before, we begin with quotations from the interviews.

Patient's Quotes Related to Unconscious Conflict

Excerpt 1

MR. C.: I'm not sure when the dream started but . . . ah . . . it was last . . . last spring or last winter . . . Umm . . . well, the first time I can recall the dream happening as . . . I was . . . ah . . . I fell asleep on the couch at home . . . at my parents' house and . . . umm . . . my brother was on another couch, there's two couches, and . . . umm . . . we have a wood stove with a . . . a chimney going up and . . . ah . . . I was dreaming that someone was standing on the other side of the chimney . . . and . . . ah . . . umm . . . everyone was around me but only I could see him . . . I was on the couch . . . and . . . umm . . . I was dreaming that my brother was asleep like he was, on . . . the other couch too . . . and the person . . . umm . . . I knew he was there and he kept peeping over and looking at me *(chuckle)* . . . and . . . ah . . . and then he pulled out a gun . . . and . . . my brother said . . . or everyone in the house said that I screamed . . . right . . . right now I've got this feeling . . . right here in my throat . . . about from here to here *(indicates temple to throat)* . . . I've never had this feeling before . . . umm . . . it's . . . it's like there's one big muscle from my temples to my . . . the center of my throat . . . No, it's not uncomfortable . . .

Excerpt 2

MR. C.: Well, I was trying . . . I was trying to figure out who . . . who the person was that was looking at me . . . or the person that was staring at me in the dream . . . *(clears throat)* . . . and . . . umm . . . and what had happened . . . in the dream and . . . umm . . . it seemed like whenever I cried something . . . something new came into my mind about what happened . . . in the dream . . . and . . . umm . . . and . . . I thought that I . . . I thought that I understood the dream better . . . well, what I thought had happened was . . . umm . . . I thought I figured out who the person was . . . and he was . . . umm . . . I thought he was my best friend . . . back home . . . or my best friend during . . . my high school days . . .

Judges' Accounts of Unconscious Conflict Underlying Symptom

JUDGE 1: On the basis of the interviews and tests, the following stand out as salient aspects of this case: The patient appears to have developed a primarily hysterical defensive repertoire. **He gives much evidence of repression, denial, and minimization of the affective significance of his experiences,** particularly experiences that are sexual in nature or have an unconscious sexual meaning. He reports no awareness of sexual fantasies, no awareness of an urge to masturbate, avoidance of ejaculation through masturbation, current avoidance of sexual intercourse, current avoidance of dating; he minimizes the significance of his father's drinking, his competition with his brothers. Although embarrassed by his recent habit of sleeping with his parents, he also seems to minimize the oddness of a 20-year-old man sleeping in his parents' bed because he is made afraid by nightmares. He also repressed the wish to sleep with them by recalling that he goes to sleep in his own bed but somehow wakes up in theirs.

Turning to the symptom and unconscious conflict underlying it, I draw attention to the dreams the patient reported and to the very obviously "loaded" nature of the dream regarding the guy peeping from behind the chimney and pulling out his pistol. This dream was associated with much affect in the interview, a wish to cry and some strong sensations in his throat. He clearly associated this dream with his symptom through the parallel of people watching and the sensations in his throat represented in both. The symbolism in this dream, for example chimney, pistol, peeping, guy, and the associations to the dream, for example "one big muscle" in his throat, "it was hot," "like someone was massaging," like "blood was rushing fast," along with indications from the testing suggesting gender identity confusion, and **unconscious homoerotic wishes, suggest to me that the**

primary unconscious conflict underlying his symptom involves homoerotic wishes, possibly including a wish to suck on a penis, swallow semen, and/or be orally impregnated. Consistent with this interpretation are some suggestions of projection and mild paranoia, for example the guy peeping at him is threatening harm with his pistol, the themes of males harming or exploiting other males in the TAT. For example, the story of a young man who is being hypnotized by an older man in order to gain some information from the younger man, and a story of a man who kidnapped another man who had "swallowed" something and was being cut up by two other men. This latter story strikes me as coming very close to epitomizing the nature of this patient's unconscious conflict because it involves only males, it repeats the symptom in that one man has "swallowed" something, it repeats one aspect of the situation when the symptom started, i.e., the idea of something being "cut open"—in the cafeteria it was the fish, in the dream one of the men—and the notion that there might be something like a treasure inside the man who was cut open could suggest an oral impregnation fantasy. Perhaps the "awful smell" that came out of the fish in the cafeteria is a compromise formation that is more loaded by defensive components.

Having proposed a possible unconscious conflict underlying the symptom, I want to add two observations that lead to the conclusion that **the patient may not be appropriate for our research:** (1) his problem may more accurately be diagnosed in the DSM-III-R category of conversion disorder rather than in the social phobia category. I say this because his primary complaint really is a physical symptom—difficulty swallowing food—and although he sometimes couples this symptom with eating in public, he also decouples it from a social context by stressing that sometimes he couldn't even eat while alone. Thus, if we compare the social anxiety component in this patient with of some of our other patients, it seems rather secondary in this case and secondary to a physical symptom that is most likely the conversion of a psychological conflict; (2) **the ego weaknesses that I described as emerging on the psychological testing suggest he may be in the midst of or at least prone to a decompensation into an acute psychotic state,** whether this be a hysterical psychosis or a schizophrenia spectrum disorder. It is worth noting that the increased stress of his transferring to a more highly competitive academic environment where his verbal IQ of 99 provides him with no special advantage and may even put him at a disadvantage, has likely contributed to his current decompensation.

If a decision is made to go ahead with this patient in spite of the above observations about diagnosis and ego weakness, there are several topics it might be well to explore in a third psychodynamic interview: In connection with **my hypothesis of homoerotic wishes underlying his symptom,** I make special note that we know too little about his relationships with men; very little detail regarding his relationship with his dad except we know he is currently dad's favorite and that he probably has identified with his dad in several ways, for example the choice of a related technical field, the working together on weekends, and perhaps a slip he made regarding having "blacked out" on his tests is an unconscious identification with dad's drinking. We also have little specific detail regarding his relationship with his roommate, with whom he has been living for two years.

In a further interview, it might be well to ask him whether he has had any other experiences that have frightened him and/or puzzled him, even if these experiences are very difficult to speak of. Here I would be giving him permission and encouraging him to talk about other experiences of ego weakness that he has had that he may wish to forget or even sexual experiences he may have had that he would prefer to forget.

I would also like to ask him what he didn't like about his experiences with drugs and what drugs he has experimented with. He mentioned not liking this and I wonder whether he had some quasi-psychotic experiences when he experimented with drugs.

I would also like to know more, if possible, regarding his reactions and his parents' reactions to his sleeping with them. For example, are both parents always in the bed, does he sleep in the middle or on the side with one or the other parent, is there any physical contact, and how does he feel about it if there is.

JUDGE 2: **The patient appears to be a somewhat naive, perhaps schizoidally shy person who is struggling with developmental issues relating to masculinity and assertiveness.** If we take his major symptom to be his social phobia (i.e., eating in public), we have to explain what affect or conflict he projects and the meaning of the displacement he uses.

The psychological testing, more than the interviews, suggests that phallic–competitive and negative oedipal issues predominate **with a tendency to regression to oral sadistic and accompanying defenses against it.**

I understand the patient to have a vaguely developed sense of being a male. He left a technical institute two years ago (perhaps out of a fear of competition for girls there) and once at the university felt increasing pressures to perform well academically. As he struggled with this task, **he systematically inhibited himself from relationships with girls, casual or serious, except in fantasy.** His eating phobia, specifically a swallowing phobia, must be seen as occurring against the background of regressive pulls to earlier modes of functioning. He describes two things that are significant for deeper understanding of the symptom about to ensue. He is increasingly in the sole company of men; he takes unexpectedly and uncharacteristically a course in theater and experiences a mental block upon reading two plays which have clearly triggered underlying incestuous conflicts (*Lysistrata* and *Oedipus Rex*). He then witnesses, with horror and disgust, a male friend eating rotten fish and forthwith experiences his swallowing phobia. In view of the previous difficulties he describes, i.e., overclose relationship to mother and a chronically unsuccessful attempt at beating his brothers for father's attention except when he assumes prephallic, infantile, dependent characteristics, I believe the rotten fish represents the ambivalently loved object that he has prized for so long but felt never able to obtain one for himself—namely, a penis. This view I feel most closely matches the circumstances of the patient's history—the general inhibitions, perhaps a constitutional intellectual deficit leading to more than average concern about phallic competence, and the **rage at not being able to compete successfully for father's role.** The orality implied in the symptom I feel is best accounted for by **the patient's unconscious wish to wrest masculinity from men by orally incorporating their penises.** In a TAT story, for example, he sees a man as having swallowed a key which is retrieved by cutting open the man. This also lends support to the cannibalistic wishes the patient harbors that are represented by the phobic avoidance of meaty food as opposed to liquid food.

A primary oral fixation as the cause of the symptom seems unlikely, or at least not well supported by the material in the interviews we have so far. One thought would be that intellectual deficits, if it can be labeled that in this patient, may well predispose him to quick regression to oral satisfaction and hysterical, fleeting identifications.

JUDGE 3: The tests amply attest to the nature of the fantasies underlying the patient's conversion symptom. Moreover, they cast some doubt on my original impression from the interviews that we are dealing with a classically hysterical conversion. If one would maintain a hysterical diagnosis, one would need to qualify it in the direction of describing that the patient's repressive defenses are in the midst of breaking down and **his fantasies are infiltrated with excessively aggressive, violent, and sadistic imagery.** Much of the inhibitions visible in the interviews—his monosyllabic answers, his being close to tears at times, etc.—may now be understood as his struggling against these waves of internally disturbing fantasies. **Mainly, as part of the regressive picture emerging in the tests, we see an emphasis on the violent sadistic teasing infighting among siblings, plotting and counterplotting in various subgroupings against each other.** The prize or treasure that is the reward for the one who will triumph is only dimly hinted at. In other words, **the triangular nature of the oedipal conflict is almost totally obscured by the regression into violent, sadistic, and homoerotic battles going on between men.** From the tests, it would appear that the patient's present adjustment is sorely threatened by this surge of fantasy and repression in his defenses so that one would anticipate that he cannot continue to do well in school and will likely go under without some kind of fairly immediate help. The line of regression is fairly clear: He will return home and try to become much closer to mother in an infantile way and surrender his ambitions to triumph over brother and father. A TAT story that seems to most clearly reflect the fantasy related to the swallowing difficulty involves an account of a young man who plots to turn over another man to accomplices who cut him open in order to retrieve a key to a treasure he has **swallowed.** We can surmise that the patient is the one who has swallowed the key to the treasure, as well as being the one to attack and obtain the key to the treasure. It is reminicient of the dream with the man watching who points a gun at the patient, as well as to the element in the experience that triggered the swallowing difficulty—the fish being cut open and the awful smell coming out.

Careful note should also be taken concerning the very widespread, voyeuristic elements in the dream that at times results in an effort to cover up the eyes and not see, and at other times, it is related to more paranoid and homoerotic impulses. Speculatively, one might relate this to his primal scene experiences that are not only likely fantasies but have some reality to them.

Careful consideration should be given to the possibility of a psychotic process underlying his current problems. Looking back at the interviews from the vantage point of the tests, one would see the patient's readiness at the age of 20 to sleep with his parents when frightened as a highly pathological act.

The questions raised in my mind for the third evaluation interview are as follows: (1) greater detail concerning the patient's relationship to his mother in particular; (2) more history as to what happened when he was on spring break before the phobia appeared; (3) more information about his early relationships with his siblings and, in particular, his older brother and his sister; (4) diagnostically, one would need to be worried about this young man right now in terms of the precariousness of his current adjustment and we should consider some effort to get him into treatment fairly quickly.

JUDGE 4: It would appear that swallowing something symbolically associated with a bad fishy odor, having a muscle in your head, in the presence of men **threatens his homosexual defenses.**

The multiple leveled aspect of his symptom is further complicated by his association to the time he blocked on a test when having to write about *Oedipus Rex* and *Lysistrata*. We do not know what aspects of these two plays he was reacting to, however, the major theme of *Oedipus Rex* is typically heterosexual and oedipal though the punishment aspect is very strong and primitive.

It appears that he experienced his father as being bossy with older brothers but not him. In fact, he is thought to be the favorite. Further, his older brothers were bossy and controlling of him and he had a passive role thrust on him in the sibship. Did his brothers pass on to him an even more primitive version of parenting than they received from their father? It sounds like father receded more into the background for him than for his oldest brother.

In his history, he reveals a fairly sadistically deprecated view of women (sister slave, mother selfless) that would possibly make a lively sexual involvement with women too threatening to his defenses against his sadism ("sex ruins relationships"), which may in turn heighten his homoerotic interest.

His father's alcoholism could attest to an atmosphere not conducive to working through oral issues.

What further kinds of sexual acting out could be expected to occur in a situation where a college-level son would be invited to share the parental bed without it seeming to be a notable occasion? It is clear that he is a fairly inhibited young man, though he seemed to have been more outgoing in high school.

The testing reveals a much more serious pathology than was evident in the interviews. In general, the testing reveals—to the extent that people really matter, an almost exclusive overriding oral-sadistic fixation to the male phallus, which in turn fires intense murderous competition with males who might get or have what he wants. Women do not appear to have or be much to him except as possessions of another man that may be taken.

Boredom, a sense of loss, helping someone who has lost something, revenge, are the only feelings acknowledged. **Remorseless murder, mutilation, rape, sneakily taking advantage of, all in the service of greed and revenge constitute the range of human actions, with men as the main players.**

Women are not depicted as offering anything or as having emotions even during upsetting events. Even murderous impulses, so rampant in men, are denied in women.

The Rorschach depicts a stark, nightmarish peopleless world of fragile, frayed, torn, worn, malformed, or, at best, poorly defined percepts.

Clinical Questions

1. What about the possibility that *Lysistrata* and *Oedipus Rex* caused the block?
2. Has he had any homosexual relationships or times when he felt uneasy around men?
3. Has he had any instances of being selfish and cunning?
4. What's it like when his father is drunk?
5. What makes sex so disruptive?
6. Regarding the associations to elements of the gunman and rolling-stone dreams, why did he have those dreams when he did?

7. Did anything else happen around age 7–8?
8. His parents have money, and he works. Yet his parents take his car. How dependent is he currently on his parents and in what ways?

Diagnostic Questions

1. WAIS scores were lower than would have been anticipated from his high school activities, his acceptance at the university, and the manner in which he expressed himself in the interviews. Further, the profile of subtests did not indicate regression from a higher level of functioning.
   a. Do his tests reflect an intense "brother transference" to the tester? If this were so, by its instantaneous and highly regressive nature it would still *bespeak severe pathology.*
2. Has the patient used more drugs than he has claimed?
3. Is there so little about women because he is repressing intense, developmentally higher-level feelings?
   a. "Divorce" was one form of revenge, as if he had a fantasy that his mother's divorce would avenge his oedipal disappointment.
   b. Is he repressing intense rage at the image of a murderous mother (perhaps a projection) and thus needing to get his supplies from the man's breast/penis?
   c. Is his sexuality for men and women repressed or are his sexual yearnings preempted by his hate and perhaps an early developmental arrest?
   d. Is the whole testing picture a massive, regressive, defensive position against homoerotic feelings?

Consensus Following First CET Meeting

In this evaluation, we were all struck by the considerable discrepancy between the patient's way of presenting himself in the interviews and what appeared on the psychological tests. In the interviews, there was general agreement that the patient presented himself as a greatly inhibited, repressed youngster suffering from a social phobia in the form of a conversion reaction. Although there were hints of something more serious—in particular, the patient's readiness to accept the parents' invitation to share their bed when he became frightened recently, after the dream mentioned above—on the whole, the picture seemed to point to an intense, competitive struggle with older brothers. The competition with the older of the two brothers had both phallic–oedipal and sadistic overtones. On the other hand, the psychological tests revealed a starker picture of a young man struggling to keep afloat in the midst of powerful sadistic fantasies and conflicts. The tests also showed evidence of marked disturbance in his thinking, suggesting the possibility that he was struggling against a psychotic decompensation, possibly schizophrenic or paranoid.

We agreed that, unless the third psychodynamic evaluation interview would clarify the nature of his severe decompensatory potential, it would be unwise to have him continue in the experiment and we should work out a treatment recommendation for him as quickly as possible. The possibility exists that some traumatic episode in his recent experience might account for the severity of his current psychological status. One candidate might be some sort of homosexual episode that happened during his recent vacation in February, just preceding the appearance of the symptom. Another possibility is a pathological grief reaction to a loss. If it can be determined that there has been a recent trauma, a different light may be cast on the patient's psychological status. If, for example, some abreaction could be obtained in the interview and the possibility of further helpful abreaction could be assessed, then he might be considered as a subject for the laboratory. However, it is unlikely that this would prove to be the case.

The judges decided that the approach in the third interview would be to initially present him with our concerns about his current status and to elicit from him any further information that might clarify what is going on with him now. If the same kind of resistance is encountered as in the previous interviews, namely his monosyllabic responses, a mild transference interpretation might be used along the following lines: "It seems like it is hard for you to talk, perhaps because these are tough things to talk about, especially with an older man. It might be easier for you to talk about them with a woman, since you are able to talk about these things with your mother." This approach may not succeed, but it might have a chance. In any case, the major purpose of the interview would be to discover quickly the extent of the patient's current pathology and his awareness of it, possibly to determine what the specific etiology might be (e.g., traumatic) and to work out a treatment recommendation with the patient. If necessary, a fourth interview might prove useful.

A number of areas might be pursued if it seems useful to do so.

1. The current status of his symptom.
2. The social aspects of his symptom.
3. The parental relationship with the patient, in particular the father's alcoholism and the context in which he so readily can be invited into their marital bed.
4. More associations to the "chimney" dream.

5. Something more about the plays that caused him to go blank and seem to have been the beginning of his difficulties.
6. What exactly happened on his vacation.
7. Some exploration of the nature of his current ability to think.
8. Evidences about this person who died, as reported on the Texas Grief Inventory,[2] and what this might lead to.
9. Greater probing into the early tempestuous relationships with his two older brothers and younger sister—in particular, aspects of their sexual play, if any.

Judges' Accounts of Unconscious Conflict Following Third Psychodynamic Interview

JUDGE 1: The following are the pieces of material that seemed most important from the third psychodynamic interview. First, there were the new associations that emerged in his emotional talk with his resident assistant. Here, he identifies the person in his dream as a best friend from high school who used his "key" to get into the house, stuck something into the patient's mouth and over his nose, and proceeded to kill everyone in the house. It is very interesting that the "key" which was so central in a TAT story shows up again here in association to the dream. It is also of note that the patient makes a slip or a negation of the idea that his brother was asleep "next to me." The dream also has a kind of paranoid tinge in that the fellow who sneaked into the house was out to hurt people and was "glad to see me in pain." In his relationship with the girl who was both his girlfriend and his friend's girlfriend, he again shows us that he has some unconscious motive for avoiding sexual intercourse. He provides another interesting but unclear association to the dream when he tells us that something is missing from his memory regarding the dream, that he knows something that happened before, but he can't recall it and this something that he knows is the reason why John was mad at him. I noticed in the context of this association he made another slip, saying "he woke up" and later changing it to "I woke up." This may suggest again the idea of sleeping with another man, i.e., if both he and the other fellow woke up they were both asleep and perhaps together. This is consistent with the negation mentioned earlier of the idea that his brother was asleep next to him. **Although there are suggestions of competitive issues with men, somehow in this material they seem quite secondary to suggestions of homoerotic conflicts. Although they could be related, somehow the homoerotic material and the paranoid tinges surrounding it,**

---

[2] A questionnaire used regularly in our initial screening of all subjects.

as well as the suggestions of ego weakness and potential psychotic decompensation seem most salient to me. Speaking of ego weakness, I would call attention to what seems to be a confusion in his mind between dreaming and perceiving: he talks about being able to "see" John sticking something into his mouth and over his nose while he is crying with the resident assistant— he says that when he was crying "it seemed real, like it happened." Because I believe that this material regarding John sticking something into his mouth and covering his nose so that he couldn't breathe is probably very close to the heart of the unconscious fantasies he is currently in conflict about, it makes sense that more regressive experiences like that just cited would be connected with it. I recalled that some peculiar references to where things breathe occurred a couple of times on the Rorschach and his reference to having something stuck over his nose in the dream and to his difficulty with the sinuses and his nostrils being clogged up I intuit to be unconsciously significant but I am not sure of precisely what the significance for him is. **His reference again to a "hot sensation" in his throat while exploring the dream seems consistent with a homoerotic interpretation.** I note that he interrupted the interviewer to tell another anecdote about suppression of aggression between himself and another fellow with whom he had been friends since childhood. However, whether this material has a primarily phallic competitive or disguised homoerotic significance is not clear and as I said above, in this case I am not comfortable with merely facilely linking the two. I might add here that I was not impressed with the significance of the death of his two grandmothers as potentially relevant to his current most salient unconscious conflict. I noticed that when the interviewer again approached the topic of his relationship with his father, there was not a lot of new material forthcoming and yet the patient's statement that he was "always asleep when he came home" may be a parallel with the dream. The context here was exploring the patient's feelings about his father coming home drunk. It might have been interesting to draw a parallel for the patient between the idea that he was always asleep when his father came home drunk and in the dream he is asleep when a menacing guy comes into their home, just to see whether this elicited any associations. I note the further associations that he produced about his difficulty falling asleep at home when he is upstairs in his room alone and feels like someone evil is there with him. Again, this underlines **the paranoid tinge to this patient's conflicts and further corroboration of associated homoereotic issues** are suggested when he says that the menacing individual is "behind me" and says that his fear is greater if he "lays on his back." He needs to turn over with his backside up to be somewhat more comfortable.

My conclusion from this interview is not much different from the prior interviews and testing. **I am impressed with the salience of homoerotic conflicts** that I suspect are quite directly related to his conscious symptom of difficulty swallowing. There is further quite a bit of suggestion of paranoia associated with these conflicts and **very worrisome suggestions of the possibility of a psychotic regression.** Although there are indications of hostile competitive issues regarding men and some suggestions of triangular oedipal material, **the pull toward the homoerotic seems most salient in his associations.** Moreover, I saw nothing in the third psychodynamic interview to overturn the massive evidence on the testing that severe regression was a potentiality. Indeed, I felt that the suggestions of paranoia and the suggestions of possible confusions between merely dreaming something and experiencing it as really happening underline the possibility of decompensation. Finally, I believe that even setting aside the issue of his apparently significant ego weakness, I still believe that his symptomatic problem more closely fits the spirit of the DSM-III-R diagnosis of conversion disorder than it fits the spirit of the diagnosis of social phobia. Although it might be possible to say that he meets the criteria for both, my clinical judgment is that he really more closely satisfies the spirit of the conversion disorder category.

JUDGE 2: The third psychodynamic evaluation interview enlarges on two issues previously brought up in the CET discussion and answers some questions **but leaves unclear the level to which this patient regresses, how psychotic and distorted his thinking can be, and illustrates the massive denial the patient uses to avoid facing homoerotic or, for that matter, any sexual issues.**

The issues that seemed more clear included the patient's openly paranoid distortions of reality with an accompanying feeling or belief about the presence of evil forces around him. This, together with the superficial and bland quality of his answers, suggests **serious problems with reality testing that fall short of psychosis,** I can explain only by invoking an extreme degree of naïveté and simple-mindedness. The term "inadequate personality" comes to mind in attempting to describe this clinical presentation. I would recommend a full mental status examination that would tap into any other existing psychotic symptom or distortion in order that we can more definitively put to test the degree of pathology this patient has and his ability to be a workable subject in the lab.

Another issue that is more clear is the **centrality of the homoerotic conflict in this patient** and his reliance on a regression to oral ties with a maternal figure in order to keep himself going. His clarification of the dream provides good evidence of the homoerotic conflict and the resulting paranoia. The way he tells about the dream, however, again leads to **questions about how well he tests reality.** I had the impression that his description of the dream mirrored the description of an actual event, even in his own mind. This brings up the issue of a traumatic occurrence in the past involving **homosexual seduction.** I wonder if the patient, as a result of his evaluation here, is proceeding to abreact, in more or less neurotic ways, via dream screens and so forth, and getting a fair amount of relief from the abreaction. This, incidentally, would bear on treatment recommendations, i.e., a carefully guided abreactive and supportive technique might be the most helpful therapy this patient can handle at this time. I would also not rule out the possibility of medications to contain this anxiety when he is with people.

The two instances of massive denial occur when the interviewer asks him about the real feelings he had during the time he was breaking up with John's former girlfriend. The patient gives a most confusing, muddled, and defensive answer—to the effect that all ended well and that he was not sexually involved.

A second occasion is when the interviewer attempts to question the patient about his experiences on spring break and he changes the subject to his conflicts about going into a profession related to his father's.

JUDGE 3: This young man poses some remarkable diagnostic questions. From the material in the third psychodynamic evaluation interview we learn that he has succeeded in unburdening his heart to a female residential assistant in his dormitory following the last interview. Mainly he talked for two hours about the dream that disturbed him so about the young person staring at him from behind the chimney who ended by pulling a gun. In the course of this abreaction, he was able to recall other details of the dream and in the course of the interview with me to further clarify the relationship of the dream to his current life. Essentially it comes down to this: The young person in the dream was a good friend of his, John, a young man his older brother's age who had moved into the parental home for two years after having been kicked out of his own place. The patient and he were fast friends. Indeed, the patient introduced John to a girl who was to become John's girlfriend. However, when John broke up with her ostensibly to go on to college, the patient picked up with her for a period of some four months, until he too left. It was evident from his description that he never quite thought of her as his girl, and he balked at having sexual intercourse with her, the one girl in high school he was close to with whom he did not. He turned out to be prophetic, because not long afterward John once again picked up with the girl. He was able to convey that the reason he identified the figure in the dream with John might have been that John was so mad at him and actually in the dream killed the family, was perhaps that he, the patient, had taken up with the girl. He denied any current feelings of regret over breaking up with her, nor does he talk about any strained relationships with John, although here again it was during the summer when all this happened that he did speak of some strains with John. Thus, on the level described so far, it would seem to be clearly oedipal in nature, in which the patient undertook to take a woman away from an older man (brother/father) to whom he was very close and then to anticipate this person's revenge on him. But, it is when we consider the nature of the revenge that the picture becomes more cloudy. The unusual event that happens in the dream, as the patient was able further to elaborate it during his talk with the residential assistant, was that at a certain point the figure in the dream attempted to stick something into his mouth and over his nose, as if to suffocate him (I am thinking of the several "mask" responses on the Rorschach). **Clearly this aspect of the dream bespeaks the anxiety or wish for a homosexual attack on him with the attendant anxiety.** If one were to pursue further an underlying homoerotic theme, one would need then to think of the patient's interest in John's girlfriend as the "female bridge" to John. It thus becomes clearer that not far behind the positive oedipal strivings is a **regressive, negative, oedipal solution in which he becomes the passive "female" victim of John's homosexual assault on him that is both exciting and revolting.** The emphasis in the dream on John having the key to the house so that he can get in is another level to the homoerotic aspect of this young man's worries. (Also recall the TAT story in which two men cut open another man in order to retrieve a key to a treasure.)

One can best put together the negative and positive oedipal aspects by arguing that the negative oedipal regression is an effort to forestall a castrative assault of the older, stronger male on the younger male who attempts to get the woman away from them. And, in this negative oedipal position, the patient strives to protect his genitals. He has to give up heterosexuality in order to protect his penis.

All this seems to make a bit more sense than it did before this interview, but, still, we have the disconcerting evidence that the patient at certain times, usually at home or in his mother's relatives' homes, experiences a sense of evil surrounding him as he goes to sleep. This **bespeaks a further regressive potential bordering on the psychotic.** He also hints that he has this experience of evil surrounding him under other circumstances as well. We may very well not know the whole story, as yet, about how disturbed he can become under the impact of his homosexual panic. Thus, it continues to be advisable to proceed very slowly and carefully with this young man, although one is impressed with the strength he has to pursue a psychological solution to his emotional dilemmas.

Very little further was learned about how he feels about sleeping in the parents' bed at his age. It seems to be acceptable to him, only a little embarrassing, but little more feeling of conflict than that. It would be wise to pursue this further in a fourth interview.

We also learn about his struggles at school and how he is considering changing his major, which would be a step away from outright competition with the older brother and perhaps with father. This again might be a protective move, a yielding up of the game to avoid attack.

At this point, I am not altogether convinced that we should rule out the laboratory procedure. He might very well be able to go through it without any difficulty. Also, I am reasonably convinced that he can benefit from psychotherapy with or without some kind of adjunctive medication for possible thought disorder. It is also probably a good idea to consider a woman as his therapist because it is apparent that he can speak much more fully and openly to women than he can to men.

JUDGE 4: The fourth judge did not change his previous impressions and questions (see pages 245–247).

Consensus Following Second CET Meeting

The third psychodynamic evaluation interview served to confirm further the seriousness of this young man's disturbance, although it did not settle the diagnostic issue altogether. There was no doubt among the four judges that the main unconscious conflict was a homoerotic one and that it was associated with disturbances in reality testing. We considered the likely diagnostic alternatives: (a) The patient has been struggling with and on the brink of a psychotic break for at least 2 years, since he left home for college; and (b) the patient is suffering from the consequences of a trauma involving some kind of homosexual experience that is considerably clouding the diagnostic picture at this time. We hoped that a fourth psychodynamic interview would help us decide between these two alternatives. A strategy for approaching the patient was agreed on: The interviewer should continue to convey his great concern about the patient and encourage him to talk more about any unusual experiences that he has had, like feeling a sense of evil or an evil presence at his bedside. If this line of inquiry results in eliciting more in the way of patent psychotic symptomatology, then the matter would rest there. If, on the other hand, this line did not produce any further support for a psychosis, then the approach would be to present to the patient our concern that he might have had some experience that has been greatly disturbing him and to explore the possibility of a trauma.

After discussion, we decided that the suitability of the patient as a subject in the laboratory would depend on the outcome of the fourth interview. If the patient gave explicit evidence of a psychosis or of being on the brink of a psychotic episode, this evidence would contraindicate his suitability for the lab. On the other hand, if it seemed to be traumatic in origin or revealed itself as a severe neurotic difficulty (quite unlikely), then we would go ahead with the laboratory. The interviewer agreed to check with the other three judges for their vote on the basis of material in the fourth interview.

*Judges' Accounts of Unconscious Conflict Following Fourth
Psychodynamic Interview*

JUDGE 1: My main overall reaction to the fourth interview is that it underlines the well-known insight that clinicians gradually learn more and more about the unconscious conflicts of patients that they interview for long periods of time. It is often noted in our meetings that we would only really know the unconscious fantasies and conflicts underlying a symptom after one or more years of analysis. Specifically, with regard to this subject, I noticed that my perspective on his unconscious conflicts and the level of severity of his psychopathology fluctuates depending on which piece of information I've most recently read. I think it would be a very interesting thing if we decided that the most accurate assessment of this patient was very, very far different from that which would have been based on the testing alone. To me this calls into question whether the testing by itself is sometimes quite misleading. What I am leading up to with regard to this patient is my sense, based on the fourth psychodynamic interview, that **perhaps oedipal-level conflicts are quite salient.** First, let me enumerate the most important pieces of information I gleaned from the fourth interview.

I thought **the patient convincingly denied psychotic experiences.** On the question of the possibility of actual trauma, it is very interesting that he lost his concentration when the interviewer asked him about this. Nonetheless, this does not mean that he did experience a trauma, rather his loss of concentration might well be explained if the interviewer's question activated his need for repression because it came close to an unconscious fantasy of his rather than a memory of an actual trauma. The subject very nicely reports a free association to this loss of concentration—the memory of being scared when Tom Sawyer was chased by a big evil looking man in a movie he saw as a boy. This underlines again the fact that the evil presence this patient is consciously and unconsciously afraid of is male. Earlier in the interview he elaborates a bit more on his experience of being threatened by an evil presence in the room when he is at home and falling asleep. He says that the fear is that an evil presence will stab him or stick a sword through his neck. So far, these pieces of information tend to give less weight to the possibility of a psychosis and I think somewhat less weight to the possibility of an actual trauma. They are, however, **quite consistent with my previous formulation of homoerotic fantasies and fears tinged with paranoia.** However, prior to this interview I was more reluctant to link homoerotic themes with phallic competitive and oedipal themes. **In the latter part of this interview the salient pieces of information seemed to me to point more toward oedipal and phallic competitive issues.** For example, he tells about taking the girl back to his house and then when he sensed that he might successfully make sexual advances to her, he abruptly fell asleep. He identifies a pattern of finding a girl who doesn't know him or he feels perhaps doesn't like him, getting her to like him, and then losing all interest in her. **This could clearly be interpreted as oedipal material.** I would like to note, parenthetically, that he uses a very peculiar phrase in talking about this girl he brought back to his house, one that my intuition tells me probably is related to some salient unconscious fantasy of his, though I am not entirely sure what it is. The phrase is: "I was afraid to open up to the girl." **Also suggestive of oedipal conflicts** is the fact that his voice dropped noticeably when the interviewer asked about close physical contact in his parents' bed, and, after this, he came up with an association regarding having sex with his mom, but consistent with his need to see the threat as coming from another male he externalized the source of this idea onto the interviewer.

To sum up, even after the fourth interview the **words and phrases that I feel most certainly relate to his unconscious conflict are words and phrases that reflect the homoerotic themes.** However, I would probably also raise my ratings of words and phrases that reflected phallic competitive themes, castration anxieties, and **oedipal fantasies.**

JUDGE 2: The fourth psychodynamic interview again shows no **gross evidence of psychotic features** except for the feeling of evil forces around him and a continuing fear of sleeping, for fear that someone might be in the room with him. As in previous interviews, there was a lack of clear discrimination in his mind as to whether these experiences were real or unreal. I did not see any material that indicated the patient clearly and unhesitatingly rejected distortions in reality testing.

On the whole, however, **I do not think he is psychotic nor do I feel he has any immediate danger of becoming psychotic.**

Otherwise, the interview material confirms the centrality of **negative oedipal issues** and the **strong feminine identification** that we saw in previous interviews. Phallic and oral issues remain in the forefront but seem unclear as to their relationship to the symptom picture the patient presents.

JUDGE 3: As a result of the fourth psychodynamic interview, it seems like **we can eliminate the presence of an active psychosis** at this time, as well as the role of a trauma overtly available to the patient's awareness. There was, in fact, a hint in the fourth psychodynamic interview that there may be some repressed traumatic event, something that happened during his sleep, or as he was falling asleep, which can be inferred from the nature of the frightening dreams he has reported, including the most recent one of being stabbed through the neck as he was lying in bed asleep. Also, there is an interesting TAT story in which the hypnotist extracts information from the young man on the bed without his knowing it. But, there is considerable repression, if indeed such an experience occurred. It is possible that it is linked to a previous roommate. Unfortunately, I forgot to explore further what happened between these two young men that led to the patient deciding to leave that teaching institution. However, I somehow doubt that anything more would have been obtained.

The fourth psychodynamic interview leads me to give greater weight than before to conflict centered around women and, presumably, the mother. There is enormous hostility toward women, as evident in the pattern he identifies in his relationship to women; he tries to get them interested in him and once they are he loses interest in them. Indeed, he loses any sexual excitement at that point. The possibility of premature ejaculation also suggests that there is much conflict, aggression, and anxiety surrounding close and intimate relationships with women, even though he describes an overt good and close relationship (perhaps overly close) with his mother. Although it is tempting and makes good sense to identify the conflict as basically an early pre-oedipal one centering around oral issues and perhaps beginning around the time that the patient's younger sister was born, **there seems so much else in the material of a clearly oedipal and phallic nature that clouds the picture.** Nor does it seem as easy as with some other cases to resolve the difficulty by considering the patient as having defensively regressed into an earlier position. There is too much evidence, in particular on the tests, of thought pathology that ordinarily would not go along with this kind of picture. **It is evident that the patient is struggling with an enormous amount of sadistic rage and aggression that is directed both at women and at men in what would appear to be a defensive regressive position to protect against homosexual attack.** There do not seem to be any reliable defenses against such hostility except for the evident repression and avoidance. We do not see strong evidences for reaction formation or isolation. His main presentation is that of a pleasant, compliant, agreeable, and stressed young man.

JUDGE 4: Although many initially vague impressions and questions remained the same, I felt that the indications for oedipal-level functioning found in the fourth psychodynamic interview made it much more likely that the patients current level of functioning was a regression from a higher level of functioning due to some, perhaps homosexual, trauma.

Final Consensus Following Third CET Meeting

The judges generally agreed that a *psychotic regression could be ruled out* and that the patient could safely be put through the laboratory procedure. Stronger evidence emerged for an oedipal-level conflict with a regressive pull toward a negative oedipal solution with prominent homoerotic features. Specifically, support for this hypothesis was provided by the patient's account of how he took up with the girlfriend of his best friend (John) and then refused to have sex with her when she indicated her readiness to do so.

Further support is provided by the patient's identification of a threatening figure behind the chimney in his anxiety dream as John, who in the dream thrusts a sword under the bed the patient is lying on and penetrates through the patient's throat. Although the homoerotic regression was clear enough by this point, some concern remained about a possible early trauma and persistent underlying sadistic impulses and violent fantasies, mainly emerging on the tests. The judges felt that these might largely be accounted for by the acute decompensation in defenses this young man is experiencing. On the positive side, the judges strongly felt that the patient demonstrated a capacity for psychological-mindedness and an ability to work hard in treatment, as evidenced by his persistent exploration of the chimney dream over the course of the evaluation.

Unconscious conflict words selected

Massaging muscle	On my back
Ripped apart	Stab me
Parent's bed	John
Men hugging	Evil

The words related to the unconscious conflict include words representing the feared castrative attack (ripped apart, stabbed me, evil), as well as the negative oedipal solution (massaging muscle, men hugging). Several other words might be said to condense both aspects of the conflict (parents' bed, on my back, John).

DEBRIEFING MEETING FOLLOWING LABORATORY SESSION

Record lost.

LABORATORY RESULTS

For hypothesis 1 the total percentage of classification success in the expected direction for the conscious symptom words (supraliminal greater than subliminal) and the unconscious conflict words (subliminal greater than supraliminal) was 14.57% (group average = 8.57%).

The average for the three subjects was 9.68%, slightly above the group average of 8.57%, indicating that these 3 subjects constituted a relatively unbiased selection from the larger group of 11 subjects.

CONCLUSIONS

Implications and Future Directions

> I propose we use the most natural strategy, what I call the *natural method*, to see if it can be made to work.
> Tactically, what I have in mind is this. Start by treating three different lines of analysis with equal respect. Give phenomenology its due. Listen carefully to what individuals have to say about how things seem. Also, let the psychologists and cognitive scientists have their say. Listen carefully to their descriptions about how mental life works. . . . Finally, listen carefully to what neuroscientists say . . . and examine the fit between their stories and the phenomenological and psychological stories.
> —OWEN FLANAGAN, *CONSCIOUSNESS RECONSIDERED*
> (1992, p. 11)

If we were constrained to choose a single, most important contribution our research makes, we would underscore the innovative value of our method to understanding the role of the unconscious in how the mind works. Without the three equally essential constituents of our method—psychodynamic, cognitive, and neurophysiological—we would not have discovered the pattern of convergent findings that provides independent evidence for the existence of a dynamic unconscious and unconscious conflict. As we had hoped, the strengths of each method contributed uniquely to the outcome, and the weaknesses of each method were compensated for by the complementary strengths of the others.

Notably, a method we worked out independently for our own purposes had also occurred to the philosopher of mind Owen Flanagan, who referred to it as the *natural method* in his book *Consciousness Reconsidered* (1992). As defined in the chapter opening quote, taken from a section entitled "Subjectivity, Objectivity, and the Natural Method," Flanagan offers his method as the best method for studying consciousness. The three essential constituents for Flanagan are the phenomenological, cognitive, and neurophysiological. Flanagan's three constituents closely parallel our own. The psychodynamic approach draws on the phenomenology of subjective experience; the subliminal and supraliminal laboratory approach draws on cognitive science; and the ERP measure draws on neurophysiology.

Flanagan proposes one important guideline for the application of this natural method: "The only rule is to treat all three—the phenomenological, the psychology, and the neuroscience—with respect" (1992, p. 11), by which he means that no one method is presumed to have the entire truth but each has something important to contribute to a fuller understanding. We could not agree more, and we believe that our version of the natural method, as Flanagan anticipated, pays dividends in new scientific findings and enhanced clarification of otherwise opaque concepts, such as the unconscious. Flanagan further observes that the natural method is seldom (if ever) practiced. Perhaps this is the case because most scientists and clinicians are firmly committed to only one of the three approaches and have difficulty respecting the others. We offer our application of the natural method as evidence of its potential power, and we encourage others to explore its worth for their own purposes.

In this chapter, we examine a number of issues brought to light by the application of our method and its findings, respond to possible objections and shortcomings, and point to fruitful future directions. We begin with a brief historical reprise.

The Historical Origins of Research on the Unconscious in Psychoanalysis and Cognitive Psychology

The first hint of what would later develop into the field of subliminal research, ironically, made its appearance in a footnote to a later edition (1919) of Freud's turn-of-the-century masterpiece, *The Interpretation of Dreams*. In a rare display of interest in experimental and nonpsychoanalytic research, Freud praised a method developed by his Viennese compatriot Otto Poetzl, as an "important contribution" with a "wealth of implications . . . [that] go far beyond the sphere of dream interpretation as dealt with in the present volume" (1900/1953, pp. 181–182). The "important contribution" was Poetzl's invention of the subliminal method. This method would, many years later, be successfully picked up by Fisher, a psychoanalytic researcher who launched a highly influential program of research based on the Poetzl procedure.

In the period between 1954 (when Fisher's first report appeared) and 1971, there was an outpouring of subliminally based research conducted largely by psychoanalytically oriented researchers. This body of work was described in a scholarly review of the field by Dixon, trenchantly entitled *Subliminal Perception: The Nature of a Controversy* (1971). The controversy was generated by behavioral psychologists who validly criticized the experimental design and insufficient controls in early subliminal studies. Behaviorists used these critiques to support their theoretical claim that the unconscious was a pseudoscientific concept. For behaviorists, psychology was the science of *observed* behavior, not of the unseen, unconscious entities that James (1890) had excoriated as psychological "whimsy."

By the mid-1970s, behaviorism was giving way to a new cognitive science in which it was permissible to incorporate unobserved mental entities based on the computer metaphor. If complex computations could go on inside the computer and produce the output on the screen, it seemed plausible to believe that complex mental processes could occur prior to consciousness and actual behavior. If consciousness and behavior were, in fact, preceded by mental processes, then these mental processes must be, at the very least, nonconscious. Thus was born the concept of preattentive processes, or those mental processes that precede conscious attention and are clearly psychological in nature and unconscious in status. This concept was a small but crucial methodological step to employing actual subliminal stimuli to determine whether unconscious processes could be experimentally studied.

By the end of the 1970s, two bodies of research on unconscious processes were emerging, an earlier one being developed by psychoanalytic researchers, and a later one being developed by cognitive researchers. The psychoanalytic researchers began with a technique that was based on energy masking, and the cognitive researchers tended to favor pattern masking (see Chapter 6 for a discussion of these two techniques for rendering a stimulus unconscious). Psychoanalytic investigators were interested in using subliminal stimulation as a way of studying phenomena in which emotion and desire were central—dreaming, imagery, defenses, and transference. Cognitive investigators were interested in using subliminal stimulation as a way of studying the "cooler," less emotional processes of perception and memory. The split between the cognitive and dynamic unconscious was beginning to be apparent. A call for healing the split was made by Shevrin and Dickman as early as 1980. They saw subliminal research as offering a two-way street on which psychoanalytic and cognitive researchers could meet and exchange ideas, methods, and findings. The research reported in this book continues in the same spirit in which Shevrin and Dickman issued that call. The split may still persist in the field, but, as our research demonstrates, it does not exist in the human mind, in which cognitive and dynamic processes are intermingled and interact constantly.

Our Application of the Psychoanalytic Method and Three Possible Problems

Innovators who are developing a new composite method are forced into an inescapable task: to understand each contributing method in the light of its own assumptions. This task was particularly necessary for the psychoanalytic method because, as a largely clinical praxis, little systematic effort has been devoted to this task. In our analysis of these underlying assumptions (see Chapter 2), the dynamic unconscious emerges as one of those assumptions rather than as an empirical discovery. We pointed out in Chapter 2 that this assumption undergirds all major psychoanalytic theories (Freud, 1915/1957, acknowledged this in his paper on the unconscious). The tendency to conflate empirical discovery with underlying assumption in this instance is understandable, considering how rich the clinical yield has been once we make this assumption. However, an assumption, even one that appears essential to making sense of many observations, can nevertheless be wrong. In this instance, our assumption presents three problems.

Problem 1

Many psychologists of note, including William James, took issue with this assumption, insisting that psychology was the science of consciousness; beyond consciousness lay the neurophysiological nonconscious, not a psychological unconscious. Unlike Freud, James accounted for the bizarre nature of dreams as caused by short circuits in the nervous system due to impoverished nutrition during sleep, a far cry from Freud's purely psychological explanation based on the assumption of a psychological unconscious. In our own day, the same Dixon who drew together numerous subliminal studies in two books—the first, referred to earlier, published in 1971 and the second published in 1981—agreed with James and considered that subliminal effects were caused by purely neurophysiological processes.

The key to appreciating the difference between the James–Dixon position and our own is to begin by distinguishing the psychological from the neurophysiological. The psychological or mental refers to what we ordinarily mean by perceptions, memories, feelings, desires, thoughts, images, and so on. We know them from our daily conscious experience. The neurophysiological refers to the activations and functions of our nervous system. As you consciously perceive the words on this page, your retina, your optic nerve, and the rear of your brain, where the neurophysiological visual center is located, are activated. The perceptual act, accompanied by these sequential neuronal activations, produces a *representation* of the object perceived. Perception is always *about* something—the mental content of the perceptual act—in this instance, the words on this page. Unless we subscribe to mind–brain dualism, the mental content, the "aboutness" of the perceptual act, also must have a neurophysiological instantiation or substrate. What is true of perception is also true of other psychological functions such as memory, motivation, and affect—they all are "about" something as well; they possess a mental content or *representation*. Here is where we approach the point at issue. James and Dixon need to deny that neurophysiological processes that are not accompanied by consciousness are "about" anything, for this "aboutness" is what confers psychological standing. If only the conscious can be psychological, then nonconscious neurophysiological processes must lack "aboutness," for that is what makes something psychological. However, as we will try to show below, subliminal studies, including our own, demonstrate that "aboutness" does exist in the absence of consciousness.

First, it is important to note that the James–Dixon approach would result in interpreting our brain-pattern findings solely as neurophysiological effects of our subliminal word categories, rather than being about, or representing, their categorical dynamic and conflictual significance. For example, we say that Mr. A's social phobia is explained by his unconscious rage, which is projected onto others; we do not say that his social phobia is caused by the pattern of time–frequency features we found in his brain responses to the unconscious conflict words. This level of explanation would be similar to James's explanation that dreams are due to a poor nutritional state of the brain during sleep. Rather, we look on these time–frequency features as *markers* pointing to the presence of neurophysiological processes that constitute the *representation*, or "aboutness," of the hypothesized unconscious rage. These representations would be causative and would, at the same time, constitute a *psychological* level of explanation. For these reasons, it is essential to talk about a *psychological* unconscious which is embodied in still unknown neurophysiological processes but for which we have discovered certain useful markers.

To assert that the nonconscious neurophysiological level lacks representations requires conceiving of the relationship between a psychological stimulus and its effects either on a reflex arc or on a dispositional basis. Neither model does justice to the complexity of the relationship between a stimulus and its effects, in particular those effects mediated by its representation as a mental content. According to the reflex arc model, the subliminal stimulus evokes a physiological reaction much as a hammer tap to the knee evokes a small kick. Just as the swing of the knee cannot be said to represent or stand for the hammer tap—it is simply an effect with no representational content—neither can a nonconscious neurophysiological response represent anything.

If, on the other hand, one argues that the subliminal stimulus results in a neurophysiological disposition that will assume representational status only when activated by some conscious process, then one fails to account for the immediate, active, representational effects of subliminal stimuli that have been amply documented in numerous priming studies. Subjects in such studies, for example, decide that "doctor" is a word more quickly if it is primed by the subliminal stimulus "nurse" than if it is primed by an unrelated word. To explain this effect, it is necessary to assume that the neurophysiological process activated by the subliminal word "nurse" stood for or represented the meaning of the word at the very moment it influenced the reading of the word "doctor." In its aspect as a representational event, the subliminally activated neurophysiological process is not different psychologically from a supraliminally activated neurophysiological process.

The same argument can be advanced for slips like the one cited in Chapter 2, when a patient intended consciously to say "canceling" and instead said "cancering." In the clinical context, it was apparent that the patient was unhappy with the analyst for going on vacation and canceling sessions. Unconsciously, her anger activated the representation of the phonically similar word "cancer." Simultaneously, the unconscious representation of "cancer" influenced the conscious activation of "cancel," resulting in the slip. One could say that the unconscious activation of the representation of "cancer" acted as an *internally* generated prime affecting the outcome of the consciously activated representation of "cancel." It is not sufficient to consider subliminally activated neurophysiological processes merely as dispositions; they are as fully representational (i.e., psychological) as supraliminally activated neurophysiological processes, and their representational aspect makes it possible to understand how unconscious processes can simultaneously affect conscious processes in meaningful psychological ways.

Problem 2

The second possible problem derives from concern over the validity of our clinical data. It is important to our research method that our understanding of the psychoanalytic method be correct and that our adaptation of it for our research purposes not violate its assumptions. We believe that we have achieved this goal. However, some psychoanalysts might be concerned that three or four interviews and psychological tests are not a sufficient database for inferring, with any certainty, the nature of unconscious conflicts. Indeed, Freud believed that it was only by the end of an analysis that one could be at all certain that the patient had been understood. Yet, it is also correct to say that patients in successful analyses benefit along the way and not only at the end when, presumably, the most complete understanding emerges. Freud's caution does not take into account that provisional understanding, a way station on the road to fuller understanding, may capture enough truth to be of help before the end of analysis. For our research purposes, we need only assume that we have arrived at some partially correct, provisional understanding of the unconscious conflict. In fact, we noted in Chapter 2 how the judges, while agreeing on the central features of an unconscious conflict, disagreed on other aspects—developmental features, fixation points, and so on. Presumably, these differences would be the ones for which the more complete data of an extended treatment would be decisive.

Problem 3

A third possible problem of considerable importance is the method we chose for arriving at judges' agreement. As noted and elaborated in Chapter 5, we departed from the more standard approach in the field of clinical judgment, which uses formal reliability measures extensively. Instead, we chose the Delphi method, which does not rely on reliability measures but frees the clinician to work with the clinical data in the same fashion as he or she would in daily practice. Observation, theory, and inference are intermingled, and rich qualitative accounts are encouraged. Each clinician is treated as an expert whose judgments are, to some important extent, valid. By arriving at a consensus among these experts on the basis of discussion and the discipline of selecting and rating the critical words, it was anticipated that the most valid understanding would emerge. Our three case studies were offered to exemplify the way we collected our data and arrived at our judgments. Finally, the proof is in the convergence with findings from the other two methods. But what exactly does this convergence mean?

IMPLICATIONS OF OUR CONVERGENT FINDINGS

Implications for Psychoanalytic Theory

Let us consider first the implications for the structural psychoanalytic theory on which we have drawn. At the heart of this approach are the concepts of compromise formation and conflict described in Chapter 2. Insofar as the words were selected on the basis of their relationship to these concepts, we can conclude that the convergent cognitive and neurophysiological findings support the psychodynamic inferences that were made in accordance with structural theory. This conclusion, however, does not rule out the possibility that other psychoanalytic theories might also succeed; different psychoanalytic theories are not necessarily contradictory to the extent that if one is true the others are not. It is unclear whether it would ever be possible to derive mutually contradictory predictions from these different theories.

Nonetheless, it is possible to imagine that different theories might not fare so well when tested by our method. Pragmatically, only this would be necessary: that the different sets of words selected be related to the putative underlying unconscious causes. One could then determine which set of words was better associated with the convergent cognitive and neurophysiological measures. In principle, therefore, our method could provide a means for testing different psychoanalytic theories.

Our findings support two modifications that we have introduced into structural theory: (a) the crucial importance of the conscious, preconscious, and unconscious states of a mental content and (b) the distinction between the nonconscious processes by which a compromise formation develops and the content of that compromise formation, which can be conscious, preconscious, or unconscious (Shevrin, 1991a). By the very nature of our subliminal/supraliminal method, we have been able to distinguish operationally between the conscious and unconscious states of a mental content. But how can we distinguish, within the unconscious state, between the preconscious and the dynamically unconscious conditions?

Let us start with the conscious symptom words. It is easy to judge from our interviews that the conscious symptom words *as a descriptive category* were readily available to subjects and were employed consciously and intentionally to describe their symptomatic experience. (The reader can refer to our three case studies to verify this fact.) It would follow that, when the conscious symptom word category was not in consciousness, it was *preconscious* insofar as it was readily available to consciousness, the main distinguishing characteristic of preconscious processes. On the other hand, when asked to *explain* their symptoms, subjects resorted to a variety of reasons but never came close to identifying the unconscious conflict words selected by the clinicians (see Chapters 9 through 11 for examples). Unlike the conscious symptom category, the unconscious conflict words *as an explanatory category* were not available to the subjects.

We stress the importance of category instead of individual words to underscore that we are dealing with a set of related ideas rather than with a list of individual words. For the subjects, the conscious symptom words formed a category of related descriptive terms that *together* described their symptoms. However, only the *clinicians* identified the unconscious conflict words as forming a category of related ideas accounting for the interacting aspects of the hypothesized conflict. Thus, it was possible for subjects to use individual unconscious conflict words in diverse contexts (see Chapter 11 for examples) without being aware of the relationship of these unconscious conflict words *to each other*. This same lack of *relational* awareness occurred when the unconscious conflict words were presented *supraliminally;* the brain responses failed to classify them as belonging together. Thus, it was all the more important to discover that when the unconscious conflict words were presented *subliminally*, the brain responses did classify them as belonging together. Also relevant in this regard is the finding, not previously reported, that when five of our subjects were asked to put all the words in as many categories as they saw fit, the unconscious conflict words were placed in significantly more categories than the conscious symptom words. In short, *consciously*, the unconscious conflict words did not hang together as a category; *unconsciously*, they did. The *categorical nature* of the unconscious conflict words was *dynamically* unconscious, not the individual words, which could emerge in consciousness in different contexts totally unrelated to each other. And when the words did occur in these various contexts, their individual meanings would be altogether different from their meanings in the context of the unconscious conflict category. Repression was not directed at individual word meanings as such but at their *relational* significance. Mr. C (see Chapter 11) could have nightmarish dreams in which he was physically assaulted by his good friend John, and he could describe how he took a girlfriend away from John; but he could not see the relationship between his waking actions and his dream.

Further supporting the conclusion that the unconscious conflict word category was subject to repression, and was thus dynamically unconscious, were the findings involving the Hysteroid–Obsessoid Questionnaire (HOQ). The more hysteroid the subject scored on the HOQ, the greater the difference in favor of subliminal versus supraliminal correct classification of the unconscious conflict word category. The same correlation for the conscious symptom word category was nonsignificant.

Summarizing what we have just presented, we conclude that our method makes it possible to distinguish between preconscious and dynamically unconscious mental contents. Moreover, we have shown that the difference is empirically meaningful. Brain responses demonstrate that the unconscious conflict category is not discriminated supraliminally, but is discriminated subliminally. Subjects, when asked to categorize the words, place the unconscious category words in more categories than they do the conscious symptom category words. Brain responses of subjects scoring high on the hysteroid scale of the HOQ show a greater classification difference for the unconscious conflict category in favor of the subliminal over the supraliminal condition. On the other hand, the conscious symptom category is better classified by the brain responses supraliminally and is placed by subjects in one or two categories when they are asked to consciously classify the words. We suggested in Chapter 2 that the unconscious conflict word selection is comparable to a clinical interpretation insofar as an interpretation formulates relationships concerning unconscious conflict. Our results support that conceptual parallel.

In the course of our discussion of the conscious, preconscious, and dynamic unconscious, we have referred to *mental contents*. We are now in a position to relate this notion of mental contents to what we have previously referred to as *representations*. We will then be able to show how compromise formations are best thought of as mental contents, or representations, produced by a compromise-forming process that is itself not represented as a mental content.

A mental content is what a representation is made of. When we speak of Mr. A's *unconscious* rage, Mr. C's *unconscious* desire to submit himself homosexually, or Mr. B's *repressed* perception of his father as fatally ill, we are talking about mental contents that are represented in the mind and instantiated neurophysiologically. Affects, desires, and perceptions are mental contents whether they are conscious or unconscious. Similarly, when we say that these patients' phobic symptoms are compromise formations, we mean that they are constituted of mental contents that are consciously describable as fears, perceptions of danger, and desires to avoid and flee that are caused by, but quite different from, the underlying unconscious dangers and desires. Consciously, Mr. A is in a state of conflict between desiring to go to a party and running the risk of encountering rage and suspicion; unconsciously, he is in conflict between gratifying his inordinate desire for domination and control, and running the risk of destroying those he needs and loves. The better bargain would seem to be to fear social gatherings and to avoid them rather than to risk acting on his sadistic rage.

How do these interacting conscious and unconscious layerings of mental contents come about? Perhaps an analogy that may really be a case in point can help answer this question. We are all capable of perceiving these words on the page, but we are not aware of the perceptual process creating the perception. We can certainly learn about that process through psychological and neurophysiological investigations, but we have no direct access to it. We suggest, as the reason for this inability, that these processes are not *represented;* they are not mental contents in the same way that perceptions, affects, and desires are mental contents. In some such way, as in the perceptual process, the *functions* of id, ego, and superego interact to form a particular compromise formation—for example, a social phobia, with its concrete and highly specific conscious, preconscious, and dynamically unconscious mental contents.

In summary, we believe that our method has permitted us to show that structural theory (at least as employed by us) can prove extremely useful as a basis for clinical inferences about the nature of the compromise formations constituting neurotic symptoms. However, we have also shown that the theory is incomplete as an explanation, without taking into account the conscious, preconscious, and dynamically unconscious status of the mental contents making up a compromise formation, and it fails to distinguish between the representational status of these mental contents and the nonrepresentational character of the process by which the compromises are formed. We have also suggested that the application of other psychoanalytic theories to our data might provide a test of their comparable strengths.

Implications for Cognitive Theory

Turning our attention to implications of our convergent findings for cognitive psychology, we first discuss an important methodological issue bearing on the validity of our results. Can we correctly claim that our stimuli were indeed subliminal? If we can not make this claim, then our key findings are undermined. To establish the correctness of our claim is no small matter; it requires diving into the midst of continued controversy over the exact conditions under which subliminal effects can be achieved. We believe that we have achieved that important goal, in this and in other studies conducted under the same conditions in our laboratory. How have we done so?

In recent years, the controversy has centered mainly on the difference between the so-called subjective and objective thresholds for establishing subliminal effects. This distinction was first suggested by Cheesman and Merikle (1984), who were critical of studies in which the investigators were willing to accept as truly subliminal a stimulus detection threshold between 50% and 60% above chance in a two-item forced-choice design. At this level, subjects claimed that they saw nothing and were just guessing; nevertheless, their "guesses" were significantly above chance. At the least, some conscious perception could not be ruled out. Cheesman and Merikle claimed that at the true objective threshold—detection at chance—no subliminal effect is found. They were willing, however, to concede that some kind of subliminal effect was occurring at the subjective threshold, given that subjects said they were only guessing and not really seeing anything. If it could be shown that these effects were qualitatively different from ordinary supraliminal effects, Cheesman and Merikle suggested, then an argument could be made that something different was going on at the subjective threshold.

In our own laboratory, Snodgrass, Shevrin, and Kopka (1993) were able to show that subliminal effects could be obtained while meeting all the criteria required by Cheesman and Merikle to establish the objective threshold. In addition, Van Selst and Merikle (1993) replicated the Snodgrass, Shevrin, and Kopka (1993) findings. Our conditions for achieving subliminality were exactly the same as those used by Snodgrass, Shevrin, and Kopka; thus, we can say with some confidence that our subliminal effects were at the objective threshold.

Results at the objective threshold have one important implication for our understanding of unconscious processes: A stimulus can register entirely out of consciousness and have determinable effects. A subliminal stimulus registering at the objective threshold is *perceived* unconsciously; it is not even briefly in consciousness and then forgotten. The latter phenomenon is drawn on in much research on implicit memory (Roediger, 1990). Snodgrass (1995) has explored the theoretical and methodological issues involved in research on unconscious perception and unconscious memory. He concluded that they are distinctly different phenomena and have different theoretical implications. In our research, it was important to establish that the unconscious conflict words, in particular, were never in consciousness at the time of their exposure. Only in this way could we claim that they were entirely processed unconsciously. Had they been even briefly in consciousness at the time of exposure, it would have been impossible to separate, in the brain responses, what was due to that brief conscious experience and what was due to the unconscious processing. We can, however, say with some confidence that they were entirely unconscious at the time of exposure and registration.

Earlier in the section recapitulating a brief history of subliminal research, we referred to Freud's interest in Poetzl's pioneering method—the method later picked up by Fisher. Attempting to account for subliminal findings, Fisher (1957) proposed a topographic model. A brief discussion of his model is germane at this point because it bears on both the question of unconscious perception and the role of conscious, preconscious, and dynamically unconscious mental states. This same model was drawn on by Shevrin and Dickman (1980) when they proposed that common ground existed between psychology and psychoanalysis precisely in the area of unconscious perception.

According to Fisher's model, *all* stimuli, supraliminal as well as subliminal, initially register preconsciously. In the case of supraliminal stimuli, the initial preconscious registration allows for the activation of related memory traces resulting in recognition, all of which takes place very briefly prior to the delivery of the percept into consciousness. It is also possible for dynamically unconscious mental contents to be activated by these preconsciously registered stimuli. If this happens, the delivery of the preconsciously registered stimuli to consciousness could be aborted by defensive processes because the stimuli would now be associated with dynamically unconscious mental contents that are subject to repression. In other words, according to this model, repression can occur at the boundary between preconscious and unconscious processes. The registration of a subliminal stimulus, on the other hand, remains at a preconscious level unless it too is assimilated into the dynamically unconscious contents. Lastly, the model accounts for the phenomenon of afterexpulsion, that is, when a content already in consciousness is repressed and becomes dynamically unconscious.

If we start with Fisher's premise that all stimuli register preconsciously and then may be processed along several routes, we can account for the main part of our findings. When exposed subliminally, the conscious symptom words register and remain preconscious, and the unconscious symptom words register preconsciously but are then reorganized at a dynamically unconscious level. When exposed supraliminally, the conscious symptom words register preconsciously and are immediately delivered into consciousness, where they are experienced as belonging together as a category. The unconscious conflict words also register preconsciously but, prior to their delivery into consciousness, a repressive process removes their category relatedness to each other, thus disabling their dynamic significance. Only then do they become conscious as individual unrelated words.

Fisher's model supports the topographic addition we have made to structural psychoanalytic theory. It provides a systematic way to account for the role that topographic considerations play in the interaction of id, ego, and superego functions. Motivations at the level of id impulses, with their associated mental contents, can interact with incoming stimuli at a preconscious level, modifying them and drawing their subjectively dangerous aspects into repression; or, if the stimuli are strong enough or too weakly repressed, they can become conscious and suffer afterexpulsion. In either case—repression at a preconscious level or afterexpulsion at a conscious level—ego and superego functions are operative in both the actual perceptual process, activation of memories and in the defensive processes. These functions operate silently from a psychological standpoint, that is, unlike the perceptions, memories, affects, and desires themselves, they have no mental representation. A compromise formation is a complex product of interacting id, ego, and superego functions operating on mental contents that emerge from the interplay of conscious, preconscious, and dynamically unconscious states. As such, a compromise formation is a relatively stable dynamic structure taking shape in the midst of fluid, shifting forces. A compromise formation is like a whirlpool appearing in a flowing stream. However, as with the whirlpool, its identifiable form is no indication of how long it might persist. As discussed in Chapter 2, a symptom may persist for years, disappear overnight, or be replaced by some other structure, depending on the shifting interplay of conscious, preconscious, and dynamically unconscious states set in motion by id, ego, and superego forces.

Of further interest is the relationship of Fisher's model to the two cognitive models discussed in Chapter 3—one based on the distinction between controlled and automatic processes, and the second, proposed by Allport, based on a shifting hierarchy of attention subject to motivational influences. Fisher's model, positing an interplay of topographic states influenced by motivational, defensive, and perceptual processes, would appear to fit better with Allport's model. In the controlled/automatic model, the only interplay possible is a one-way street in which controlled processes operate on automatic processes by selectively inhibiting them or directing them in accordance with some task. Because controlled processes are defined as conscious and automatic processes as unconscious, only ego functions operating at a conscious level can influence preconscious mental contents, and they can do so only by selectively inhibiting or directing those contents. Moreover, Bargh denies that truly *unconscious* intentions exist; thus, he reasons, unconscious intentions cannot influence the course of automatic processing or have any effect on consciousness (see Chapter 3). The controlled/automatic model allows for no fluid interplay of perception, intention, or defense with conscious and unconscious states.

Allport's model, on the other hand, does allow for such interplay, with the important qualification that Allport does not explicitly relate his hierarchical model to conscious and unconscious states. The model could, however, readily accommodate these concepts. The lower-priority adaptive task that, according to Allport, can quickly gain the highest priority could, without doing an injustice to his model, be unconscious, and the highest-priority task could be conscious. Allport also makes it plain that, even though at a lower priority, interaction with the surround continues so that a change in the environment that is related to the lower-priority task could quickly change its priority. Without this provision, adaptive behavior would be unacceptably slow and inefficient.

One could make further sense of Allport's model by incorporating Fisher's premise that all stimuli initially register preconsciously. Thus, the lower-priority task would continue to have access immediately to changes in the environment at the same time that the high-priority task was being pursued. Once this preconscious access is assumed, one can account for rapid shifts in priority.

Our findings make sense from a cognitive standpoint in the context of a model similar to Allport's, as further qualified by Fisher's topographic model. When the conscious symptom and the unconscious conflict words are flashed at 1 msec, each word registers and undergoes a different fate, depending on which category it belongs to. This fate is in part determined by prevailing intentions related to the presence or absence of unconscious conflictual significance. Because of their hypothesized conflictual character, the unconscious conflict words are processed as belonging together and are quickly assimilated into mental contents at a dynamically unconscious level. The conscious symptom words remain at a preconscious level. In Allport's terms, the unconscious conflict words are rendered of lower priority in the hierarchy determining access to consciousness. The conscious symptom words are higher in that hierarchy, although they too fail to enter consciousness because they are not strong enough perceptually. When the words are presented supraliminally, matters change. The time–frequency patterns turn about. Now, the conscious symptom words show the same pattern that the unconscious conflict words did when flashed subliminally; that is, they are now organized as a category, and the unconscious conflict words are not. We would suggest that now the categorical identification of the conscious symptom words becomes a high-priority task, and the categorical identification of the unconscious conflict words remains of low priority as a result of repression.

Implications for Psychophysiological Theory

Let us now consider implications for neurophysiological theory. The category-differentiating sensitivity of the ERP *t–f* feature analysis is of special importance. First, we must stress that this analysis is *not* the same as an EEG frequency analysis, in which a fairly wide time window is needed to establish a dominant frequency (see Spydell & Sheer, 1982 for work based on this approach in the study of attention). Nor is this analysis the same as a fast Fourier transform (FFT) analysis, which provides a distribution of all frequencies present in a given EEG episode and their relative power but not their sequence in time. Rather, the *t–f* feature analysis detects specific time-bound frequencies. Our results suggest that changing patterns of frequencies within relatively brief time intervals are markers for conscious and unconscious category processing of stimuli related to affect, symptoms, and conflict.

Why the particular patterns of low- and high-frequency latencies were found requires further study. For our present purposes, it would not matter what specific ERP parameters were related to the clinically selected word categories; the ERP method was used mainly to provide an objective, non-behavioral, and immediate correlate of the word categories. Nevertheless, the time–frequency findings may open the door to a uniquely sensitive brain indicator of complex processing bearing on the nature of the cognitive and dynamic unconscious.

It is, however, of some relevance that there is a fast developing neurophysiological literature based on animal studies using implanted electrodes, that provides intriguing evidence for the important role of precisely timed frequencies in brain processes associated with cognitive functioning. Recently, Jagadeesh, Gray, and Forster (1992) have reported, based on their investigation of the cat visual cortex, that "rhythmic firing can be synchronized among cells in widespread areas of the visual cortex. The visual stimulus condition under which this process occurs suggests that the synchronization may contribute to the aggregation of information across broadly displaced parts of the visual field" (p. 252). According to this view, parallel and distributed processes, in a purely psychological sense, may be integrated neurophysiologically on the basis of frequency features, a possibility that is consistent with our findings.

The adaptive Gabor transform goes beyond the time–frequency analysis by incorporating both time and frequency spreads, energy level, and phase. These parameters have received little attention in the literature, yet they seem to be, at the very least, markers for complex psychological processes. Shastri and Ajjanagedde (1993) have recently proposed a theory in which a connectionist representation of rules and variables might be accounted for neurophysiologically by the dynamic binding of networks on the basis of temporal synchrony of in-phase frequencies. The possible role of frequency spread is also intriguing. If frequencies play some role in integrating diverse networks of distributed processes, it may be that the *range* or bandwidth of frequencies may also be important. Different frequencies that are operative at the same time may play a part in integrating different subsystems of the larger whole simultaneously. This would suggest that the larger the bandwidth, the more complex the diverse processes being integrated. Perhaps the important contribution made by the highest-frequency feature in our findings speaks to this possibility. The highest frequency may mark the peak frequency of a range of frequencies. If this were the case, it would follow that the processing of the unconscious conflict words was more complex *early* subliminally and *later* supraliminally, and that the reverse was true for the conscious symptom words. In each case, the earlier complex processing was associated with more correct classification of the category in question. It would seem reasonable to suppose that the complex determination of category relationships among a group of words would require more complex processing—hence the integration of more diverse subsystems representing the various features and relationships among the category members.

We also know that the later appearance of the highest-frequency feature supraliminally for the unconscious conflict category was associated with a *failure* to classify the words together and that this failure correlated with the HOQ hysteroid end of the scale. This suggests that the greater bandwidth found supraliminally for the unconscious conflict category could be associated with the complex processing involved in *divesting* the words of their categorical significance in the service of repression, and this might also account for the delayed latency of the highest-frequency feature supraliminally. A hypothesis of this nature points to a significant current limitation of neurophysiological speculation. A given parameter may be associated with a variable such as complex processing, but, in and of itself, it does not indicate *what* specifically is being processed; for that purpose, the specifics of the psychological content are essential.

Our findings reveal certain functional relationships between the parameters of highest and lowest frequency on the one hand, and psychological categories and exposure conditions on the other. These functional relationships hold across subjects, even though the *particular* words differ from subject to subject. Indeed, we believe that it was only *because* the words were individually tailored that we were able to find the relationships holding across subjects. This suggests that certain neurophysiological patterns are invariant for unconscious conflict and conscious symptom experience, regardless of the particular content of the conflict or symptom experience. Moreover, these patterns are formed by *relative* (not absolute) frequencies. The actual frequencies are quite different from subject to subject; no one *absolute* frequency is required. This point leads us to another important implication of our findings for brain organization and functioning.

The fact that our frequency findings are relative and not absolute is predictable if we assume that each brain is different, not only genetically but because of different developmental histories and life experiences. A theory proposed by Edelman (1987) takes into account individual differences in brain organization and functioning. Edelman argues that the neural organization of functional brain systems develops on the basis of a principle of neuronal selection that is very similar to what happens in the immunological system in the development of antibodies. Because he theorizes that both of these systems operate on the basis of natural selection, he refers to his neurophysiological theory as neural darwinism. Groups of neurons begin to operate together as a function of group selection processes influenced by the organism's interaction with the environment. These neuron systems or maps do not have fixed boundaries; the actual neurons in a given functional organization may change from moment to moment, as may the boundary itself, but the function remains the same. Thus, this theory can account for intraindividual variability in brain response from time to time or from one stimulation to another.

As psychoanalysts, we find Edelman's theory quite attractive. The theory provides a neurophysiological frame of reference for explaining the inter- and intraindividual differences that are of such importance to psychoanalysts. Also, the theory allows for the specifics of experience, situationally and developmentally, to directly affect brain organization. In other theories, the brain is mainly a genetically engineered product with fixed neuroanatomical boundaries, and it changes only slowly as a function of maturation and learning. In Edelman's theory, the brain is a dynamic temporal and spatial organization capable of fluid shifts and rapid reorganizations. These characteristics are especially important to psychoanalysts for whom the mind works in a fashion very much as Edelman's account of the brain.

Our own findings fit well with Edelman's conception of the brain. The importance of relative frequencies, for example, relates to functional similarities across brains that are differently organized. Also, the finding that the same words will be processed differently, depending on whether they are presented subliminally or supraliminally, speaks to the same brains that are responding with different functional organizations across time with respect to the same stimulus.

One other implication of our ERP findings requires attention. Our results were found for the electrode pair C_zP_z/P_3 but were not found for C_zP_z, C_zP_z/P_4, P_3, and P_4. Factors shared by the left hemisphere and a more centrally placed electrode (C$_z$P$_z$) accounted for the outcome. The left hemisphere is generally considered to be involved in sequential, linguistic processing; the right hemisphere is engaged more in spatial, configurational processing. Because our stimuli are words, they would favor left-hemisphere processing. The HOQ findings with respect to percent-correct classification would be consistent with this interpretation: Repression is directed primarily against verbal, ideational representatives or derivatives of unacceptable wishes, rather than at the concrete, affective qualities associated with them. Thus, a hysterical patient might blush at a sexual reference but not recall its actual content. Similarly, in split-brain patients, Sperry has reported, as noted by Galin (1974), that when a nude figure is presented to the right hemisphere, patients will blush but not know what they are blushing about. It is inviting to hypothesize that repression acts like a functional splitting of the hemispheres.

These left-hemisphere results do not fit, however, with the Galin hypothesis that unconscious processes are mainly to be found in the right hemisphere (Galin, 1974). Rather, our results suggest that unconscious processes may also be found for left-hemisphere functions. Our results are consistent with the psychoanalytic structural view that defenses draw on a wide range of normally occurring psychological functions, such as verbalization, recall, forgetting, and attention (Brenner, 1982; Shevrin & Bond, 1994).

POSSIBLE LIMITATIONS OF OUR METHOD AND FINDINGS

An objection can be raised regarding whether the specific unconscious conflict identified by the clinicians is, in fact, *the cause* of the symptom. We may have *identified* an unconscious conflict, but our results do not *necessarily prove* a causal connection. This objection is reasonable. At the same time, it should be borne in mind that the clinicians originally selected the unconscious conflict words because they hypothesized that these words were related to the cause of the symptoms. Our results supported this hypothesis, although not conclusively. Perhaps the only way evidence for a causal connection can be gathered is in a psychodynamic treatment, during which the conflict identified previously emerges, and understanding results in symptomatic modification.

At least three alternate hypotheses can be offered to account for our results:

1. The words selected for the unconscious conflict category may simply be more unpleasant for the subject than the conscious symptoms or ordinary unpleasant words when compared to the ordinary

pleasant category, and, for some unknown reason, very unpleasant words follow the pattern of the brain responses found;

2. The results are not related to word *category* as described above but may be the outcome of several powerful affective words;

3. The unconscious conflict words may indeed be related to conflict and form a category, but they are not necessarily unique to that patient; were these words shown to other psychiatric patients, they would elicit the same pattern of findings. Or, more generally, there may simply be something about the unconscious conflict words— exactly *what* remains to be determined—that would elicit the same pattern of findings in anyone.

In response to the first hypothesis, we can report that subject ratings on the Osgood evaluative dimension, collected after the laboratory procedure was completed, showed no difference in unpleasantness between the unconscious conflict and conscious symptom words. Indeed, usually one or two unconscious conflict category words had consciously positive affect, such as the word **John** for Mr. C. **John** was hypothesized to elicit negative feelings only unconsciously; consciously, the subject considered him to be a close friend. This alternate hypothesis would be hard pressed to account for the actual pattern of findings, but the psychoanalytic hypothesis would have little difficulty.

The second hypothesis is more difficult to answer definitively. We have, in further analyses, tried to see whether our categories can be differentiated from pseudocategories that are made up of two words each (from each of the four categories). Presumably, the pseudocategories should have no category coherence because they are made up equally of words from the four categories. The results tended to support the belief that we were dealing with real categories and not with the impact of several powerful words (Kushwaha, Williams, & Shevrin, 1992).

In response to the third hypothesis, the same conflict was not found in every patient or even among patients who had the same symptom (e.g., social phobia). For this reason, it is unlikely that the unconscious conflict words would elicit the same pattern of findings in every patient. Although it is logically possible that, for some unknown reason, the unconscious conflict words for a given patient would elicit the same pattern of findings in everyone, it is highly unlikely, given that some of the words could have no meaning at all to anyone other than the patient (e.g., **John** for Mr. C).

We are planning to correct one limitation in our design in future research. We employed only one duration order: subliminal/supraliminal. Our results may not generalize to the reverse order. Practical time limitations imposed by our method made it difficult to incorporate a balanced design; another comparable group of patients would need to have been evaluated and tested in the reverse duration order. However, there was an advantage in starting with the subliminal/supraliminal order. The order ensured that the words were exposed subliminally to subjects in the absence of any prior awareness of these words. Had we started with the reverse order (supraliminal/subliminal), the subjects would have already been exposed consciously to the words, and the subliminal results would have been more difficult to interpret. Against the background of our current findings, however, results with the reverse duration order could be more easily understood. For example, if the results were the same, it would strongly suggest that subliminal processing is relatively insulated from prior conscious exposure and that the same conflict-related words can be responded to differently subliminally and supraliminally, as our present results suggest and clinical experience supports. A patient may talk, as our patients did, about their symptoms, dreams, and fantasies, employing the words used in the laboratory, without being aware of their unconscious significance. However, additional research will be required to answer this question.

APPENDIX A

Word Selection Algorithms

Clinicians should be afforded a readily interpretable set of metrics to measure convergence or divergence of opinion on word selections and, at the same time, allow for the assessment of relative degrees of belonging and nonbelonging to the categories of interest.

These considerations have led to a technique of quantifying the various aspects of the word selection process. "Belonging" is quantified for each word in terms of each of four categories (U, C, E−, E+) on a scale from +9 to −9, thus creating a multivariate metric space in which the orthogonal axes are the measures of "belonging" for each category. In this manner, the joint properties, as well as the individual properties, of the words may be analyzed. These rankings may also be thought of as measures of "belief" and "disbelief" in the sense described by Shortliffe (1976), enabling the modeling of the decision process in production rules as in MYCIN.

Properties of interest in word selection are several, and they are not easily confined in a single meaningful metric. An important property is closeness to an ideal category. This implies a distance metric and is readily expressed as a Euclidian distance of the multivariate word ranking from the ideal ranking—that is, a ranking of +9, −9, −9, −9 for a four-category space. Coupled to this property is the distance from other categories. Combining these two distances in a single function serves to provide a meaningful measure of "closeness" to the ideal ranking and "distance" from other categories. In other words, it is a combined or simultaneous measure of "belonging" and lack of ambiguity. The most promising measure among the many available seems to be the mean square distance for the distance metric and a form of likelihood ratio for the function (Sneath & Sokal, 1973). A promising function is a product of distance to ideal category and the sum of inverse distances to other categories. The following formula has been developed to capture these dimensions:

APPENDIX A

$$D_c - D_u$$

where

$$D_c = 1 + \sqrt{(9 - C_{mn})^2 + (9 + U_{mn})^2}$$
$$D_u = 1 + \sqrt{9 + C_{mn})^2 + (9 - U_{mn})^2}$$

D_c = category distance of conscious symptom words;
D_u = category distance of unconscious conflict words;
C_{mn} = mean of conscious symptom word ratings;
U_{mn} = mean of unconscious conflict word ratings.

A P P E N D I X   B

Time–Frequency Distributions

There are a number of ways of representing the energy present in a signal in terms of the relative contributions of the various frequency components at a specific time. The spectrogram method commonly used in speech analysis and the Wigner distribution are two well-known time–frequency energy distributions of Cohen's class of distributions (Cohen, 1966). Cohen's class of time–frequency energy distributions is defined for a signal waveform $f(t)$ to be, for a given kernel $\phi(\xi,\tau)$:

$$C_f(t,\omega,\phi) = \frac{1}{2\pi} \iiint e^{j(\xi t - \tau\omega - \xi\mu)} \phi(\xi,\tau)f(\mu + \frac{\tau}{2})f^*(\mu - \frac{\tau}{2})d\mu d\tau\, d\xi \quad \text{(B.1)}$$

This is the energy content of the signal $f(t)$ as a conjoint function of time (t) and frequency (ω). If two signals, $f(t)$ and $g(t)$ are considered then:

$$C_{fg}(t,\omega,\phi) = \frac{1}{2\pi} \iiint e^{j(\xi t - \tau\omega - \xi\mu)} \phi(\xi,\tau)f(\mu + \frac{\tau}{2})g^*(\mu - \frac{\tau}{2})\, d\mu d\tau\, d\xi \quad \text{(B.2)}$$

This form reflects the shared or cross energy distribution between the two signals as a function of time and frequency. The well-known Wigner distribution results when $\phi(\xi,\tau) = 1$. The Wigner distribution has many desirable characteristics, but suffers from the fact that multiple signals produce strong cross-terms as well as the individual signal contributions. Although mathematically desirable and correct in a theoretical sense, the cross-terms are difficult to interpret visually when a plot of the energy surface as a function of time and frequency is viewed. It is also difficult to apply pattern recognition techniques in the presence of these cross-terms since they result from interactions of significant features in the data and are not unique to a given signal component in and of itself. A new distribution (termed the reduced interference distribution, or RID) obtained by careful design of $\phi(\xi,\tau)$ yields a result that retains the contributions of individual signal components while significantly reducing cross terms (Choi & Williams, 1989; Williams & Jeong, 1989). This has made the pattern recognition and classification approach utilized in this report possible. Formulas incorporating the new RID kernel were used to obtain time–frequency features for signals derived from two electrodes (e.g., C_zP_z and P_3, C_zP_z and P_4; see formula B.2).

References

Abend, S. (1989). Countertransference and psychoanalytic technique. *Psychoanalytic Quarterly, 58*(3), 374–395.

Abend, S. (1990a). Psychotherapeutic processes: Motives and obstacles in the search for clarification. *Psychoanalytic Quarterly, 59*(4), 532–549.

Abend, S. (1990b). Unconscious fantasies, structural theory and compromise formation. *Journal of the American Psychoanalytic Association, 38*(1), 61–73.

Allers, R., & Teler, J. (1960). On the utilization of unnoticed impressions in associations. *Psychological Issues, 2,* 121–154. (Original work published 1924)

Allison, T., Wood, C. C., & McCarthy, G. (1986). The central nervous system. In M. G. H. Coles, E. Donchin, & S. W. Porges (Eds.), *Psychophysiology: Systems, processes, and applications* (pp. 5–25). New York: Guilford.

Allport, A. (1989). Visual attention. In M. I. Posner (Ed.), *Foundations of cognitive science* (pp. 631–682). Cambridge, MA: MIT Press.

American Psychiatric Association. (1987). *Diagnostic and statistical manual of mental disorders* (3rd ed. rev.). Washington, DC: Author.

Arlow, J. (1969). Unconscious fantasy and disturbances of conscious experience. *Psychoanalytic Quarterly, 38,* 1–27.

Arlow, J. (1975). The structural hypothesis—theoretical considerations. *Psychoanalytic Quarterly, 44*(4), 509–525.

Arlow, J. (1979). Metaphor and the psychoanalytic situation. *Psychoanalytic Quarterly, 48,* 363–385.

Arlow, J., & Brenner, C. (1964). *Psychoanalytic concepts and the structural theory.* New York: International Universities Press.

Baars, B. J. (1992). *Experimental slips and human error.* New York: Plenum.

Bargh, J. A. (1989). Conditional automaticity: Varieties of autonomic influence on social perception and cognition. In J. S. Uleman & J. A. Bargh (Eds.), *Unintended thought* (pp. 3–51). New York: Guilford.

Barkoczi, I., Sera, L., & Komlosi, A. (1983). Relationships between functional symmetry of the hemispheres, subliminal perception and some defense mechanisms in various experimental settings. *Psychologia, 26,* 1–20.

Beres, D. (1965). Structure and function in psychoanalysis. *International Journal of Psycho-Analysis, 46,* 3–63.

Boesky, D. (1982). Acting out: A reconsideration of the concept. *International Journal of Psycho-Analysis, 63*(1), 39–55.

Boesky, D. (1983). The problem of mental representation in self and object theory. *Psychoanalytic Quarterly, 52*(4), 564–583.

Boesky, D. (1988). Comments on the structural theory of technique. *International Journal of Psycho-Analysis, 69*(3), 303–316.

Bond, J. A. (1974). Behavior therapy, learning theory and scientific method. *Psychotherapy: Theory, Research and Practice, 11*, 118–132.

Bond, J., Hansell, J., & Shevrin, H. (1987). Locating transference paradigms in psychotherapy transcripts: Reliability of relationship episode location in the core conflictual relationship theme (CCRT) method. *Psychotherapy, 24*, 736–749.

Bower, G. H., & Clapper, J. P. (1989). Experimental methods in cognitive science. In M. I. Posner (Ed.), *Foundations of cognitive science* (pp. 245–300). Cambridge, MA: MIT Press.

Brakel, L. A. W. (1991). Psychoanalytic data: Two problems contributing to our evidential difficulties. *American Psychological Association Meetings, Division 39.*

Brakel, L. A. W. (1993). Shall drawing become part of free association: Proposal for a modification in psychoanalytic technique. *Journal of the American Psychoanalytic Association, 41*(2), 359–394.

Brakel, L. A. W. (1994). On knowing the unconscious: Lessons from the epistemology of geometry and space. *International Journal of Psycho-Analysis, 75*(1), 39–49.

Brandeis, D., & Lehmann, D. (1986). Event-related potentials of the brain & cognitive processes: Approaches and applications. *Neuropsychologia, 24*(1), 151–166.

Brenner, C. (1976). *Psychoanalytic technique and psychic conflict.* New York: International Universities Press.

Brenner, C. (1982). *The mind in conflict.* New York: International Universities Press, Inc.

Brown, M. L. (1994). *Optimal representation of transient signals using the adaptive Gabor transform.* Unpublished doctoral dissertation. Ann Arbor: The University of Michigan.

Brown, M. L., Williams, W. J., & Hero, A. O., III. (1993). Non-orthogonal Gabor representations of event-related potentials. In *IEEE-EMB International Conference on Engineering in Medicine and Biology, 1*, 314–315.

Brown, M. L., Williams, W. J., & Hero, A. O., III. (1994). Non-orthogonal Gabor representations of biological signals. *IEEE-SP International Conference on Acoustics, Speech and Signal Processing, 4*, 305–308.

Brown, M. L., Williams, W. J., Shevrin, H. (1995). *Automatic classification of event-related potentials using the adaptive Gabor transform.* Manuscript submitted for publication.

Brown, W. S., Lehmann, D., & Marsh, J. T. (1980). Linguistics and meaning related differences in evoked potential topography: English, Swiss-German, and Imagined. *Brain and Language, 11*(2), 340–353.

Caine, T. M., & Hawkins, L. G. (1963). Questionnaire measures of the hysteroid/obsessoid component of personality: The HOQ. *Journal of Consulting Psychology, 27*, 206–209.

Caine, T. M., & Hope, K. (1967). *Manual of the Hysteroid/Obsessoid Questionnaire (HOQ)*. London: University of London Press.

Callaway, E., & Harris, P. R. (1974). Coupling between cortical potentials from different areas. *Science, 183,* 873–875.

Chapman, R. M. (1979). Connotative meaning and averaged evoked potentials. In H. Begleiter (Ed.), *Evoked brain potentials and behavior.* New York: Plenum.

Cheesman, J., & Merikle, P. M. (1984). Priming with and without awareness. *Perception and Psychophysics, 36,* 387–395.

Choi, H. I., & Williams, W. J. (1989). Improved time–frequency representation of multicomponent signals using exponential kernels. *IEEE Transactions on Acoustics, Speech, Signal Processing, 37,* 862–871.

Choi, H. I., Williams, W. I., & Zaveri, H. (1987). Analysis of event-related potentials: Time–frequency energy distribution. *Proceedings of the Rocky Mountain Bioengineering Symposium,* 251–258.

Claasen, T. A. C. M., & Mecklenbrauker, W. F. G. (1980a). The Wigner distribution—a tool for time–frequency signal analysis: Part I. Continuous-time signals. *Philips Journal of Research, 35,* 217–250.

Claasen, T. A. C. M., & Mecklenbrauker, W. F. G. (1980b). The Wigner distribution—a tool for time–frequency signal analysis: Part II. Continuous-time signals. *Philips Journal of Research, 35,* 276–300.

Claasen, T. A. C. M., & Mecklenbrauker, W. F. G. (1980c). The Wigner distribution—a tool for time–frequency signal analysis: Part III. Continuous-time signals. *Philips Journal of Research, 35,* 372–389.

Cohen, L. (1966). Generalized phase-space distribution functions. *Journal of Mathematical Physics, 7,* 781–786.

Cohen, L. (1989). Time–frequency distributions: A review. *Procedures IEEE, 77,* 941–981.

Colby, K. M., & Stoller, J. R. (1988). *Cognitive science and psychoanalysis.* Hillsdale, NJ: Erlbaum.

Crews, F. (1995). *The memory wars: Freud's legacy in dispute.* New York: New York Review of Books.

Dahl, H. (1979). *Word frequencies of spoken English.* Detroit, MI: Verbatim Books.

Dalkey, N. (1975). Evaluation, Part B. In H. A. Linstone & N. Turoff (Eds.), *The Delphi method: Techniques and applications* (pp. 236–261). Reading, MA: Addison-Wesley.

Daubechies, I. (1990). The wavelet transform, time–frequency localization, and signal analysis. *IEEE Transactions on Information Theory, 36,* 961–1005.

Devijver, P. A., & Kittler, J. (1982). *Pattern recognition: A statistical approach.* London: Prentice-Hall.

de Weerd, J. P. C., & Kap, J. I. (1981). Spectro-temporal representations and time-varying spectra of evoked potentials: A methodological investigation. *Biological Cybernetics, 41,* 101–117.

Dixon, N. F. (1971). *Subliminal perception: The nature of a controversy.* London: McGraw-Hill.

Dixon, N. F. (1981). *Preconscious processing.* London: Wiley.

Donchin, E. (1986). Cognitive psychophysiology and human information. In M. G. H. Coles, E. Donchin, & S. W. Porges (Eds.), *Psychophysiology: Systems, processes, and applications* (pp. 244–267). New York: Guilford.

Donchin, E., Ritter, W., & Cheyne, W. (1978). Cognitive psychology: The endogenous components of the ERP. In P. T. E. Callaway & S. Koslow (Eds.), *Event-related brain potentials in man* (pp. 349–412). New York: Academic Press.

Eagle, M., Wolitzky, D. L., & Klein, G. S. (1966). Imagery: Effect of a concealed figure in a stimulus. *Science, 15*, 837–839.

Edelman, G. M. (1987). *Neural Darwinism*. New York: Basic Books.

Edelson, M. (1975). *Language and interpretation in psychoanalysis*. New Haven, CT: Yale University Press.

Edelson, M. (1984). *Hypothesis and Evidence in Psychoanalysis*. Chicago: University of Chicago Press.

Edelson, M. (1988). *Psychoanalysis: A theory in crisis*. Chicago: University of Chicago Press.

Eriksen, C. W. (1960). Discrimination and learning without awareness: A methodological survey and evaluation. *Psychological Review, 67*, 279–300.

Eysenck, H. J. (Ed.). (1960). *Behavior therapy and the neuroses*. New York: Pergamon.

Fisher, C. (1954). Dreams and perception: The role of preconscious and primary modes of perception in dream formation. *Journal of the American Psychoanalytic Association, 2*, 389–445.

Fisher, C. (1957). A study of the preliminary stages of the construction of dreams and images. *Journal of the American Psychoanalytic Association, 5*, 60–67.

Fisher, C. (1960). Introduction: Preconscious stimulation in dreams, associations, and images. Classical studies. *Psychological Issues, 2*, 1–40.

Fisher, C., & Paul, I. H. (1959). The effect of subliminal visual stimulation on imagery and dreams: A validation study. *Journal of the American Psychoanalytic Association, 7*, 35–83.

Flanagan, O. (1992). *Consciousness reconsidered*. Cambridge, MA: MIT Press.

Forgas, J. P., & Moylan, S. (1987). After the movies: Transient mood and social judgments. *Personality & Social Psychology Bulletin, 14*, 146–158.

Freud, S. (1950). Project for a scientific psychology. In J. Strachey (Ed. and Trans.), *The standard edition of the complete psychological works of Sigmund Freud* (Vol. 2, pp. 281–347). London: Hogarth Press. (Original work published 1895)

Freud, S. (1953). The interpretation of dreams. In J. Strachey (Ed. and Trans.), *The standard edition of the complete psychological works of Sigmund Freud* (Vol. 5, pp. 1–630). London: Hogarth Press. (Original work published 1900)

Freud, S. (1955). Studies on hysteria. In J. Strachey (Ed. and Trans.), *The standard edition of the complete psychological works of Sigmund Freud* (Vol 2). London: Hogarth Press. (Original work published 1893)

Freud, S. (1957). The unconscious. In J. Strachey (Ed. and Trans.), *The standard edition of the complete psychological works of Sigmund Freud* (Vol. 14, pp. 159–216). London: Hogarth Press. (Original work published 1915)

Freud, S. (1958). Formulations on the two principles of mental functioning. In J. Strachey (Ed. and Trans.), *The standard edition of the complete psychological works of Sigmund Freud* (Vol. 12, pp. 213–226). London: Hogarth Press. (Original work published 1911)

Freud, S. (1959). Inhibitions, symptoms and anxiety. In J. Strachey (Ed. and Trans.), *The standard edition of the complete psychological works of Sigmund Freud* (Vol. 20, pp. 77–178). London: Hogarth Press. (Original work published 1926)

Freud, S. (1961). The ego and the id. In J. Strachey (Ed. and Trans.), *The standard edition of the complete psychological works of Sigmund Freud* (Vol. 19, pp. 1–68). London: Hogarth Press. (Original work published 1923)

Galin, D. (1974). Implications for psychiatry of left and right cerebral specialization: A neurophysiological content for unconscious processes. *Archives of General Psychiatry, 31*, 572–583.

Gersch, W., Yonomoto, J., & Naitoh, P. (1977). Automatic classification of multivariate EEG's using an amount of information measure and the eigenvalues of parametric time series model feature. *Computational Biomedical Research, 10*, 297–318.

Ghiselin, B. (1952). *The creative process.* New York: New Atheneum Library.

Giddan, N. S. (1967). Recovery through images of briefly flashed stimuli. *Journal of Personality, 35*, 1–19.

Goldiamond, I. (1958). Indicators of perception. 1. Subliminal perception, subception, unconscious perception: An analysis in terms of psychophysical indicator methodology. *Psychological Bulletin, 55*, 373–411.

Grossman, W., & Kaplan, D. M. (1988). *Oedipus complex.* Manuscript in preparation.

Haber, P. N., & Erdelyi, M. H. (1967). Emergence and recovery of initially unavailable perceptual material. *Journal of Verbal Learning and Verbal Behavior, 6*, 618–627.

Harashima, H., Kamatake, T., & Miyakawa, H. (1976). A theory of information flow in time series: An analysis of information flow in multiple series with applications. *Technical Group for Communication Systems,* C76–98.

Hartmann, H. (1958). *Ego psychology and the problem of adaptation.* New York: International Universities Press.

Holender, D. (1986). Semantic activation without conscious identification in dichotic listening, parafoveal vision, and visual masking: A survey and appraisal. *Behavioral & Brain Sciences, 9*, 1–23.

Inouye, T., Yagasaki, A., Takahashi, H., & Shinisaki, K. (1981). The dominant direction of interhemispheric EEG changes in the linguistic process. *Electroencephalography and Clinical Neurophysiology, 51*, 265–275.

Jagadeesh, B., Gray, C. M., & Forster, D. (1992). Visually evoked oscillations of membrane potential in cells of cat visual cortea. *Science, 257*, 552–554.

James, W. (1890). *Principles of psychology.* New York: Holt.

Jeong, J., & Williams, W. J. (1992). Kernel design for reduced interference distributions. *IEEE Transactions on Signal Processing, 40*, 402–412.

Kahneman, D., & Henik, A. (1981). Perceptual organization and attention. In M. Kuborg & J. R. Pomeranz (Eds.), *Perceptual organization.* Hillsdale, NJ: Erlbaum.

Kamitake, T., Harashima, H., & Miyakawa, H. (1984). A time series in electronics analysis method based on the directed transformation. *Electronics Communication, 67*–A.

Kawabata, N. (1973). A nonstationary analysis of the electroencephalogram. *IEEE Transactions on Biomedical Engineering, BME-20,* 444–452.

Keppel, G. (1982). *Design and analysis: A researcher's handbook* (2nd ed.). Englewood Cliffs, NJ: Prentice-Hall.

Klein, G. S., Spence, D. P., Holt, R. R., & Gourevitch, S. (1958). Cognition without awareness: Subliminal influences upon conscious thought. *Journal of Abnormal Social Psychology, 54,* 167–170.

Kostandov, E., & Arzumanov, Y. (1977). Averaged cortical evoked potentials to recognized and non-recognized verbal stimuli. *Acta Neurobiologiae Experimentalis, 37,* 311–324.

Kuhn, T. (1962). *The structure of scientific revolutions.* Chicago: University of Chicago Press.

Kushwaha, R. K., Williams, W. J., & Shevrin, H. (1992). An information flow technique for category related evoked potentials. *IEEE Transactions on Biomedical Engineering, 39*(12), 165–178.

Kutas, M., & Hillyard, S. A. (1989). An electrophysiological probe of incidental semantic association. *Journal of Cognitive Neuroscience, 1*(1), 38–49.

Libet, B., Alberts, W. W., Wright, E. W., & Feinstein, B. (1967). Responses of human somatosensory cortex to stimuli below threshold for conscious sensation. *Science, 158,* 1597–1600.

Libet, B., Wright, E. W., Jr., & Gleason, C. A. (1982). Readiness potentials preceeding unrestricted "spontaneous" versus preplanned voluntary acts. *Electroencephalography and Clinical Neurophysiology, 54,* 322–335.

Linstone, H. A., & Turoff, N. (1975). *The Delphi method: Techniques and applications.* Reading, MA: Addison-Wesley.

Luborsky, L. (1988). Recurrent momentary forgetting: Its content and context. In M. Horowitz (Ed.), *Psychodynamics and cognition* (pp. 223–251). Chicago: University of Chicago Press.

Luborsky, L., Blinder, B., & Schimek, J. (1965). Looking, recalling & GSR as a function of defense. *Journal of Abnormal Psychology, 70,* 270–280.

Luborsky, L., & Shevrin, H. (1956). Dreams and day residues: A study of the Poetzl observation. *Bulletin of the Menninger Clinic, 20,* 135–148.

Ludolph, P. S. (1981). *The dissociative tendency, its relationship to personality style and psychopathology.* Unpublished doctoral dissertation, Ann Arbor: The University of Michigan.

Marcel, A. (1983). Conscious and unconscious perception: Experiments in visual masking and word recognition. *Cognitive Psychology, 15,* 197–257.

Mars, N. J. I., & van Arragon, G. W. (1982). Time delay estimation in non-linear systems using average amount of mutual information analysis. In *Signal processing* (pp. 139–153). Amsterdam: North-Holland.

Merikle, P. M. (1992). Perception without awareness: Critical issues. *American Psychologist, 47*(6), 792–795.

Moore, B., & Fine, B. (1990). *Psychoanalytic terms and concepts.* New Haven and London: The American Psychoanalytic Association and Yale University Press.

Moser, J. M., & Avnon, J. I. (1986). Classification and detection of single evoked brain potentials using time–frequency amplitude features. *IEEE Transactions on Biomedical Engineering, BME-33-12,* 1096–1106.

Murray, H. A. (1971). *Thematic Apperception Test.* Cambridge, MA: Harvard University Press.

Nagel, T. (1994). Freud's permanent revolution. *New York Review of Books, 41*(9), 34–38.

Nagera, H. (1966). *Early childhood disturbances, the infantile neurosis, and the adult disturbances.* New York: International Universities Press.

Osgood, C. E., May, W. H., & Miron, M. S. (1975). *Cross-cultural universals of affective meaning.* Urbana: University of Illinois Press.

Paul, I. H., & Fisher, G. (1959). Subliminal visual stimulation: A study of its influence on subsequent images and dreams. *Journal of Nervous and Mental Disease, 129,* 315–340.

Pierce, C. S., & Jastrow, I. (1884). On small differences of sensation. *Minnesota National Academy of Science, 3,* 73–83.

Pine, F. (1960). Incidental stimulation: A study of preconscious transformation. *Journal of Abnormal Social Psychology, 60,* 68–75.

Poetzl, O. (1960). The relationship between experimentally induced dream images and indirect vision. *Psychological Issues, 2,* 41–120. (Original work published 1917)

Polanyi, M. (1958). *Personal knowledge.* Chicago: University of Chicago Press.

Polanyi, M. (1967). *The tacit dimension.* Garden City, NY: Anchor Books.

Posner, M. I. (1982). Cumulative development of attentional theory. *American Psychologist, 37,* 168–179.

Posner, M. I., & Boies, S. L. (1971). Components of alteration. *Psychological Review, 78*(5), 391–408.

Pribram, K. H., & Gill, M. M. (1976). *Freud's "project" re-assessed.* New York: Basic Books.

Pylyshyn, Z. (1989). Computing in cognitive science. In M. I. Posner (Ed.), *Foundations of cognitive science* (pp. 49–92). Cambridge, MA: MIT Press.

Rapaport, D. (1967). The scientific methodology of psychoanalysis. In M. M. Gill (Ed.), *The collected papers of David Rapaport* (pp. 165–220). New York: Basic Books.

Reinke, W., & Dickman, V. (1987). Uncertainty analysis of human EEG spectra: A multivariate information theoretical method for the analysis of brain activity. *Biological Cybernetics, 57,* 379–387.

Roediger, H. L. (1990). Implicit memory: Retention without remembering. *American Psychologist, 45*(9), 1043–1056.

Rubenstein, B. (1976). On the possibility of a strictly clinical psychoanalytic theory: An essay in the philosophy of psychoanalysis. In M. M. Gill & P. J. Holzman (Eds.), *Psychology versus metapsychology* (pp. 229–264). New York: International Universities Press.

Rumelhart, D. E. (1989). The architecture of mind: A connectionist approach. In M. I. Posner (Ed.), *Foundations of cognitive science* (pp. 133–160). Cambridge, MA: MIT Press.

Satio, Y., & Harashima, H. (1981). Tracking of information within multichannel EEG records. In N. Yamaguchi & K. Fujisawa (Eds.), *Recent advances in EEG and EMG data processing* (pp. 133–146).

Sayre, K. M. (1986). Intentionality and information processing: An alternative for cognitive science. *Behavioral and Brain Sciences, 9,* 121–166.

Schafer, R. (1954). *Psychoanalytic interpretation in Rorschach testing*. New York: Grune & Stratton.

Searle, J. R. (1970). Consciousness, explanatory inversion and cognitive science. *Behavioral and Brain Sciences, 13*, 585–642.

Seitz, P. (1966). The consensus problem in psychoanalytic research. In L. Gottschalk & A. Auerbach (Eds.), *Methods of research in psychotherapy* (pp. 209–225). New York: Appleton-Century-Crofts.

Shannon, C. E., & Weaver, W. (1963). *The mathematical theory of communication* (2nd ed.). Urbana: University of Illinois Press.

Shapiro, D. (1965). *Neurotic styles*. New York: Basic Books.

Shastri, L., & Ajjanagedde, V. (1993). From simple associations to systematic reasoning: A connectionist representation of rules, variables and dynamic bindings using temporal synchrony. *Behavioral and Brain Sciences, 16*, 417–494.

Shevrin, H. (1973). Brain wave correlates of subliminal stimulation, unconscious attention, primary- and secondary-process thinking and repressiveness. *Psychological Issues, Monograph 30, 8*(2), 56–87.

Shevrin, H. (1984). The fate of the five metapsychological principles. *Psychoanalytic Inquiry, 4*(1), 33–58.

Shevrin, H. (1986, Spring/Summer). Subliminal perception and dreaming. *Journal of Mind and Behavior, 7* (2&3), 379–395.

Shevrin, H. (1988). Unconscious conflict: A convergent psychodynamic and electrophysiologic approach. In M. Horowitz (Ed.), *Psychodynamic and cognition* (pp. 117–167). Chicago: University of Chicago Press.

Shevrin, H. (1990). Subliminal perception and repression. In J. P. Singer (Ed.), *Repression and dissociation: Implications for personality theory, psychopathology, and Health* (pp. 103–119). Chicago: University of Chicago Press.

Shevrin, H. (1991a). *The conscious symptoms and unconscious conflict: Convergent psychoanalytic, cognitive and neurophysiological findings*. The Charles Fisher Memorial Address, New York Psychoanalytic Society, New York.

Shevrin, H. (1991b). *The nature of the psychoanalytic method: Clinical and research implications*. Paper presented at the First International Conference on Psychoanalytic Research, International Psychoanalytic Association, London.

Shevrin, H. (1992a). The Freudian unconscious and the cognitive unconscious: Identical or fraternal twins? In J. W. Barron, M. N. Eagle, & D. L. Wolitzky (Eds.), *Interface of psychoanalysis and psychology* (pp. 313–326). Washington, DC: American Psychological Association.

Shevrin, H. (1992b). Subliminal perception, memory, and consciousness: Cognitive and dynamic perspectives. In R. F. Bornstein & T. S. Pittman (Eds.), *Perception without awareness: Cognitive, clinical, and social perspectives* (pp. 123–142). New York: Guilford.

Shevrin, H., & Bond, J. A. (1993). Repression and the unconscious. In N. E. Miller, L. Luborsky, J. P. Barber, & J. D. Docherty (Eds.), *Psychodynamic treatment research* (pp. 307–325). New York: Basic Books.

Shevrin, H., & Dickman, S. (1980). The psychological unconscious: A necessary assumption for all psychological theory? *American Psychologist, 35*, 421–434.

Shevrin, H., & Fisher, C. (1967). Changes in the effects of a waking subliminal stimulus as a function of dreaming and nondreaming sleep. *Journal of Abnormal Psychology, 72*, 362–368.

Shevrin, H., & Fritzler, D. (1968). Visual evoked response correlates of unconscious mental processes. *Science, 161*, 295–298.

Shevrin, H., & Luborsky, L. (1958). The measurement of preconscious perception in dreams and images: An investigation of the Portal phenomena. *Journal of Abnormal and Social Psychology, 56*, 285–294.

Shevrin, H., & Luborsky, L. (1960). The rebus technique: A method for studying primary process transformations of briefly exposed pictures. *Journal of Nervous and Mental Disease, 133*, 479–488.

Shevrin, H., & Rennick, P. (1967). Cortical response to a tactile stimulus during attention, mental arithmetic, and free associations. *Psychophysiology, 3*, 381–388.

Shevrin, H., Smith, W. H., & Fritzler, D. (1969). Repressiveness as a factor in the subliminal activation of brain and verbal responses. *Journal of Nervous and Mental Disease, 149*, 261–269.

Shevrin, H., Smith, W. H., & Fritzler, D. (1970). Subliminally stimulated brain and verbal responses of twins differing in repressiveness. *Journal of Abnormal Psychology, 76*, 39–46.

Shevrin, H., Williams, W. J., Marshall, R. E., Hertel, R. K., Bond, J. A., & Brakel, L. A. W. (1992). Event-related potential indicators of the dynamic unconscious. *Consciousness and Cognition, 1*, 340–366.

Shortliffe, E. H. (1976). *Computer-based medical consultations: MYCIN.* New York: Elsevier.

Sidis, B. (1898). *The psychology of suggestion.* New York: Appleton.

Simon, H. A., & Kaplan, C. A. (1989). Foundations of cognitive science. In M. I. Posner (Ed.), *Foundations of cognitive science* (pp. 1–48). Cambridge, MA: MIT Press.

Smokler, I., & Shevrin, H. (1979). Cerebral lateralization and personality style. *Archives of General Psychiatry, 36*, 949–954.

Sneath, P. H., & Sokal, R. R. (1973). *Numerical taxonomy.* San Francisco: Freeman.

Snodgrass, M. (1995). *Unconscious perception at the objective threshold: Positive evidence and theoretical significance.* Paper presented at the American Psychological Society Meeting, New York City, New York.

Snodgrass, M. (1996). *Theory and method in the study of unconscious processes.* Manuscript in preparation.

Snodgrass, M., Shevrin, H., Brakel, L. A. W., & Medin, D. (1995). *Qualitative differences in the principles of organization for conscious and unconscious categorization.* Poster presented at the American Psychological Society Meeting, New York City, New York.

Snodgrass, M., Shevrin, H., & Kopka, M. (1993). The mediation of intentional judgments by unconscious perceptions: The influences of task strategy, task preference, word meaning, and motivation. *Consciousness and Cognition, 2*, 169–193.

Spydell, J. D., & Sheer, D. E. (1982). Effects of problem solving on right and left hemisphere 40 hertz EEG activity. *Proceedings of the Society for Psychophysiological Research, 19*(4), 420–425.

Stevens, J. (1986). *Applied multivariate statistics for the social sciences.* Hillsdale, NJ: Erlbaum.

Tomkins, S. S. (1962). *Affect, imagery, consciousness.* New York: Springer.

Tomkins, S. S. (1963). *Affect, cognition, and personality: Empirical studies.* New York: Springer.

Uleman, J. S., & Bargh, J. A. (1989). *Unintended thought.* New York: Guilford.

Van Selst, H., & Merikle, P. M. (1993). Perception below the objective threshold? *Consciousness and Cognition, 2,* 194–203.

Vidal, W. J. (1977). Real time detection of brain events. *Proceedings of the IEEE, 65,* 633–641.

Williams, W. J., Brown, M. L., Zaveri, H. P., & Shevrin, H. (1994). Feature extraction from time–frequency distributions. In C. Dagli, B. R. Fernandez, J. Ghosh, & R. T. Saunder-Kumara (Eds.), *Intelligent engineering systems through artificial neural networks: Proceedings of the Artificial Neural Network in Engineering (ANNIE 1994) Conference, November 13–16, St. Louis.* New York: ASME Press.

Williams, W. J., & Jeong, J. (1989). New time–frequency distributions: Theory and applications. *IEEE Transactions,* 1243–1247.

Williams, W. J., & Jeong, J. (1992). Reduced interference time–frequency distributions. In B. Boashash (Ed.), *Time–frequency signal analysis: Methods and applications.* Melbourne, Australia: Longman Chesire–Wiley.

Williams, W. J., Shevrin, H., & Marshall, R. (1987). Information modeling and analysis of event related potentials. *IEEE Transactions on Biomedical Engineering, BME-34*(12), 928–937.

Winer, B. (1971). *Statistical principles in experimental design* (2nd ed.). New York: McGraw-Hill.

Wong, P. S., Shevrin, H., & Williams, W. (1994). Conscious & nonconscious processes: An ERP index of an anticipatory response in a conditioning paradigm using visually masked stimuli. *Psychophysiology, 1,* 87–101.

Wong, P. S., Shevrin, H., Williams, W. J., & Marshall, R. E. (1988). *The psychophysiology of voluntary movement: Awareness of an intentional act and the obsessional personality.* Paper presented at the Society for Psychophysiological Research Meeting, San Francisco, California.

Zaveri, H. P., Williams, W. J., Iasemidis, L. D., & Sackellares, J. C. (1992). Time–frequency representation of electrocorticograms in temporal lobe epilepsy. *IEEE Transactions on Biomedical Engineering, BME-39,* 502–509.

Zaveri, H. P., Williams, W. J., & Sackellares, J. C. (1992). Cross time–frequency representation of electrocorticograms in temporal lobe epilepsy. Paper presented at the IEEE EMB Conference, Orlando, Florida.

Index

Abandonment, impact of, 155, 160, 175, 181
Abuse, impact of, 150
Activation, connectionist network, 44
Adaptive Gabor transform (AGT):
  development of, 127
  formal mathematical description of, 127–128
  time–frequency distributions and, 134
  unconscious conflict research study, 139, 143
Adaptive logon transform, 275–276
Additivity, 113–114
Affect:
  cognitive psychology, 7
  historical perspective, 92
  unconscious and, 2
Afterexpulsion, 272–273
Aggression:
  fear of, 182–185
  sadism and, 169, 257
Agoraphobia, 151, 158
Alienation, 151–152
Allport, A., 46–49, 51–54, 273–274
Anal phase, 26
Anal sadistic conflict, 172, 182
Anhedonia, 172
Anticipatory anxiety, 196, 201
Anxiety:
  anticipatory, 196, 201
  castration, 20, 173, 213, 218
  discontinuity and, 5
  predisposition to, 160
  signs of, 196, 237
  as symptom, 16, 24
Artificial intelligence (AI), 42, 51
Assumptions, underlying, 6
Attention:
  defenses and, 8, 278
  motivation system, 45–48
  selective, 47
Authoritarian parents, impact of, 189, 205, 225

Authority, rebellion toward, 217–219
Automatic processes:
  cognitive architecture, 40
  goal-oriented, 50
  selection-for-action theory, 45–46
  social cognitive perspective, 49–50
  spreading activation, 55
Avoidance, case illustration, 176
Avoidant personality disorder, 156, 158
Axis I/Axis II diagnoses, case illustrations, 155–156, 158
Axons, 42

Bandwidths, time–frequency distributions, 119–120
Bargh, J. A., 48–54, 56, 275
Biological level, cognitive architecture, 39
Boundary:
  connectionist network, 44–45
  social phobias, 157–158
Bound cathexis, 55
Brain, generally:
  effects, 16
  hemispheric research, 277–278
  melodies, 133
  processes, psychophysiological theory and, 59–60
  rhythms, 127

Castration anxiety, 20, 173, 213, 218
Cathexis, 55
Causality, unconscious, 7
Character traits, 25, 28
Childhood, generally:
  dangerous situations, 20
  Oedipal complex, 26–27
  psychosexual stages, 26
Clinical cases:
  conscious symptoms/unconscious conflict words, 146, 149–186
  eating phobia, 231–258
  interviews, overview, 145–147
  psychodiagnostic tests, 147

295

Clinical cases (*continued*)
  psychodynamic method, 187–230
  structure of, 146–147
Clinical evaluation team (CET):
  agreements/disagreements among,
    31–32
  function of, *see specific clinical cases*
  psychodynamic formula, word selection
    procedure, 75, 79–81, 86–87,
    89–90
Cognitive control, cognitive architecture,
    40
Cognitive Psychology (Marcel), 102
Cognitive theory:
  attention motivation system, selection-
    for-action theory, 45–48
  computation, 38–39, 51–52
  connectionist view, 42–45
  conscious process, 54–56
  controlled/automatic distinction, 52–54
  frame of reference, 6–8
  information processing, 39
  research:
    historical origins of, 262–263
    implications for, 56–57, 271–275
  social cognitive perspective, 48–51
  symbol-based architecture, 39–42
  unconscious process, 54–56
Competition:
  fear of, 183
  phallic, 169, 213, 226, 255
Compromise formations:
  case illustration, 22
  defined, 21
  nature of, 21–22
  problems with, 22
  symptoms as, 23–25
  transference manifestations, 25–26
  unconscious conflicts, 20, 23
Compulsions, 16
Computational view:
  connectionists and, 42–43
  overview, 51–52
  symbol-based cognitive architecture, 41,
    43
Condensation, 17, 36
Conflict, unconscious, *see specific types of
    conflicts*
  psychoanalytic theory, 14–15, 20–21,
    60
  word selection and, 83–84
Congenial mentor, 169

Connection theory:
  elements of, 42–45
  research implications, 276
  spreading activation, 55–56
Connotative meaning, 8
Conscious, in psychoanalytic theory, 14
Consciousness Reconsidered (Flanagan),
    261–262
Continuity, psychological, 4–6
Controlled/automatic dichotomy, 46–47,
    52–54, 273
Controlled processes:
  boundaries, 45
  cognitive architecture, 40
  connection theory, 45
  selection-for-action theory, 46, 48
  social cognitive perspective, 49
Convergent research, 73
Conversion disorder, 242, 244, 251
Copernicus, 1
Crews, Frederick, 1–2

Darwin, Charles, 1
Daydreams, diagnostic technique, 28
Delirium, 16
Delphi method, 77–78, 146, 267
Delusions, 16
Dendrites, 42
Denial, in case illustrations, 218, 241, 252
Depression, 16, 24
Descriptive category, conscious symptom
    words, 268
Desensitization, in vivo, 147, 214, 220
Desires, 91
Developmental concepts, 27
Direct associations, 30
Discontinuity:
  case illustration, 16–17
  defined, 5–6
Displacement:
  case illustration, 24
  function of, 17
  unconscious conflict formulation,
    30–31
Disposition, historical perspective, 92
Divorce, impact of, 172, 174, 181, 247
Dixon, N. F., 93–94, 263–265
Dogs, fear of, 24–25
Dreams:
  anxiety in, 238–239, 253
  in cognitive psychology, 7
  diagnostic technique, 28, 30

function of, generally, 2
latent, 30
manifest, 30
nightmares, 241
paranoia in, 249
subliminal perception research,
    97–98
symbolism in, 241
as symptoms, 24
DSM-III-R:
psychoanalytic theory and, 19
social phobia, 69
Dysthymic disorder, 155

Early/late selection, 46–47
Eating phobia, case illustration:
debriefing meeting, 258
evaluation:
    interviewer's perspective, 233–234
    procedure, 231
laboratory results, 258
psychodynamic formulation:
    conscious symptoms, 235–240
    unconscious conflict symptoms,
        240–258
psychosocial history, 232–233
referral, nature of, 231
subject presentation, 231
ED, time–frequency distributions, 126
Edelman, G. M., 277
EEG, time–frequency distributions, 119
Ego:
assessment of, 31
controlled processes, 273–274
defined, 20–21
factors, 53
function of, 270
posturing, 178
structural approach, 11
weakness, 242, 250
Ego maniac, case illustration, 151
Embarrassment, 87–88
Embarrassment/sweating fear, case
    illustration:
debriefing meeting, 229–230
evaluation:
    interviewer's perspective, 191–193
    procedure, 188
laboratory results, 230
psychodynamic formulation:
    conscious symptoms, 193–204
    unconscious symptoms, 205–221

psychosocial history, 188–191
referral, nature of, 187
subject presentation, 187–188
unconscious conflict words selection,
    221–229
Emotional reactions, defined, 91
Endogenous components, event-related
    potentials (ERPs), 62–63
Energy masking, 263
Eternal flame, 88
Event-related potentials (ERPs):
amplitude voltage, 109–110
bias and, 61–62
brain processes and, 59–60
contributions of, 62
defined, 4, 59
diagnosis and, 29
identification of, 61
information technique and, 117
limitations of, 61–62
production of, 61
psychophysiological assumptions and,
    8–9
real time character of, 62
studies review, 63–64
subliminal processes research, 64–66
word selection and, 37, 73
Exhibitionism, 31–32, 181, 214
Exogenous components, event-related
    potentials (ERPs), 62–63
Expectancy wave, 66
Explanatory category, unconscious
    symptom words, 268
Externalization, case illustration, 180

Fantasies:
fear of, 182–183
homosexual, 213, 226
impact of, 7, 20
Oedipal phase and, 26–27
primal-scene, 31
transference and, 25
unconscious conflict and, 30
Femininity, 26
Fisher, C., 95–101, 272–274
Fixation:
defined, 31
oral sadistic, 243, 246
points, 27
Flanagan, Owen, 261–262
Focal psychotherapy, 214
Forgetting, 278

Fourier transform, time–frequency
    distributions, 119–120, 122–123, 127
Frame of reference:
    cognitive psychological method, 6–8
    psychoanalytic method, 4–6
    psychophysiological assumptions and,
        8–9
Free association:
    case illustration, 17, 255
    conditions of, 18
    connections, 17
    purpose of, 6, 14, 19
    subliminal perception research, 101
Freud, Sigmund:
    dream interpretation and, 262
    Oedipal complex, 26
    unconscious motivation, 1
    validity issues, 266

Gabor transform, 8, 68
Galin hypothesis, 278
Grandiosity, 179

Hallucinations, 16
Hard science, 58
Helplessness, 152
Heredity, as causal factor, 16
Homoerotic conflict, 234, 242, 245–246,
    248–251, 254
Homosexual fantasies, 213, 242
Honesty, 54
Humiliation, fear of, 158
Hysteria, 16
Hysterical conversion, 244
Hysteroid-Obsessoid questionnaire
    (HOQ), 139, 142–143, 269, 276, 278

Id:
    defined, 20–21
    function of, 270
    impulses, 273
    structural approach, 11
Idealization, primitive, 179
Ideation, primary, 55
Identifications, 25
Imipramine, 156, 159
Implicit memory, 272
Impulsivity, 223
Inaccessible causative psychological
    unconscious, 6
Inadequate personality, defined, 251
Inderal, 147, 214, 220

Individual differences, in psychoanalysis,
    2, 14
Inferences, of clinician:
    cognitive psychology and, 7–8
    in psychoanalysis, 2–3
Information processing, 39, 110
Information-theoretic approach:
    additivity, 113–114
    applications of, 117–1119
    benefits of, 112–113
    bias, 116
    description of, generally, 8, 110–112
    information:
        estimation of, 115–116
        formal description of, 114–115
        problems with, 116
Intentions:
    repressed, 53
    in unconscious processes, 50–51
Internal flame, 87–88
Interpretation of Dreams, The (Freud), 59,
    95, 262
Intersubjectivity theory, 13
Interviews:
    in case illustrations, *see specific case
        illustrations*
    open-ended, nonstructured, 19
    word selection procedure, 78–79
Involuntary processes, 45–46
Iodine, radioactive, 7–8

James, William, 1, 264–265
Judgments, *see specific case illustrations*
    purpose of, 7, 20
    word selection, 73–74, 78, 83–89

Kleinian school, psychoanalytic method,
    14–15
Knowledge level, cognitive architecture,
    39–40

Latency phase, 27
Latent dreams, 30
Lateral neglect, 47
Law of exclusion, 100, 105
Links, connectionist network, 44
Logic machine, 41
Loss of object/object's love, 20

Major depression, 16
Manifest dreams, 30
MANOVA program, 141

Marcel, A., 102–103
Markers, neurophysiological processes, 60, 265
Marr, David, 52
Marshall, Robert, 81
Masculinity, 26
Maternal relationship, impact of, 160, 170, 172, 177, 210
Memory:
    in cognitive theory, 7
    implicit, 272
    repressed, 17
Meninger Foundation, 96, 100
Mental contents, 269
Mentor-savior relationship, case illustration, 178–180
Merikle, P. M., 104–105
Messenger, cognitive architecture, 41
Mobile cathexis, 55
Motivation, 1, 7. *See also specific theories*
Motivational importance, 48
Multidetermination:
    case illustration, 36–37
    defined, 14, 27–28
Multivariate analyses, 140
MYCIN, 81

Narcissism, case illustration, 156, 168–169
Neediness, 152
Negative image, fear of, 199
Neostructural theory, 267, 270
Neural Darwinism, 277
Neurons, connectionist view, 42
Neuroses, 254
N400, event-related potentials (ERPs), 64
Nightmares, 241
Nodes, connectionist network, 44
Nonrapid eye movement (NREM), 107

Object identification, 47
Object relations theory:
    evolution of, 2, 15
    structural theory and, 13
    transference manifestations, 25
Obsession, case illustration, 171
Obsessive-compulsive defenses, case illustration:
    decompensation, 177
    types of, 174
Oedipal complex, *see* Oedipal phase
    defined, 14, 26–27
    structural theory issues, 14

Oedipal phase:
    case illustration, 172, 174, 180
    subliminal perception research, 94–95
Oedipal triangle, 27, 173, 225, 244
Oral sadistic fixation, 243, 246
Oral/tactile phase, 26–27
Organic brain syndrome, 16
Organic causality, 16
Overdetermination, 14, 27–28

Panic attacks, case illustration, 150, 156, 158, 160
Paranoia, case illustration, 154, 157, 177, 249, 251
Parapraxes, 24
Parental approval, significance of, 213
Parental loss, impact of, 160, 170
Parenting style, impact of, 189, 205, 225
Part for whole, 17
Paternal relationship, impact of, 160, 170, 175, 189, 205, 210–211
Pathological grief reaction, 28
Pathology, cognitive psychology and, 7
Pattern masking, 102, 263
Perception:
    defined, 7
    distortions, 180
    processes of, 264
Personal knowledge, 73
Personal meaning, 2
Phallic competition, 169, 213, 226, 255
Phallic-exhibitionism, 226
Phallic phase, 27
Phallic-stage conflict, 225
Phobias, 16, 24. *See also* Agoraphobia; Social phobias
Physical level, cognitive architecture, 39
Plato, 91
Pleasure principle, 20
Poetzl, Otto, 95–97, 99–101, 105, 262
P100/P200/P300, event-related potentials (ERPs), 63–65
Preattentive processes, 54–55, 263
Preconscious:
    automatic processes, 49–50
    in psychoanalytic theory, 14
    symptom, 272–273
Preoedipal conflicts, 27
Primary ideation, 55
Primary processes, 55
Principles of Psychology (James), 1

Prioritization, adaptive, 48
Priority systems, high-/low-, 47, 52–53,
    56, 274–275
Project for a Scientific Psychology (Freud),
    58–59
Projection, case illustration, 180, 182
Projective identification, 175–176
Pseudocategories, 279
Pseudo-Wigner distribution (PWD), 126
Psychic continuity, 14–15
Psychic determinism:
    case illustration, 16–17
    defined, 14–15
Psychic reality, 20, 27
Psychoanalysis:
    brain processes and, 59
    decentered consciousness, 1
    process of, overview, *see* Psychoanalytic
        process
    psychoanalyst role, 14, 18, 59
    validity of, 266
Psychoanalyst:
    role of, 14, 18, 59
    transference strategies, 25
    word choice, 34
Psychoanalytic method:
    basic assumptions of, 14–19
    clinical applications:
        conscious symptoms description,
            29–30
        data, agreement/disagreement levels,
            31–32
        diagnosis, 28–29
        team contributions, 34
        unconscious conflict, formulating,
            30–31
        word selection, 32–34
    clinical theories, 14, 19–20
    compromise formations, 21–23
    evolution of, 13
    frames of reference, 4–6, 14
    Freud's two theorems/basic pillars, 18
    motivations, generally, 53–54
    multideterminism, 27–28
    Oedipal Complex, 26–27
    overdeterminism, 27–28
    research:
        application of, sample problems,
            264–267
        historical origins of, 262–263
        implications for, 267–271
    symptoms, 23–25

    transference manifestations, 25–26
    unconscious conflict, 20–21
Psychoanalytic process:
    clinical data, agreement/disagreement
        levels, 31–32
    conscious symptoms description, 29–30
    diagnosis, 28–29
    team contributions, 31–32, 34
    unconscious conflict, formulating,
        30–31
    word selection, 32–34
Psychoanalytic theory, *see* Psychoanalytic
    method
Psychological continuity, 4–5
Psychological unconscious, existence of,
    14
Psychophysiological theory:
    adaptive Gabor transform, 126–129
    event-related potential *see* Event-related
        potentials (ERPs)
    frame of reference, 8–9
    information-theoretic approach, *see*
        Information-theoretic approach
    overview, 59–63
    research implications, 275–278
    time–frequency distributions (t-f):
        discrete, 126
        feature analysis, 120–122
        information theory, combined with,
            126
        new distributions, 122–126
        overview, 119–120
Psychoses:
    active, 256
    underlying, 177
Psychosexual stages, 14, 27
Pylyshyn, Z., 39–42, 51–52

Rage:
    management of, 181
    narcissistic, 168–169, 178
    projected, 175
    sadistic, 168–169, 178, 257
Rapid eye movement (REM), 107
Reaction formation, case illustration, 176,
    178
Reality testing, 251
Rebus stimulation, subliminal perception
    research, 106–107
Recall, 278
Reduced interference distribution (RID),
    time–frequency distributions, 125

Regression:
  case illustrations, 171, 180, 240, 244
  function of, generally, 27, 31
Relational awareness, 268
Relative frequencies, 277
Representations, 270
Repression, 241, 272–273
Research:
  historical origins of, 262–263
  implications for:
    cognitive theory, 271–275
    psychoanalytic theory, 267–271
    psychophysiological theory, 275–278
  limitations of, 278–280
Research Center for Mental Health, NYU,
  96
Response, to stimuli, 8
RID, time–frequency distributions,
  125–126
Rorschach Test, 69, 147
Rubenstein, B., 59–60
RWED, time–frequency distributions, 126

Scare cues, case illustration, 151–152
Scatterplot, 81–82
Secondary processes, 55
Selection-for-action theory, 45–48
Selective attention, 47
Self-consciousness, 150
Self psychology, evolution of, 13–15
Self-regard, loss of, 20
Semantic level, cognitive architecture, 39
Separation-individuation conflict, 210,
  228
Sexual difficulties, case illustrations,
  171–172, 257
Sexual identity, problems with, 176, 212,
  227
Sexual wishes, fear of, 183
Shyness, case illustration, 201, 243
Slip "cancering," 16–17
Slip of the tongue, 16–17, 87–88
Social event fears, case illustration:
  debriefing meeting, 185–186
  evaluation:
    interviewer perspective on, 152–153
    procedure, 149–150
  laboratory results, 186
  psychodynamic formulation:
    conscious symptoms, 153–163
    unconscious symptoms, 163–185
  psychosocial history, 150–152

  referral, nature of, 149
  subject presentation, 149
Social isolation, case illustration, 157
Social phobia(s):
  boundaries, 157–158
  case illustrations:
    eating phobia, 231–258
    embarrassment/sweating fear,
      187–230
    overview, 29–31, 84–86
    social event fears, 149–186
  diagnosis of, 28
  unconscious conflict, 31, 84, 87
  word selection procedure, 84–86
Soft story, 87–89
Spectral analysis, 119–120
Stimulation, subliminal:
  cognitive psychology, 7–8
  psychoanalytic method, 4
  psychophysiological assumptions and, 9
Stimulus onset asynchrony (SOA),
  102–103
Studies on Hysteria (Freud), 50
Subliminal cognitive method,
  conscious/unconscious processes
  study:
  cognitive implications, 107–108
  criticisms, response to, 104
  overview, 93–104
  relevant contributions, 105–107
Subliminal exposure, 9
Subliminality, criteria for, 104–105
Subliminal perception:
  historical perspective, 2
  research studies, 93–104, 146
*Subliminal Perception: The Nature of a
  Controversy* (Dixon), 263
Subliminal processes, event-related
  potentials (ERPs) research, 64–66
Subliminal research, nature of, 263
Subliminal stimulation, *see* Stimulation,
  subliminal
Subliminal stimulus, 271–272
Subliminal/supraliminal duration order,
  279–280
Superego:
  defined, 20–21
  function of, 270
  structural approach, 11
Swallowing phobia, 243–244
Symbol-based cognitive architecture,
  39–42

Symbolic representation, 17
Symbol level, cognitive architecture, 39
Symptoms, generally:
  compromise formations:
    case illustration, 24–25
    impact of, 23–24
  conscious, 29–30
  development and, 35–36
  environment factors and, 35–36
  neurotic, 36
  unconscious, 272–273
  word selection criteria, 32–33, 82–83
Synapses, 42

t-f distributions, see Time–frequency
    distributions
Thematic Apperception Test (TAT), 69,
    147, 152, 176, 208–209, 244–245,
    253, 256
Thought, 7
Time–frequency distributions:
  defined, 122–123
  discrete, 126
  feature analysis, 120–122
  information theory, combined with, 126
  new distributions, 122–126
  overview, 119–120
  research implications, 275
  unconscious conflict research study,
    139–140
Time–frequency feature analysis, 8, 68,
    138
Tip-of-the-tongue phenomenon, 50
Topographic model, 273–274
Transference:
  case illustrations, 152, 228, 247–248
  manifestations, 25–26
Transformation, hypothesized principles
    of, 17
Transinformation, 115, 118
Trauma, impact of, 16, 31, 50, 254
Triangular dynamics, 171
Tripartite psychic structural symptoms, 20

Unbound cathexis, 55
Unconscious:
  conflict, see Unconscious conflict
  inaccessible causative psychological, 6
  motivation, 1
  motives, cognitive theory, 54–56

in psychoanalytic theory, 14–16
  symptom, cognitive theory, 272–273
Unconscious conflict:
  event-related potentials (ERPs) and, 60
  formulation, 30–31
  psychoanalytic theory, generally, 14–15,
    20–21
  research study:
    analysis methods, 138–139
    laboratory procedure, 136–137
    results, 139–143
    subject selection, 134–136
  word selection, see Unconscious conflict
    words
Unconscious conflict words, case
    illustration, 149–186
Underlying assumptions, 6
Unintended Thought, 48–49

Verbal expression, impact of, 34
Verbalization, 278
Viral illness, 16
Voluntary actions, 45–46
Voyeuristic impulses, 181

Waking behavior, diagnostic technique,
    28–29
Wants, 91
Wechsler Adult Intelligence
    Scale/Wechsler Adult Intelligence
    Scale-Revised (WAIS/WAIS-R), 69,
    147, 176
Wigner distribution (WD), 121, 123, 125
Wishes, 91
Word ratings, 80, 89–90
Word selection:
  compromise formation, 32–33, 82–83
  criteria for, 32–34
  psychodynamic clinical method:
    delphi method, 77–78
    judges' unconscious word
      nominations/word ratings, 78,
      83–89
    judgments, reliance on, 73–74
    overview, 69–74
    psychodynamic formulation, 74–75
    word ratings, reliability of, 80, 89–90
    word selection procedures, 78–83

Xanax, 147

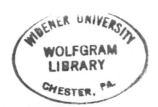
WIDENER UNIVERSITY
WOLFGRAM
LIBRARY
CHESTER, PA.